No Man's
Land

ALSO BY WENDY MOORE

The Knife Man: Blood, Body Snatching,
and the Birth of Modern Surgery

Wedlock: The True Story of the Disastrous Marriage and
Remarkable Divorce of Mary Eleanor Bowes,
Countess of Strathmore

How to Create the Perfect Wife:
Britain's Most Ineligible Bachelor and His
Enlightened Quest to Train the Ideal Mate

The Mesmerist: The Society Doctor
Who Held Victorian London Spellbound

No Man's Land

THE TRAILBLAZING WOMEN WHO RAN BRITAIN'S MOST EXTRAORDINARY MILITARY HOSPITAL DURING WORLD WAR I

WENDY MOORE

BASIC BOOKS
New York

Basic Books
Hachette Book Group
1290 Avenue of the Americas, New York, NY 10104
www.basicbooks.com

Printed in the United States of America

Originally published in 2020 by Atlantic Books in the UK

First US Edition: April 2020

Published by Basic Books, an imprint of Perseus Books, LLC, a subsidiary of Hachette Book Group, Inc. The Basic Books name and logo is a trademark of the Hachette Book Group.

The Hachette Speakers Bureau provides a wide range of authors for speaking events. To find out more, go to www.hachettespeakersbureau.com or call (866) 376-6591.

The publisher is not responsible for websites (or their content) that are not owned by the publisher.

The Cook-Dickerman Collection is held at the Eleanor Roosevelt National Historic Site, National Park Service, New York State.

Pictures belonging to the Anderson family and Annie Fox are held at the London School of Economics (LSE) Women's Library.

Print book interior design by Jeff Williams.

Library of Congress Cataloging-in-Publication Data
Names: Moore, Wendy, 1952– author.
Title: No man's land : the trailblazing women who ran Britain's most
   extraordinary military hospital during World War I / Wendy Moore.
Identifiers: LCCN 2019041778 | ISBN 9781541672727 (hardcover) | ISBN
   9781541672734 (ebook)
Subjects: LCSH: Murray, Flora. | Anderson, Louisa Garrett, 1873–1943. |
   Women's Hospital Corps—History. | Endell Street Military
   Hospital—History. | World War, 1914–1918—Hospitals—Great Britain. |
   World War, 1914–1918—Medical care—Women. | Women in medicine—Great
   Britain—History—20th century. | Women surgeons—Great
   Britain—Biography. | Suffragists—England—Biography. | Covent Garden
   (London, England)—History—20th century. | BISAC: HISTORY / Women
Classification: LCC D629.G7 M66 2020 | DDC 940.4/7642132—dc23
LC record available at https://lccn.loc.gov/2019041778

ISBNs: 978-1-5416-7272-7 (hardcover), 978-1-5416-7273-4 (ebook)

LSC-C

10 9 8 7 6 5 4 3 2

To Jennian

Guide, mentor, and friend

And for all the women who worked at
Endell Street and all the men and women
who were treated there

Contents

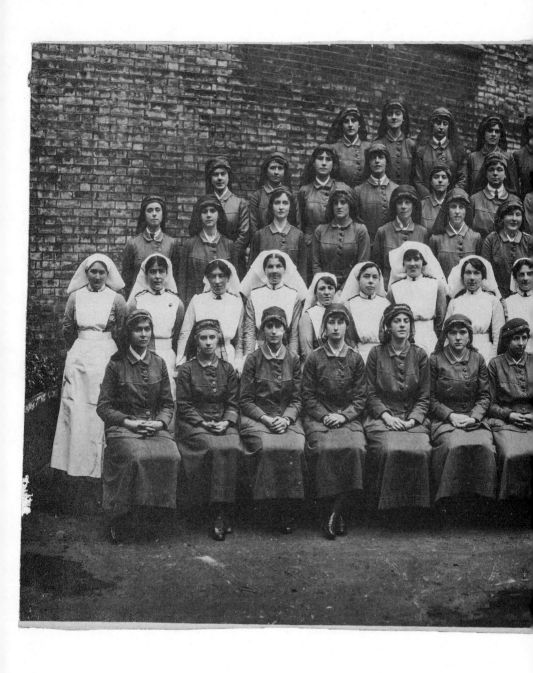

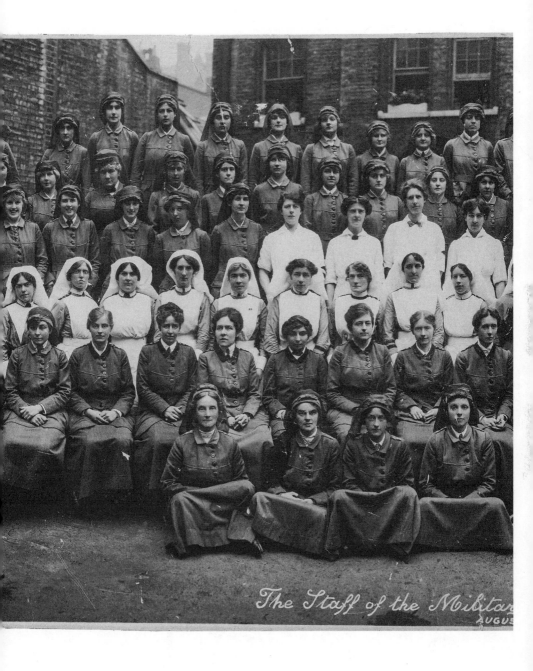

The Staff of the Military
AUGUS

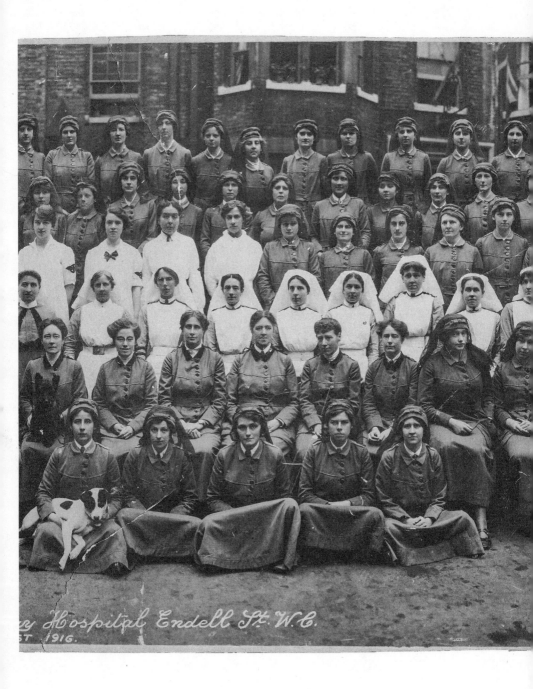

...y Hospital Endell St. W.C.
...ST 1916.

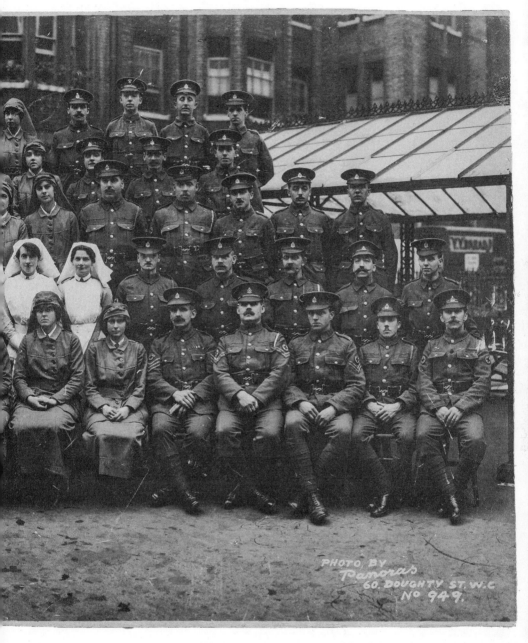

The Staff of the Military Hospital Endell St., August 1916

(BY KIND PERMISSION OF ANNIE FOX.)

Arrivals

Covent Garden, London, 1915

It was like slipping into a dream. Or waking from a nightmare. They had grown used to the constant thunder of shelling, the crackling of rifles and machine guns, the screams and groans of their comrades. Now all they could hear was the gentle thrum of the city at night as they rumbled through dark, deserted streets. For months, they had known only the rural landscapes of France and Flanders, where every living thing had been crushed and obliterated into the mud of the trenches and shell holes. Now they were being driven down a narrow street between tall buildings that blotted out the night sky. They had been living in a world peopled by men. But now they would enter a world run solely by women.

Most of them were young men in their twenties and thirties; some were just boys in their late teens. Officially, they were supposed to be at least nineteen to fight overseas, but some had lied about their age. Many had signed up in bands of friends in a fit of patriotic zeal, or shown up shamefaced at a recruitment office after being challenged with a white feather by a stranger in the street. For some, being injured had come as a blessing—a "Blighty wound" that allowed them to escape the death and devastation of war. For others, their injuries meant a new kind of terror and fear for the future: the prospect of never working, perhaps never walking again,

1

the possibility of perpetual pain, of permanent disfigurement. They had suffered long and agonizing journeys, having been scooped up from the battlefield by regimental stretcher-bearers, sometimes after lying abandoned for hours in "no-man's-land" before being shuttled back to casualty posts in tents and dugouts for basic first aid, a shot of morphine, and perhaps a hurried operation. They had been transported in ambulance trains to one of the French ports, crammed into hospital ships to cross the Channel, then packed into Red Cross trains bound for London. Arriving at one of the main-line stations, they had been collected by volunteers who drove them in ambulances or private cars across town. If the men asked their drivers where they were being taken the answer came: "To the best hospital in London."

When they pulled up outside the old workhouse building in Endell Street, in the heart of London's Theatreland, the great black iron gates were opened by a woman in a military-style jacket and ankle-length skirt. The ambulances juddered to a halt in the dimly lit courtyard, and women stretcher-bearers, wearing the same military-style uniforms, carried them to a lift. When they arrived on one of the wards, they saw a room bright with colored blankets and fragrant with fresh flowers. Rows of patients watched, their heads resting on crisp white pillows, as the new arrivals were lifted onto coarse blankets protecting the beds from their muddied and bloody uniforms.

The men were surrounded, naturally enough, by female nurses, orderlies, and clerks. Then the doctors arrived. And all of these were women, too. From the physician who assessed the condition of the patients to the surgeon who inspected their wounds, from the radiologist who ordered X-rays to the pathologist who took swabs, from the dentist who checked their teeth to the ophthalmologist who tested their sight, every one of the doctors was female. Other than the burly policeman at the entrance and a handful of male orderlies who were too old or too infirm for combat, the Endell Street Military Hospital was staffed entirely by women.

For some of the men who arrived at Endell Street on one of those dark nights, the stink of the trenches still clinging to their uniforms, to enter this female world after living in the hell wrought by men was a glorious relief. But for others it was a threatening, shocking, even distressing experience. Women nurses were one thing. Many of the men had already had their wounds dressed by female nurses in field hospitals and on ambulance trains. Women doctors were something else entirely. None of them had ever been treated by a female doctor in civilian life—the idea of women providing medical care to men was simply unknown—and they knew full well that women doctors were not ordinarily employed in the army. Some of the men had wounds in intimate places; others had contracted venereal diseases after sexual encounters with women in France. A few were convinced they had been sent to Endell Street to die, that they were hopeless cases. For why else would the army dispatch them to a hospital run solely by women—and not just any women, but suffragettes, former enemies of the state?

Yet, as the women doctors listened sympathetically to the men's fears, and as trained nurses gently tended their bodies and friendly orderlies comforted their spirits, the men began to change their minds. Before long, they all agreed that Endell Street Military Hospital was, indeed, the best hospital in London.

I

A Good Feeling

Victoria Station, London, September 15, 1914

Louisa Garrett Anderson and Flora Murray waited to board their train.[1] Tall, slim, and erect in the midst of the fourteen younger women who were going with them, they exuded calm authority. Everyone had come to see them off—family, friends, and comrades from the suffragette movement—and to ply them with gifts. One well-wisher had arrived with three boxes packed with provisions for the journey, while others had brought fruit, chocolates, or flowers. Surrounded by the luggage they would take onto the train, the women looked awkward in their stiff new uniforms. Their "short" skirts, grayish-brown, just covered the tops of their ankle boots, and their matching belted tunics were buttoned firmly up to their necks. Their main luggage had already been stowed and would be waiting for them upon arrival—or so they thought.

Victoria Station was bustling.[2] In the six weeks since war had been declared, the railway terminus had been transformed. Along with commuters pouring off the trains for their daily drudgery, there were now Belgian refugees, who had fled the invading German Army carrying pitiful bundles of belongings, their frightened children in tow. Traumatized and bewildered, they were met by women volunteers who had set up emergency canteens on the concourse. There were other British travelers, too, people who had found themselves stranded in Europe and farther afield when war broke out and who were only now straggling home.

Departures were relatively few. Thousands of soldiers had already passed through Victoria on their way to France and Flanders. Weighed down by kitbags and buoyed up by patriotic songs, they had exchanged farewells with their families and sweethearts before boarding their trains. One traveler, aware that many who said their goodbyes would never see each other again, called Victoria the "Palace of Tears."[3] More would follow in the ensuing weeks and months. While the soldiers of the British Expeditionary Force, made up of the regular army and reservists, were already mired in the thick of battle on the Western Front, hundreds of thousands more men had since enlisted in response to the "call to arms" declared by the new secretary of state for war, Lord Kitchener. So far, at least, the casualties which had begun to stream back from the first battles had arrived at London stations under cover of night.[4] Many, indeed, had never returned at all; the army's medical services had been so overwhelmed already by the sheer scale and severity of the injuries that thousands had perished before they could be treated.

Yet for all this, the atmosphere at Victoria Station that morning was predominantly cheerful—especially among the party of women waiting to board their train for France. For them, one war had ended as another had begun.

JUST AS POLITICIANS of all stripes had buried their differences to fight the common enemy on the outbreak of war, so, too, had a truce been declared between women and men. After years of escalating militancy in the battle for women's voting rights, the leaders of the suffragists and suffragettes had put aside their demands immediately when war began.[5] Millicent Fawcett, president of the non-militant National Union of Women's Suffrage Societies (NUWSS), had led the way by calling on her supporters—the suffragists—to offer their services to their country. "Women, your country needs you," she exhorted her members within days of war being declared, even before Kitchener's iconic poster made the same appeal to men.[6] Emmeline Pankhurst, the steely matriarch of the Women's Social and Political Union (WSPU), had followed her example a few days later, urging her militant members—the suffragettes—to suspend all activism and divert their energies and organizational skills into supporting the war effort. In return, the government had announced an amnesty and released all suffragettes from prison—some several hundred women—within a week of declaring war.

Although some stalwarts of the women's movement had joined pacifist campaigns, most women threw themselves into the new cause in a rush of patriotic fervor. One group of suffragettes had already launched the Women's Emergency Corps to recruit women into jobs vacated by men who were now enlisting. Women had flocked to its headquarters to volunteer as drivers and motorcycle dispatch riders, or to run soup kitchens and refugee shelters.[7] Aristocratic women and society ladies, until recently some of the loudest voices demanding the vote, were now offering their homes in London as convalescent hospitals for the wounded and raising funds to send medical units to France. And women everywhere, whether they identified themselves as suffragists or not, were signing up to play their part as volunteers at home and overseas.

Louisa Garrett Anderson and Flora Murray, who were waiting to board their train at Victoria that morning, had been among the first to recognize the unique opportunity that war presented to women. They knew that war with Germany posed a terrifying threat to Britain, but it also offered women a once-in-a-lifetime chance. Both Anderson and Murray were qualified doctors of many years' standing. Anderson, forty-one, was a surgeon, and Murray, four years older, a physician and anesthetist. Yet despite the fact that each woman had more than ten years of experience in her chosen profession, neither had enjoyed a significant spell of work in a major general hospital. Hospital boards were almost entirely controlled by men, and women doctors were effectively excluded from training or working in mainstream hospitals or attaining high-status medical positions. Women were likewise barred from becoming army doctors regardless of the current need. Although their medical qualifications were exactly equivalent to those of their male colleagues, Murray and Anderson had been restricted to treating women and children. Through necessity as much as desire, they had worked in hospitals run by women for the treatment of women and children alone.

War had changed everything. Despite their complete lack of experience in treating men or in dealing with war injuries, the two women had decided to set up their own emergency hospital to treat wounded soldiers plucked from the battlefields in France. Gathering together a team of young recruits, including three more women doctors, eight nurses, three women orderlies, and four male helpers, they were bound for Paris.[8] It was a gamble. They were not only heading for unknown dangers in a war zone with eighteen young people under their command, but their medical inexperience meant they were seriously unprepared for the challenges ahead. Both, however, were as committed to the women's cause as they were to each other. They saw the unfolding drama in France as their first chance to prove that women doctors were equal to men.

FOR ANDERSON, ENTERING the medical profession had always seemed a foregone conclusion. Born in 1873, the eldest child of Elizabeth Garrett Anderson, the first woman to qualify in Britain as a doctor, and James Skelton Anderson, a Scottish shipping owner from a family of medics, Louisa had grown up in a world suffused by medicine.[9] Although she had been looked after by a nanny for much of her childhood, Louisa had vivid memories of riding in her mother's carriage—holding out her hand to catch raindrops—when her mother made her doctor's rounds from their house in London's West End. Occasionally she had even accompanied her mother to the New Hospital for Women, which her mother had founded in a poor part of west London, where Louisa had romped on the beds. A lively and imaginative child, Louisa was described by her mother as a "bright, skipping little creature, full of character and intelligence."[10]

Growing up with all the comforts of middle-class Victorian life, Louisa had enjoyed an idyllic childhood. While her parents worked long hours in London, Louisa ran wild with her younger brother, Alan, in the sprawling grounds of their family home near the seaside town of Aldeburgh in Suffolk, albeit with their nanny keeping a close eye.[11] In summer, they played in the sea and sailed paper boats in rock pools, and in winter they skated on frozen ponds. From the age of eight Louisa wrote fond letters to her parents, nicknamed "Moodle" and "Poodle," relating tales of derring-do and make-believe while lamenting how much she missed them. The carefree childhood nurtured a rebellious streak, so that "Louie," as she was known, became quietly determined to get her own way—in stubborn opposition to her mother, who fussed and worried over her children's health.

After being tutored at home and briefly attending a day school in London, Louisa had been sent to a girls' boarding school, St Leonard's, in St Andrew's on the east coast of Scotland, at fourteen.[12] One of the first big private schools for girls, St Leonard's modeled itself on the country's top boys' schools. Although the girls wore long, demure skirts and long-sleeved blouses, they learned Greek, Latin, French, and mathematics and played cricket and tennis, just as their brothers might do at Eton or Rugby. Clever and bookish, with a pretty face, pale complexion, and auburn hair, Louisa made friends easily and chaffed at her mother's fretting. "I must really expostulate against these sudden outbursts of excitement," she replied pompously when her mother feared she was ill.[13] At first, Louisa had been drawn to the arts: she edited the school magazine and took leading roles in school plays. Yet by the age of seventeen she had decided to follow in her mother's footsteps and embark on a career in medicine. This, even for the daughter of Britain's most famous medical woman, was no small feat.

LOUISA'S MOTHER, ELIZABETH Garrett Anderson, had succeeded in becoming the first woman qualified in Britain to join the Medical Register through a combination of iron will and stealth. In the mid-1800s, when Elizabeth was growing up, the daughters of middle-class families were raised with one ambition: to marry well.

Since women were regarded as physically, intellectually, and emotionally inferior to men, a serious education was considered not only unnecessary but decidedly unfeminine. Most girls from well-to-do families were allowed only rudimentary instruction at home, followed by a few years at boarding school, if they were lucky, to prepare them for married life. If they remained single over the age of thirty, women were written off as "old maids" and regarded as a financial burden on their fathers or brothers. There were only two routes to paid employment for middle-class women—becoming a governess or a lady's companion—and both were widely despised as scarcely above the rank of a servant.

Louisa was well aware of the obstacles her mother had battled. Born into a prosperous family in Suffolk, Elizabeth had enjoyed just two years of formal education at a girls' school in London from the age of thirteen.[14] But in her early twenties, she fixed on the idea of becoming a doctor after meeting Elizabeth Blackwell, an English-woman brought up in America who had obtained a medical degree at Geneva Medical College in New York State.[15] When she returned briefly to England in 1858, Blackwell had become the first woman to enter her name on the newly established UK Medical Register. In a pattern that would become wearily familiar to women who dared to follow in her footsteps, this door was immediately closed as the General Medical Council (GMC) ruled that doctors who qualified overseas were ineligible for the register. When Elizabeth Garrett announced her ambition, her mother shut herself in her room crying. Her father, initially repulsed by the idea, became one of her strongest allies.

Over the next six years, Elizabeth had battled every conceivable medical organization and educational institution in her mission to achieve her aim. Initially, she trained as a nurse for six months at the Middlesex Hospital, London, where she persuaded the hospital apothecary to accept her as a pupil. She even attended medical lectures, until she angered the male students by answering a question nobody else could answer, and was barred from future classes. One by one, every medical school and university in England and Scotland refused to admit her. But after completing her five-year apothecary apprenticeship, in 1865 she passed the examination of the Society of Apothecaries and in that way added her name to the Medical Register, thus becoming the first woman qualified in Britain to do so. The society immediately amended its rules to prevent other women from following her example.

Having qualified to practice as a doctor in Great Britain, Elizabeth also obtained a medical degree in Paris—the first woman to do this—then slowly built up a viable practice in London. When Elizabeth married Louisa's father, James Skelton Anderson, a partner in the Orient Steamship Line, friends assumed she would give up her career. Far from surrendering her independence, Elizabeth not only continued her private practice but opened ten beds above the dispensary she had founded, creating the New Hospital for Women. This infirmary would treat impoverished women and provide clinical experience for other would-be female doctors. Yet since every door that Elizabeth had pried open had just as quickly been slammed shut by the male medical establishment, other women who aspired to study medicine had been barred from following her—despite determined efforts.

Some women obtained medical degrees at universities on the Continent, which were gradually opening their doors to female students—but this did not permit them to practice in Britain. Refusing to be defeated, one enterprising woman, Sophia Jex-Blake, founded a medical school exclusively for women, the London School of Medicine for Women (LSMW), which opened in 1874. Elizabeth Garrett Anderson became the only woman on the otherwise entirely male teaching staff. Yet none of the nineteen medical examining bodies would grant the school accreditation.

Hostility to the idea of women becoming doctors intensified during the 1870s. One prominent doctor declared that he would rather follow his only daughter to the grave than allow her to study medicine.[16] The *British Medical Journal* feared the "Temple of Medicine" was being "besieged by fair invaders," and the leading medical journal, *The Lancet*, warned of a potential "invasion of Amazons."[17] The barriers were finally breached when Parliament passed the Medical Act of 1876, which enabled—though it did not compel—universities to admit women.[18] That same year, the Royal College of Physicians of Ireland agreed to recognize the LSMW and examine its students, providing them with a route to qualify for the Medical Register. A year later, the LSMW struck a deal with the cash-strapped Royal Free Hospital to provide its students with clinical experience on the wards in return for handsome fees. Soon after that, the school was incorporated as a college of the University of London. Other British universities slowly followed suit in admitting women as medical students, although Oxford and Cambridge would continue to bar women from studying medicine even in 1914.

The battle for women's entry into medicine had been won. By the time Louisa Garrett Anderson set her sights on becoming a doctor in 1890, women were theoretically permitted to study medicine and qualify to practice—albeit chiefly through the LSMW. Some one hundred women doctors had added their names to the Medical Register by 1891.[19] Obtaining postgraduate training and hospital experience was another matter. The route for men who wished to climb the medical career ladder was generally straightforward. After training at a reputable medical school, they were normally offered a junior post in the hospital attached to that school. Given the right connections, they would then progress to a senior post in a specialty such as surgery or gynecology. Hospital jobs were honorary and unpaid—hospitals were charities that treated only the poor, while wealthier patients were attended at home or in private nursing homes—but they usually led to lucrative private practice in the chosen field. With no access to these male networks, women were denied this route.

None of the major medical schools accepted women, and the royal medical colleges in London and Edinburgh barred women from taking the specialist examinations required to progress up the surgical and medical ladders.[20] Apart from at the Royal Free and one or two hospitals elsewhere, women were simply never considered for junior posts by the all-male appointment boards. Effectively blocked from working in surgical or medical specialties, and likewise prevented from treating men, women were unable to take the first step on the career path leading to prominent hospital positions and successful private careers. Women doctors, therefore, had little choice but to take low-paid and low-status jobs as medical officers in schools, prisons, and asylums, to work in hospitals set up and run by women to treat women and children, or to head overseas for jobs men did not want in medical missions—about a third of LSMW graduates went abroad. Committing herself to medicine at the age of seventeen, Louisa Garrett Anderson therefore knew that the obstacles would be considerable and the opportunities few.

LEAVING ST LEONARD'S at eighteen, Anderson had enjoyed a vacation in Paris with her mother and brother and then stayed on alone with a French family to brush up her French. Her mother was still fretting about her daughter's health, remarking, "She will turn into a sweet, delightful woman if she lives, but I should much like to see her stronger."[21] Clearly more robust than her mother believed, Anderson survived her French leave and spent the next year at the women-only Bedford College in London, studying the sciences in preparation for medical school. The following year, in the autumn of 1892, she enrolled at the LSMW, where her mother was now dean, along with thirty other women students. She worked hard, winning several prizes, to qualify as Bachelor of Medicine at the end of the five-year course, and achieved Bachelor of Surgery the following year. Now legally entitled to practice as a doctor, she faced the scramble for her first hospital job.

Since there was no point in applying to a major general hospital, Anderson took junior posts at two charitable hospitals in poor areas of south London in 1898 and 1899.[22] She gained her Doctor of Medicine degree from London University in 1900, aged twenty-seven. Already she had determined on becoming a surgeon. Her mother had never enjoyed operating, Anderson would later say, but Louisa was inspired by another woman doctor, Mary Scharlieb, who had worked in India. Watching her perform complex abdominal surgery at the New Hospital, Anderson was awed at seeing "her slender hands seeming to go everywhere with marvellous speed."[23] The following year, when the Royal Free designated two of its six junior doctor posts for women, Anderson was appointed house surgeon there, becoming one of the first women to obtain a junior post in a general hospital—albeit still on the women's wards and for just six months.

Eager for wider clinical experience, she was forced to look overseas. Earlier in 1901, she had spent a few weeks with a friend in Paris attending anatomy lectures and had even assisted at an operation—"both of us dressed up in Frenchman's operating pinafores," she told her mother.[24] In December, she and another friend sailed for the United States to attend lectures at two of America's most prestigious medical schools.

Arriving in Baltimore, Louisa enrolled as a postgraduate student at the Johns Hopkins Hospital Medical School, which admitted women students on the same basis as men. Though she found Baltimore a "sleepy" town, she was impressed by the school's professor of medicine, Dr. William Osler, who emphasized the importance of listening to patients—a novel concept—in forming a diagnosis.[25] It was a practice Louisa would take pains to follow. Moving on to Chicago, she was shocked at the "bustling and dirty" city with its seventeen-story "houses," but the clinical lectures of Dr. Nicholas Senn, professor of surgery at Rush Medical School, made it all worthwhile. Crammed into the lecture theater with up to five hundred other students, Louisa was transfixed as Senn exhibited some thirty patients in turn and then—after downing a glass of milk and beaten eggs—performed five or six major operations and the same number of minor ones. Having served as a surgeon in Cuba in 1898 during the Spanish-American War, Senn was an expert in military surgery and wound management. It is possible he also instilled an appetite in Anderson for war surgery. Her experience in America confirmed her ambition to become a surgeon, and yet she was no nearer a permanent hospital post. In London, Paris, and Chicago, she had watched operations on men, women, and children—and even assisted at a few—but she lacked direct experience of performing operations herself.

ANDERSON RETURNED TO London in 1902 as the Victorian era gave way to the twentieth century, but her prospects were not promising.

Her brother, Alan, had followed his father into the family shipping firm after studying at Eton, then Oxford. After Alan got married in 1902, his future was settled. Louisa was still living at home in London with a generous private income from her parents. Yet although her training and experience were equal to those of her male contemporaries, she had no chance of securing a post as a consultant surgeon in a major hospital to provide the professional status she craved. There were now more than two hundred women doctors on the Medical Register, but almost all of them worked in women-run hospitals or dispensaries treating only women and children. One enterprising female doctor ran two sanatoria, which treated both men and women for tuberculosis, and a handful of medical women had West End consulting rooms, where they attracted society ladies who chose to be examined by a woman rather than a man.[26] Such a preference was not only regarded as eccentric, but was fiercely opposed by male consultants eager to protect their profitable gynecological practices. Attitudes toward "lady doctors" were as hardened as ever. Anderson, therefore, had no choice but to take a post in a hospital run by women that treated women and children.

Anderson joined the staff of the hospital her mother had founded, the New Hospital for Women, in 1902, around the same time her mother retired. The hospital had recently moved into larger premises in Euston Road. She would work there as a surgical assistant, and later senior surgeon, until the outbreak of war.[27] With forty-two beds and a busy outpatient department to run, the fourteen members of the medical staff were in constant demand. Working-class women from all over London flocked to the New Hospital to be treated by women doctors, and many of them were seriously ill after waiting months or years for medical aid. One patient had been in pain for four years while her male doctor insisted to her husband that she was suffering from "hysteria"; she underwent a successful operation at the New Hospital.[28] By 1913, the hospital had expanded to include a cancer ward, an isolation ward—for venereal disease—and an X-ray department. That year the staff treated nearly 900 inpatients, attended 300 women giving birth at home, and saw more than 32,000 outpatients.

At the New Hospital Louisa was kept busy performing gynecological operations as well as some general surgery. She approached her work with a rigorous scientific method, judging from a research paper she published jointly with the hospital's pathologist in 1908, analyzing 265 cases of cancer of the uterus over the previous twelve years.[29] The paper, which included results for some of her own operations for hysterectomy, emphasized the importance of following up with patients after their operations to assess which surgical methods were the most successful, but it also made clear the need for surgeons to work closely with pathologists. Meanwhile, she set up consulting rooms in a house her father had bought her in Harley Street—London's most popular medical address—in 1903.[30] The family name drew some prominent patients: in 1910, she signed the death certificate of Florence Nightingale.[31]

Yet despite the family connections, Anderson was completely blocked from advancing in surgery so long as men still held the keys to all the major London hospitals and specialist positions. While her mother's generation—the pioneers—might have accepted their confinement to women-only hospitals, Louisa and her contemporaries—the second generation of medical women—would not.[32]

IT WAS LITTLE wonder, given the injustice and discrimination she faced, that Anderson had been drawn to the battle for women's rights. Here, too, she was following in her family's footsteps, since her mother had supported women's suffrage since its earliest days. Indeed, her mother had presented a petition to Parliament demanding votes for women as far back as 1866.[33] But it was Louisa's aunt, her mother's younger sister, Millicent Garrett Fawcett, who had taken up the banner for women's right to vote most forcefully. In 1897, Aunt Millie had become founding president of the NUWSS, which campaigned for the vote through democratic means. By the time she was thirty, in 1903, Louisa was active in several organizations affiliated with the NUWSS. But by 1907, she had become impatient with the suffragists' moderate tactics, which had achieved nothing but lip service from the Liberal government. So she joined the newly formed and much more confrontational WSPU—the suffragettes—led by the formidable Emmeline Pankhurst and her charismatic daughter Christabel. Compared with the demure earnestness of the suffragists, the suffragettes provided a far more exciting and radical prospect. Hearing Christabel speak, one recruit declared, "It thrilled me through and through."[34] Louisa made large donations to the WSPU and joined its protest rallies, speaking at several meetings and leading women medical graduates on one of its marches.[35]

AS THE PROTESTS escalated, with mass arrests of women who chained themselves to railings and ambushed election rallies, Louisa applauded the WSPU's policy of civil disobedience and even tried to persuade Aunt Millie to join its forces. Exasperated at the slippery twists and turns of the Liberal prime minister, Herbert Asquith, in 1908, she urged her aunt to support the WSPU in "more militant action." Despite two enormous NUWSS and WSPU demonstrations that summer, the government remained intransigent. "Surely we must do <u>something</u>," she told Aunt Millicent. "They [the WSPU] mean to protest at once & on a large scale & unless we can protest constitutionally & effectually I think it is the duty of everyone who is able to do it to join them." To do nothing, she insisted, is "really too feeble."[36] Her appeal was fruitless—Millicent Fawcett would become increasingly opposed to the WSPU's uncompromising approach—but Louisa had more success with her mother. That summer, Elizabeth Garrett Anderson joined the WSPU—a major coup for Emmeline Pankhurst—and spoke at several rallies. A few months later, Louisa was among the crowd when suffragettes attempted to invade the House of Commons, and she later gave evidence in support of the action when Pankhurst was tried for incitement.[37]

The following year, in October 1909, as suffragettes on hunger strike were being force-fed by prison doctors for the first time, Louisa Garrett Anderson hosted the inaugural meeting of the Women's Tax Resistance League in her Harley Street house.[38] Refusing to pay income tax on the basis that they were denied representation, its members included several women doctors. And a year later, when Asquith provoked fury by blocking a promised new bill, Louisa was ready to act on the WSPU's motto of "Deeds not Words."

After warning the New Hospital board that she might be arrested, on November 18, 1910, she joined her mother on the platform of a huge rally in central London at Caxton Hall, along with Emmeline Pankhurst and other leading suffragettes.[39] After Pankhurst spoke, the Garrett Andersons followed her out of the hall to lead three hundred women in a march on the House of Commons. In Parliament Square, they were met by ranks of police and hired hooligans who blocked their way. Although Pankhurst and Elizabeth Garrett Anderson were allowed to pass, other women were jostled and assaulted. "I nearly fainted," said one supporter, "and Louie Garrett Anderson succeeded in making them let me through."[40] In the pitched battle, more than one hundred women were arrested and scores were injured and sexually molested. Louisa herself was arrested but released without charge. The day would become known as Black Friday. Undeterred by the increasing violence, Louisa was prepared, two years later, to take her support of the women's cause a crucial step further.

On March 4, 1912, Louisa joined a mass protest of suffragettes who marched through London's West End, smashing windows with hammers and stones. They had been motivated by the jibes of a Liberal Member of Parliament (MP) who had proclaimed that if the suffrage campaign really enjoyed popular support, then women would be breaking the law like the men who had agitated for the 1832 Reform Act. Anderson was arrested for throwing a stone through the window of a house in Knightsbridge and sentenced to six weeks of hard labor in Holloway Prison. Pleading guilty, she said her action was a "political protest" prompted by the MP's remark about the 1832 campaign. She added, "We are fighting the same battle as was fought then, and if it is the only argument that the country can understand we are obliged to use it."[41] It was a bold and dangerous step. As a doctor, she was risking her reputation by engaging in militant—indeed criminal—activity. Seizing on her status as a high-profile figure, newspapers broadcast her conviction under headlines such as "Lady Doctor Sentenced"—although one at least felt the need to point out that it was not her mother, who almost approached the status of a national treasure, in the dock. Aunt Millie was not pleased: the report of Louisa's sentence in *The Times* was juxtaposed with an article reporting Millicent Fawcett's condemnation of the suffragettes' actions.

Anderson gamely resigned herself to a spell behind bars in the notorious Holloway women's prison, where inmates were kept in solitary confinement in tiny cells for up to twenty-three hours a day and hunger-striking suffragettes were physically restrained while they were force-fed. Despite the captivity, she smuggled out several letters to her mother written in pencil on tissue-thin paper. Although Elizabeth had now severed links with the WSPU, Louisa told her mother she was "glad & proud" of her actions because she believed that "this kind of fighting . . . is necessary to win our Cause."[42] Regardless of the hard beds, plain food, and lack of freedom, she made light of her situation, likening the prison to "a badly kept hotel with cold monotonous food & bells that no one answers!" In a demonstration of the sense of irony that would stand her in good stead in years to come, she described her enforced break as "a complete holiday."

Far from deterring her from future militancy, Anderson's imprisonment reinforced her loyalty to the women's cause and gave her a taste for being in the midst of the action. "This is the most wonderful experience I have ever had," she enthused, adding, "It is enormous luck to be alive just now & in this thing, really in the centre of it." The sight of desperately poor women in jail for petty theft and prostitution, some of them with babies, reduced her to tears and made her all the more determined to improve women's lives. "I never knew so clearly before why I was a suffragist," she wrote. Through it all, the camaraderie among the suffragette inmates maintained morale. While Emmeline Pankhurst kept up their spirits, the composer Ethel Smyth conducted the women in a rendition of the suffragette anthem by waving her toothbrush from her cell window. One fellow prisoner described Anderson dancing a Highland fling with another inmate and organizing games of cricket with pieces of wood. Another, who kept a secret diary, said of Anderson, "It amused me so much to see her running hard today playing . . . under the shadow of a high prison wall."[43] Meanwhile, her brother used his business influence to persuade the Home Office to release her five days early, on the understanding that her family would encourage her to temper her rebellious ways. The home secretary, Reginald McKenna, sanctioned her release before Easter, so she was home by the time her fellow prisoners began a hunger strike.[44] Anderson protested at her special treatment, telling a suffragettes' meeting two weeks later that on account of her social standing, "the Home Office found that I might like to spend Easter with my family," while other prisoners had spent the holiday behind bars.[45]

Although Anderson left the WSPU a few months later, along with others objecting to Emmeline Pankhurst's increasingly autocratic conduct, her prison sentence made her more radical rather than less so. It was in this atmosphere of intense political agitation that she had come to know Flora Murray.

BORN IN DUMFRIESSHIRE in the Scottish borders in 1869, Flora Murray was the daughter of a retired naval commander with a long Scottish heritage and a sizable country estate.[46] A prominent local family, the Murrays had lived at their home, Murraythwaite, for almost five hundred years. Flora, the fourth of six children, had grown up in a grand mansion amid lush gardens surrounded by farmland and woods. Yet her childhood was not without strain. Her father, John Murray, the sixteenth laird, had died when she was three, leaving her mother, Grace, to bring up six children and manage the estate alone. Although there was income from tenant farmers and shares, there was little left for luxuries. Nonetheless, Flora had been educated by private tutors in Edinburgh and attended girls' boarding schools in London and Germany. When she was home, she rubbed shoulders with the local gentry at hunting events and county balls, escorted by her eldest brother, William, the seventeenth laird.

Although she was four years older than Anderson, Murray had embarked on her medical career later. At twenty-one she had signed up for six months' training as a nurse at the London Hospital, Whitechapel, before deciding she wanted to become a doctor. She enrolled at the LSMW in 1897, the same year Anderson left, at the comparatively mature age of twenty-eight. Just over two years later, in January 1900, her second-eldest brother, Fergus, a captain in the Scottish Rifles, was killed in action in the Boer Wars, aged thirty-one. Despite being wounded in four places, Captain Murray had continued to command his troops before he finally expired. His death in battle may well have inspired Murray to serve in some military capacity. That same year she left the LSMW, perhaps to be closer to her grieving family, and finished her training at Durham University. She qualified in medicine and surgery in 1903 before gaining her Doctor of Medicine degree in 1905.

Facing the usual brick wall confronting women doctors, Murray took a junior post at Crichton Royal Institution, a vast Victorian asylum near her family home, in charge of female patients. Moving to London in 1905, she had no choice but to follow the path of other women doctors in taking honorary posts in small hospitals for women and children. Murray worked as a house surgeon at Belgrave Hospital for Children in south London and assistant anesthetist at Chelsea Hospital for Women. Taking a keen interest in children's health and anesthesia, she published an article in *The Lancet* in 1905 on the safest form of anesthetic for infants. She also championed the idea of "health visitors" who would offer advice on child welfare to poor mothers in their own homes.[47]

Yet despite her personal ambitions and determination to improve health care, Murray was as stymied as any other woman doctor in pursuing her goals. With only a small income from private patients, possibly supplemented by an allowance from her family, she was not well off. "Her early life was a struggle against hard conditions and financial stress," Anderson would later say.[48] The problems plainly rankled. Observing male colleagues of equal or lesser abilities rise effortlessly through the ranks, Murray grew increasingly angry. In an impassioned article in the *New Statesman* in 1913, she railed against the inequalities and discrimination. Women were denied entry to medical schools, blocked from postgraduate training, and refused jobs in hospitals, she wrote. "Staff appointments are professional prizes. They are made by the council or governing body, generally consisting entirely of men, upon the advice of a medical staff composed entirely of men. They are usually given to men."[49]

Like Anderson, Murray had thrown herself into the battle for women's rights, joining Fawcett's NUWSS soon after arriving in London and later Pankhurst's WSPU.[50] Murray never engaged in overt militant activity or went to prison like Anderson, but her involvement with the suffragettes was potentially far more dangerous. Not only did she speak at rallies and join marches, but she also organized first aid posts to treat women bloodied and battered in the clashes with police, as well as tending Pankhurst and other suffragettes when they were released from prison, emaciated from hunger strikes, at a nursing home she helped run near Notting Hill Gate. Murray was regarded as "honorary physician" to the WSPU; according to Christabel Pankhurst, she "devoted herself to the medical care of Mother and of all our many prisoners."[51]

After the government sanctioned the force-feeding of hunger-striking suffragettes in 1909, Murray had become one of the most vociferous opponents of the practice. While most of the medical profession maintained that forcible feeding was safe, she rallied sympathetic doctors who protested that it was both dangerous and inhumane. Within weeks, she had organized a petition to Asquith signed by 116 doctors. She continued to campaign against force-feeding by writing pamphlets and articles outlining the medical dangers in graphic detail. From her experience treating Pankhurst and other force-fed suffragettes, Murray declared that "teeth may have been broken or loosened, the body is black and blue, the marks of nails are visible on the hands and arms of the victim." In the most serious cases, a woman had contracted pneumonia after food entered her lung, and a man had become insane.[52]

Many suffragettes would later write with fond affection of Flora Murray's care. One activist, who was force-fed 232 times, said, "It was a joy and comfort to be received and cared for by our own splendid Dr. Flora Murray."[53] Another woman, who worked at the nursing home, said, "All the women who were being forcibly fed were brought to that house. Some were brought there on stretchers, and looked after until they were well again."

The government grew increasingly alarmed at the prospect of a suffragette dying and being hailed a martyr, and legislation was introduced in 1913 allowing prisoners to be released for short periods in order to recover from their hunger strikes before being rearrested to continue their sentences. Murray was quick to condemn the law, dubbed the "Cat and Mouse Act," as "brutalising and degrading." Writing in *The Suffragette*, the WSPU's newspaper, she described how Emmeline Pankhurst and others had been released from prison in a precarious state of health and then rearrested before they had fully recovered, only to be released again a few days later "on a stretcher, half-killed." She declared, "The true meaning of it all is murder—murder by Act of Parliament."[54] By this point, in 1913, Murray was looking after Pankhurst and other activists on an almost full-time basis. She frequently gave evidence in court attesting to defendants' medical conditions. On their temporary releases, many prisoners were discharged into her care, and when their time expired, the warrants for their rearrest were often issued to her.[55] In one series of photographs, Murray is pictured with Catherine Pine, a redoubtable nurse who cared for many suffragettes, accompanying Pankhurst as she was apprehended by a detective before she sank fainting into Pine's arms.[56] Another time, Pankhurst was returning from Paris with Murray and Pine when two detectives boarded the train at Dover and arrested her. Pankhurst and other activists were being shadowed constantly by officers from Scotland Yard, and by 1913 Murray was herself under surveillance. Detectives suspected her of aiding and abetting her patients as they attempted to outwit the police and commit further outrages.

By this stage, the WSPU campaign had reached unprecedented levels of violence. Suffragettes and their supporters set private property on fire, poured chemicals into public mailboxes, and cut telegraph wires. A cottage belonging to the chancellor of the exchequer, the Liberal Party statesman David Lloyd George, was badly damaged by explosives, and a tea room in Regent's Park burned to the ground. It was "guerrilla warfare," said Pankhurst.[57] Meanwhile, the suffragettes had become adept at evading rearrest by adopting elaborate disguises during their time out of prison and affecting ingenious getaways.

Murray was plainly complicit in some of these great escapes. One of her suffragette patients described how a friend had dressed as her "double" and left a nursing home in a taxi to trick detectives into following her; meanwhile, the woman the detectives thought they were following boldly walked out of the nursing home just minutes later and boarded a bus, having been dosed by Murray with strychnine to "brace me up."[58] At times Murray's own house was watched by detectives and she was followed as she went about her duties. When Edwy Clayton, a chemist who supported the WSPU, was tried in 1914 for conspiracy to bomb government buildings and other targets, a detective giving evidence said he had followed Clayton to Murray's house. He kept watch for three days before Murray told police Clayton had left and the surveillance was lifted.[59]

In colluding with the suffragettes' increasingly violent tactics, Murray was making powerful enemies in the Home Office and among other authorities. By the summer of 1914, she found herself under attack within the medical profession too.[60] Murray and a fellow physician, Frank Moxon, had accused doctors at Holloway of drugging prisoners with bromide to make them more docile for force-feeding, and published results of laboratory tests on three women to back their claims. In July, the Holloway doctors sued Murray and Moxon for libel.

MIXING IN MEDICAL circles sympathetic to the suffragettes, Murray and Anderson had become friends. Before long, this connection deepened. Tall and slim with red hair, sharply defined features, and a boyish figure—one friend described her as "flat-chested" and "hipless"—Murray, known as "Flo" to friends, was a taciturn but forceful personality who kept calm under pressure. Acquaintances regarded her as "cool and reserved"—one described her as "very Scottish & harsh"—but friends thought her "tender and gentle" with a pervading aura of composure.[61] One colleague said that "even the fractious baby in a children's hospital ceased its crying when Dr Murray spoke." Murray found common cause with the more demonstrative, more impulsive, more gregarious Anderson. Both were ambitious to succeed in medicine. Together, they raised funds to open a small hospital for children in two terraced cottages in Harrow Road, a desperately poor area of west London, in 1912.[62] Proudly brandishing their political affiliations, they adopted the WSPU slogan—"Deeds not Words"—as the hospital's motto.

Since hospitals for children were still a rarity, the Harrow Road outpatient department had been quickly overwhelmed by demand from needy families all over London. As many as one hundred children crowded the clinic on a single afternoon, and the hospital treated more than seven thousand patients in its first eighteen months. Raising funds from well-heeled friends, Anderson and Murray expanded into the neighboring house and opened a ward with four beds and three cots in 1913. A female journalist, shown round by Anderson in the summer of 1914, was touched by the scene. She found the wards brightly decorated with red, blue, and white bedspreads and liberally supplied with toys. Anderson had ended the tour by picking up "a stout and aggressive toy donkey," which she introduced as "Bodkin." Others were less impressed. *The Hospital* magazine, which took a dim view of women doctors, thought the building "wholly inappropriate" for inpatients with its primitive bathroom and tiny operating room. At the center of this clamor, Murray is pictured in a photograph calmly writing a prescription in a crowded clinic; nearby, a mother bounces her baby on her knee and a girl holds up two dolls to the camera.[63]

Jointly running their modest hospital, Anderson and Murray juggled the demands of their other medical posts as well as their suffragette activities. By this stage, they were not only partners in their medical work; they had also become partners in their private lives.

BY EARLY 1914, Murray and Anderson were living together at 60 Bedford Gardens, a semidetached Victorian villa in Kensington that Anderson had bought the previous year.[64] Handy for the children's hospital and the suffragette nursing home, the house boasted four bedrooms, a library, wine cellars, and a walled garden. They also jointly owned a weekend cottage they had built in the village of Penn in Buckinghamshire a few years earlier. Murray and Anderson were not unusual in setting up house together as two unmarried women in the early twentieth century. For many single professional women, sharing a home provided not only financial convenience but also social independence. Styled "Boston marriages" after two female characters in Henry James's novel *The Bostonians*, these arrangements particularly suited medical women, who valued the mutual support of working and living together in a hostile male environment.[65] As many as 80 percent of women doctors were unmarried in the early 1900s. Marriage and medicine "did not mix," said one female doctor, who believed "a wedding-ring led to the graveyard of a medical woman's ambitions."[66]

For some women doctors—and a number of suffragettes—living together was part of a loving relationship as well as a convenient partnership. Unlike male homosexuality, lesbian relationships were not illegal, and were so little discussed they were rarely even suspected; it was deemed perfectly respectable for two professional women to share a home without a hint of scandal. Murray and Anderson therefore made no attempt to keep their arrangement secret. Yet by 1914, it is clear they were effectively living as a married couple.

While in prison, Anderson had applied to the Home Office for permission for a visit from Murray—ostensibly "on business"—a request that was refused. In later life, Murray would refer to Anderson as "my loving comrade," and Anderson would tell her sister-in-law "we hate being apart."[67] They wore identical diamond rings. One friend, a journalist and fellow suffragette named Evelyn Sharp, would later say she had enjoyed a close relationship with Anderson until Murray "came between us," adding that their "friendship seemed broken" just before the outbreak of war.[68] Anderson and Sharp had spent two summer vacations together in 1910 and 1911 at a cottage in the Scottish Highlands belonging to Anderson's mother. Sharp fondly described their "great times together climbing the easier mountains." Writing to Sharp after one of these trips, Anderson said their fortnight together had brought her "great happiness," but she urged Sharp not to hate the Penn cottage that she and Murray had recently bought, pledging that it "isn't going to come between us." Despite Anderson's protestations, however, by early 1914 a rift had developed. Henry Nevinson, a veteran war correspondent and suffragette sympathizer who was Sharp's devoted companion, though married, revealed that in January Evelyn had shown him "an appealing, passionately loving letter" from Anderson arguing against Sharp's resolve not to meet. Sharp, however, had told him the situation was hopeless owing to "Dr. F.M.'s bullying absorption of the other." While Anderson seemed anxious to maintain her close friendship with Sharp, Murray was apparently too possessive.

It is impossible to say whether Murray and Anderson enjoyed a sexual relationship—no letters between them have survived—but by August 1914, when they set off for France, they had certainly forged a lifelong loving bond. For both of them, the partnership was inextricably bound up with their commitment to women's rights and their determination to prove the worth of women doctors. The success of their medical mission to France was crucial in this cause.

THEY HAD ACTED quickly. During the summer of 1914, few people in Britain had anticipated war.[69] Anxieties, if any, were focused closer to home on the threat of civil war in Ireland, the spate of strikes beginning to paralyze the country, and the new round of vandalism being wreaked by suffragettes. Although by the end of July the tensions in the Balkans had made war in mainland Europe look increasingly likely, most people still believed this would not involve Britain. During the bank holiday weekend of August 1 to 3, many Britons were enjoying seaside outings and countryside excursions under cloudless blue skies: they returned to their homes that Bank Holiday Monday to news that Germany had declared war on France. The following day, August 4, as Germany invaded Belgium, and with Britain's ultimatum on Belgian neutrality running out at 11:00 p.m., most people were still in shock. Waking up the next morning to news that Britain was at war, one prominent suffragette said, "The world in which we lived and dreamed and worked was shattered to bits."[70]

Yet within a week of Britain declaring war on Germany, as troops were being hastily mobilized for France and recruitment posters were being pasted on walls, Murray and Anderson had decided they, too, would go to war. Just as male doctors in reserve units were being called up to serve in the army's medical corps, so they resolved to dedicate their medical skills to the war effort. This was not only a chance to do their duty for their country; it was a unique opportunity to gain vital surgical experience and prove that women doctors were every bit as good as men.

They did not waste time approaching the army or the British government. As suffragettes with records of political protest and criminal defiance, they knew they were regarded in government circles effectively as public enemies. Besides, they were well aware there was no point in offering their services to the War Office. One fellow surgeon, the Scottish suffragist Elsie Inglis, had already volunteered her skills to army medical chiefs in Scotland and been smartly rebuffed by an official who told her, "My good lady, go home and sit still."[71] Another woman doctor, Florence Stoney, who had set up the first X-ray departments at the Royal Free and the New Hospital for Women, had offered to take herself and her mobile X-ray unit to the front. But the War Office had spurned her, too. Instead, on August 12, 1914—two days after the government set all the suffragette prisoners free—Murray and Anderson called at the French embassy in London.

They had been received by one of the embassy secretaries in an "absolutely airless room" reeking of "stale cigar smoke," Murray later wrote.[72] In "somewhat rusty French" they offered to organize a surgical unit for France. In retrospect, Murray would admit, the official had probably assumed they simply wanted to finance and equip a unit—in the manner of other women volunteers—rather than actually treat any wounded soldiers themselves. In France, women doctors were no more welcome in the army than in Britain. Nevertheless, they were referred to the London headquarters of the French Red Cross, which accepted their offer immediately and gave them less than two weeks to raise funds, recruit staff, and organize supplies.

Friends, family, and fellow suffragettes had immediately rallied to the cause. Within a fortnight, subscribers had raised a colossal £2,000 (about £200,000 today, nearly US$250,000) to finance the "Women's Hospital Corps" (WHC). Half the money was immediately laid out on medicines, hospital equipment, and general supplies, including camp beds, blankets, chests of tea, invalid foods, surgical instruments, and chloroform. Packed up in more than one hundred bales and boxes, all emblazoned with the Red Cross symbol, the baggage weighed eighty tons. As it piled up outside the suppliers—Barker's department store, on Kensington High Street—the sprawling cargo attracted a crowd of sightseers. Meanwhile, Murray and Anderson had issued appeals for staff and been inundated with applications from young women eager to serve as doctors, nurses, and orderlies.

Volunteering to serve without pay, all the women who answered the call came from the same middle- or upper-class backgrounds as Murray and Anderson. They had been brought up by nannies and nursemaids, taught by governesses, and waited on by servants before being packed off to boarding schools. After leaving school, their social lives had revolved around tennis parties and costume balls, where they had been allowed to mix for the first time with men outside their immediate families, albeit under strict chaperone supervision. When war was declared, they had seen their brothers, cousins, and young male escorts rush to obtain commissions as junior officers heading for the front. Now they were determined to serve their country as well.

The three other doctors—Hazel Cuthbert, Gertrude Gazdar, and Grace Judge—were all younger and even less experienced than Murray and Anderson, having qualified in medicine within the previous six years.[73] At thirty-five, Gazdar was the eldest, although her petite figure and elfin face made her look years younger. Judge, who was attractive and self-assured, was thirty-one, and Cuthbert, with bright blue eyes and dark glossy hair, was twenty-eight. All three had only ever worked with women and children; Cuthbert and Judge had both held junior posts at Harrow Road. The eight nurses who accompanied them, including a nurse from Harrow Road, had probably served more time in general hospitals and had more experience of male patients than the doctors.

The three female orderlies had virtually no experience of working in any situation—let alone in a hospital. One of them, Galantha Cuthbert, was Dr. Cuthbert's younger sister, while the other two, Mardie Hodgson and Olga Campbell, were Murray's cousins by marriage. All three were in their early twenties. It was just as well then, perhaps, that Murray and Anderson had also recruited four male nurses to act as stretcher-bearers. Racing to meet the French Red Cross timetable, the two women speedily organized passports and vaccinations, made travel arrangements, and ordered uniforms for the sixteen women members of the corps.

The uniforms were chosen with care. Anderson and Murray had picked the ankle-length skirt—daringly short by 1914 standards—and belted, button-through tunic so they would be practical yet feminine. The durable fabric, which Murray described as "greenish-grey," but was closer to a greyish-brown, mimicked British army khaki, so the women would be taken seriously in a military situation.[74] The outfit was topped off with red shoulder straps—white for the orderlies—which were embroidered with the WHC initials, a hat with a veil, and an overcoat. Yet for all their efforts at femininity, Murray and Anderson wore their purple, white, and green suffragette badges on the fronts of their tunics with pride.

The French Red Cross was not nearly so efficient. While the French organizers searched for a suitable hospital location, and the St John Ambulance brigade arranged passports and transport, the corps' departure was delayed by two weeks. "We have spent weary hours with one incompetent official after another each contradicting what the last said," Anderson grumbled to her mother, "& all of them losing papers & letters which they assured us had to pass thro' their hands."[75] But at last the paperwork was completed, the arrangements finalized, and the baggage stowed. The day of departure had come.

THE THRONG OF well-wishers had swelled as the station clock neared 10:00 a.m. Henry Nevinson, the war journalist, who had come to watch the women leave, was thrilled to see a "great crowd of suffragettes like an old-time meeting."[76] Among them was Anderson's mother, who had made a special trip to bid her daughter farewell. Now seventy-eight, she was widowed, frail, and confused, not entirely sure where her daughter was going or even which war she was heading for. Her last words to the group, according to Murray, were, "My dears, if you go and if you succeed you will put forward the women's cause by thirty years." Given that Anderson later said she could not see her mother in the crowd, the story may be apocryphal. As the veteran of many wars, Nevinson read out the roll call of names and the onlookers cheered as the women boarded their train.

For all the optimism, as they settled into their saloon carriage and the whistle blew, Murray and Anderson must have felt apprehensive. A few days earlier, Anderson had assured her mother there was "no danger at all" in Paris, despite the fact that thousands of Parisians, including the entire French government, as well as the staff of the British Embassy, had fled the city. Many more citizens were even now packing their bags, since the German Army was encamped within sixty miles northeast of Paris and had launched air attacks on the city. Yet what the women lacked in experience they made up for in enthusiasm.

"We are a very gay young party except for Dr M. & me," Anderson wrote to her mother from the train, "and we feel we have a great chance which is a reason for joy."[77] The three orderlies were "very attractive capable girls who speak French well and know how to look after themselves." Even the men, including a boy who had left his job in a grocery shop to join them as a stretcher-bearer, were hopeful about their chances, she told a colleague. This gave them all "a good feeling" from the moment they left Victoria, and they knew they were "in for a 'big thing,'" she added. "This is just what you would have done at my age," Anderson told her mother, adding, "I hope I will be able to do it half as well as you wd have done." Murray was just as optimistic. When war was declared, women doctors knew "instinctively that the time had come when great and novel demands would be made upon them," she later wrote. War meant that "a hitherto unlooked-for occasion for service was at their feet."[78]

Although other women doctors—such as Elsie Inglis and Florence Stoney—had also begun to organize medical units to go abroad in the few weeks since Murray and Anderson had launched their mission, the Women's Hospital Corps was the first to leave for France. It was a departure in more ways than one. Leaving their old lives behind, the women were embarking on a daring, exhilarating, and dangerous new path. As their train steamed out of Victoria, they looked forward to all that lay ahead of them.

2

A Sort of Holiday

Paris, September 17, 1914

In its commanding position on the Champs-Élysées the brand-new Hôtel Claridge made an impressive sight.[1] The grand seven-story edifice had been outfitted with marble staircases, luxury furnishings, and crystal chandeliers in anticipation of the millionaire set its owners hoped to attract.[2] Yet just as the hotel was ready to welcome its first guests, the war had broken out and the building had been requisitioned by the French government.

Standing in the hotel's mirrored foyer, the women looked around with dismay at the bare salons and dining rooms, the whitewashed windows, and the workmen's debris littering the mosaic floors. The builders had left so recently that the plaster on the walls was still damp. The lighting and central heating were not yet working, and there was no hot water. Everywhere was cold, dark, and dirty. It was not a promising start. Indeed, it seemed as if the Women's Hospital Corps had been dogged by problems ever since leaving Victoria.

On arriving in Paris two days earlier, after twelve hours of travel, the women had found the Saint-Lazare railway terminus in near darkness, with no porters to be found. The door from the concourse to the Grand Hôtel Terminus, where they had rooms booked, was locked, on account of the nightly curfew imposed on the city. What was worse, they had discovered upon arrival in Dieppe that their

main baggage, £1,000 worth of supplies they had painstakingly organized, had not been loaded onto the boat they had boarded for
the Channel crossing, following their journey by train. Undaunted
by these setbacks, Mardie Hodgson and Olga Campbell, the two
Scottish orderlies, had immediately taken charge of the situation.
Despite protestations from officials, they had commandeered a trolley and trundled the remaining luggage round to the hotel's front
entrance. Then, since the lift was not working, they heaved their bags
up three flights of stairs to the bedrooms.[3] When they discovered that
the kitchens were closed, so that not so much as a *chocolat* could
be procured, the party had sat down on their beds and assembled a
picnic from the leftovers in their lunch baskets. As they tucked into
bread and butter with pressed beef washed down with cups of tea,
the women laughed and chatted. For the young nurses and orderlies, it was all a big adventure. They might have been sitting in their
dorms enjoying a midnight feast out of hampers sent from home.

Mardie Hodgson was in her element. The only child of affluent
parents who owned a Scottish estate, she had spent much of her
childhood riding her pony in the local woodlands and sailing the
Mediterranean in the yacht her father skippered.[4] She was a dare-
devil with a zest for adventure. Family photographs show her as
a young girl running barefoot along the deck of her father's yacht
with the wind ruffling her bloomers and her long hair flying out
behind. After her drink-loving father died when she was nine, her
mother had married a rather more sober and sensible widower, who
was a justice of the peace. Hodgson had spent some years at an
English boarding school before settling into a life of relatively idle
pleasure. Before the war she had filled her days with theater trips
and dances during the winter "season" in London; her summers
were devoted to family motoring tours around Europe and outdoor
jaunts in Scotland. She had learned not only to sail but to drive—
still a rarity among women at the time. Spending much of her time
with her Campbell cousins, Hodgson had become close to her first
cousin Olga.

Like Hodgson, Campbell had enjoyed a privileged upbringing and
carefree childhood, sporting with her four brothers on the family's

Scottish estate and traveling with her parents overseas. She had sailed to Southeast Asia to visit the tea plantation her father owned in what was then Ceylon (modern-day Sri Lanka) in 1913 and had just returned from a long vacation in California in July 1914. Like her cousin, Campbell had learned to drive. She even smoked—also rare for women of the time—and her personality combined the ebullience of a free spirit with sensible practicality. In America, she had enjoyed the freedom to consort with men her own age without the constant surveillance of a chaperone, and decided she wanted to train as a business secretary. Both Campbell and Hodgson were twenty-three years old, and both had been pressed into joining the Women's Hospital Corps by their Aunt Evelyn, who was married to Murray's eldest brother, William. Neither had needed much persuasion.

Sharing a tiny room at the Grand Hôtel Terminus with Campbell, Hodgson had scribbled a letter to her mother the morning after they arrived. The journey had been "great fun" and they had all arrived at Folkestone in "excellent spirits" before boarding the boat for a rather damp Channel crossing, she declared.[5] On their first day in Paris, Campbell and Hodgson had been charged with taking the nurses and male orderlies sightseeing, apparently unconcerned by any potentially imminent air raids. Their uniforms had caused quite a stir on their excursions around Paris, but the women felt "rather appressed" by having to wear their jackets in the warm September weather, since "our shirt sleeves are not sufficiently military looking," wrote Hodgson. Although her private schooling had failed to polish her spelling, Hodgson had picked up fluent French and German while touring Europe with her mother and stepfather and had been appointed the corps' chief interpreter. Since their cargo of supplies had still failed to arrive, the women had kept themselves busy by organizing their identity papers and arranging inoculations for those still needing them.

THE WOMEN HAD dealt with French bureaucrats and red tape with characteristic determination. But when they arrived at the Hôtel Claridge on the morning of September 17—their second full day in

Paris—and saw for the first time the building that would serve as their hospital, it was hard not to feel downhearted. Murray, who was keeping a diary, noted that the long corridors were "gloomy" and no ray of sunlight ever entered the salons.[6] Dashing off a letter to her mother, Anderson described Claridge's as "a gorgeous shell of marble & gilt without heating or crockery or anything practical."[7]

There was no time for misgivings. Drawing on the stamina and ingenuity that had been hallmarks of the suffragette campaign, Murray and Anderson embraced the new challenge with gusto. Doctors, nurses, and orderlies all rolled up their sleeves and set to scrubbing floors and cleaning windows from morning until nightfall. Quickly appraising their surroundings, Anderson and Murray decided that the four large salons on the ground floor would best serve as wards. These were situated surrounding an open courtyard. The ladies' cloakroom, with its tiled walls and floor, plentiful washbasins, and light-reflecting mirrors, could be converted into an operating theater, and the adjoining rooms on either side would become a dispensary and a sterilizing room, with fish kettles pressed into use as sterilizing units. Sending a sketch of the arrangements to her mother at the end of the first day's work, Hodgson wrote, "I was on the run all day & very happy."[8]

The following day, the corps checked out of the Grand Hôtel Terminus and moved into bedrooms on the first floor of Claridge's. As order began to prevail, the women pasted white paper onto the glass partitions that separated the salons and made up rows of camp beds with luxury linens purloined from the hotel stores. Some Belgian refugees, already billeted on the seventh floor, were dragooned into helping. Surveying the transformation, Anderson told her mother that through "dint of mild 'militancy' & unending push things have advanced immensely." The hotel concierge had told them he thought he would have had "an easier time fighting the Germans than facing so many active English Ladies!"[9] By the end of the second day, fifty beds were ready to receive the wounded. It was not a moment too soon.

That same day a visitor called. A doctor from the American Hospital in the Paris suburb of Neuilly, he asked Murray and Anderson if they were ready to take any wounded. Originally founded for Americans living in Paris, the American Hospital had opened its doors to war casualties immediately once hostilities began.[10] Although America had declared itself neutral at the outbreak of war, staff at the American Hospital had been using their fleet of motor ambulances to collect wounded soldiers from the battlefront. Less than two weeks later, they were already overwhelmed by French, Belgian, and British casualties.

Murray, who had assumed the role of medical director at Claridge's, did not hesitate. Despite the fact that their medical supplies had still not arrived, she volunteered to take in fifty patients that night. All of them, warned the American doctor, would be severely wounded and in need of urgent surgery. The nurses and orderlies cast anxious glances at each other but said nothing. As soon as their visitor left, Campbell joked, "At any rate, they'll have lovely beds, if nothing else."[11] But it was no laughing matter.

EVER SINCE THE British Army had arrived in France in the middle of August, medical services had been in chaos.[12] As the troops had marched north toward the advancing German Army, their medical units and equipment had followed them. Under the command of Sir Alfred Keogh, the Royal Army Medical Corps (RAMC) had been completely revamped in recent years, so it was better staffed and better prepared for war than ever before. Its one thousand regular medical officers and four thousand other staff members had been boosted by civilian doctors—general practitioners and hospital consultants—and other reserves to create a total force of some twenty thousand men.[13] These were supplemented by six hundred army nurses and thousands of volunteer helpers organized by the British Red Cross and St John Ambulance.

Drawing on lessons from the Boer Wars, which had ended twelve years earlier, army chiefs had established a clear strategy for evacuating wounded soldiers from the front line. This chain of evacuation was based on the principle that casualties should be picked up from the battlefield by battalion stretcher-bearers and scuttled back to regimental aid posts a short distance behind the front line for immediate first aid before being transported farther back to dressing stations—in tents or makeshift shelters—for basic medical care, and eventually to casualty clearing stations (essentially field hospitals) for emergency treatment. If they survived this far, they would either be patched up and returned to the front or sent onward for further treatment to base hospitals at the Channel ports. From there they could, if necessary, be shipped to England. That was the plan. The reality was confusion and disorder, with fatal consequences.

Heavily outnumbered by the powerful German Army at the Battle of Mons on August 23—the first British engagement with the Germans—British troops had been forced to retreat even as their medical units were still moving forward. In the resulting mayhem, the medical units were hopelessly overwhelmed by the scale of casualties; most of the wounded were captured by the pursuing Germans or left behind to die. This chaos continued as the British fought a rearguard action at the Battle of Le Cateau on August 26, which crucially stalled the German advance but resulted in heavy casualties. One of the biggest problems was transporting the wounded. Although medical advisers had requested motor ambulances before the war, the army's commanders had decided they were an unnecessary luxury. So the RAMC was entirely dependent on horse-drawn ambulance wagons and a few motor lorries to convey all the wounded and life-saving medical equipment.

In the blistering August heat, at the start of the two-hundred-mile retreat, the horses were slow. They needed frequent stops for feeding, watering, and resting, and they often cast their shoes or went lame. Once the late summer rains began, the horses floundered in mud, so that RAMC men had to harness themselves to the ambulance wagons, or abandon them and carry the wounded on their backs. The injured soldiers who were lucky enough to be picked up at all suffered long, excruciating journeys as they were jolted over the cobbled roads of northern France in wagons or trucks. Even more were left in waterlogged shell holes or open fields without help for days. Those who did get medical help were often laid on straw or bare floors in cellars and churches, awaiting aid, but many of these also had to be abandoned as the German advance continued. One doctor was left alone in charge of fifty patients in a château when the order came to retreat. Another, working in a converted school, had a patient already anesthetized with chloroform; he was ready to amputate the man's foot when he was given five minutes to pack and leave. He had to abandon his groggy patient along with 120 more.[14] Even the large base hospitals established at Le Havre, Rouen, and Amiens had to be hurriedly evacuated as the Germans continued toward Paris.

In the pandemonium of August and early September, the roads had been choked with retreating British, French, and Belgian soldiers, the waysides littered with dead horses and dying men. Medical officers themselves came under fire as they tried to help the wounded. "It was wicked work," said one doctor. "Several of our fellows were killed by the shrapnel, and some of the wounded received worse wounds while lying helpless."[15] Faced with the German Army's hugely superior strength and firepower, the allies' chances looked hopeless. But the Germans' decision to wheel around northeast of Paris, rather than westward as expected, had enabled the French to attack them north of the capital in early September. British troops had then doubled back across the River Marne. The joint assault succeeded in halting the German advance thirty miles north of Paris, at the four-day Battle of the Marne.

Despite the "miracle of the Marne," which saved Paris, casualties had continued to mount, and evacuation arrangements remained woefully inadequate. The French railways might have offered a faster way to evacuate the wounded, but they were overwhelmed by the demand. Since transport for troops and ammunition took priority, wounded men waited on open platforms at stations outside Paris. As the French had no dedicated ambulance trains, casualties were piled into goods trucks for journeys of up to five days to reach the base hospitals. For those sent onward to England, the journey from battlefield to hospital bed could take as long as thirteen days.[16]

The result of this complete breakdown in organization was that the well-equipped base hospitals on the French coast were virtually empty in the first few months of the war, while thousands died of untreated wounds in the field. The French arrangements were no better than the British ones. Hospitals designated for the wounded in northern France overflowed with casualties, yet the authorities refused to make use of thirty thousand beds lying empty in Paris, probably fearing the Germans would soon overrun the capital. Acting on their own initiative, therefore, doctors from the American Hospital were driving to railway stations and emergency centers near the front line scouting for wounded soldiers to bring back for treatment. As one military expert remarked: "Fortunate is the man who is picked up by an American ambulance."[17]

AS SHE GATHERED information on the chaotic medical situation, Anderson had decided to survey the scene for herself. On her first day in Paris on September 16—while Hodgson and Campbell were taking the nurses sightseeing—she had accompanied a friend, a British doctor and suffragette sympathizer named Leslie Haden-Guest, to a railway station outside Paris where casualties were piling up. Four days earlier, the British had supported their French allies in a fierce attack on German troops north of the River Aisne, sixty miles northeast of Paris. Once again, army medical services had been overwhelmed by casualties. Like the American doctors, Haden-Guest was using his own motor ambulance to collect wounded soldiers and take them to a hospital; in this case, it was a French Red Cross facility that he was helping to run in another converted hotel, the Majestic, in Paris.

When she arrived at the station, Anderson found a large number of wounded British soldiers who had been lying in a shed for three days with almost no help.[18] An army surgeon who had been left in charge with virtually no supplies wrung her hand in gratitude when she offered assistance. She helped to load "the three worst," including one man with typhoid, into Haden-Guest's ambulance and accompanied them to the Majestic. One of the wounded was a twenty-year-old officer. "I sent a telegram to his family & felt I had not come here in vain," she told her mother, though she did not reveal his fate. Two of the corps' junior doctors, Hazel Cuthbert and

Gertrude Gazdar, volunteered to help at the Majestic while Claridge's was being prepared.

Despite the shock of her first encounter with the casualties of war, Anderson was determined not to lose her nerve. "There is not an atom of danger & no discomfort," she assured her mother. "We are having a wonderful time & I hope we are going to be of use." Rather more candid to her sister-in-law, Alan's wife, Ivy, she admitted, "There is nothing ready for us & still less for a hospital."[19] Becoming rapidly aware of the devastation unfolding all around, she telegraphed friends in London to send more staff, an ambulance, a car, and X-ray equipment. She had already bought a basic operating table in Paris. Still, it was, she told Ivy, "excellent training."

They would need more than training to cope with the fifty patients who were due to arrive at Claridge's by the end of the second day. Fortunately, the missing supplies turned up in the nick of time. After hours negotiating with French customs, Hodgson returned triumphantly with the vital equipment just as the first stretchers bearing the wounded began streaming through the doors. The orderlies hurriedly unpacked the surgical instruments and medicines while the nurses transferred the casualties to their beds. A handful of the men were officers, who were placed in a small separate ward according to army etiquette, but most were ordinary British soldiers, or "Tommies," as they were popularly known. Wounded during the Battle of the Aisne, many had waited days for hospital care.

At their first sight of the injured men, with their gray, unshaven faces and mud-stained uniforms, the staff reeled in horror. The men were all exhausted, dehydrated, and in shock; they had mangled and shattered limbs, gaping head wounds, and horrific flesh injuries. Most, if not all, were professional soldiers or reservists, already enlisted in the army or called up as soon as war had been declared, who had set off with the British Expeditionary Force for France, healthy, vigorous, and full of bluster, a few weeks earlier. Some were barely conscious, others screamed or sobbed in pain and terror, and some were beyond hope. "As those first stretchers with their weary burdens were carried in, a thrill of pity and dismay ran through the women who saw them," wrote Murray. "Here, for the first time, they touched the wastage and the desolation of war."[20] The realization of what they had signed up for was rapidly sinking in for the women: they were now the only hope for these desperately injured men. Luckily there was no time to question their resolve, for, as the American doctor had warned, most of them needed urgent surgery.

As the instruments were sterilized in the fish kettles and the chloroform unpacked in the ladies' cloakroom, Anderson and Murray donned their surgical gowns to get ready for a long night in the operating theater. Nothing in their training or experience to date had prepared them for this moment.[21] At the New Hospital, Anderson was used to performing gynecological operations, and occasionally other surgeries on women; at Harrow Road, she had sometimes operated on children and babies. But she had little experience of general surgery or major trauma, had no direct experience of military surgery, and had never before operated on men. Murray, who assumed the role of anesthetist, had previously administered anesthetics exclusively to women and children, who needed significantly smaller doses of anesthetic agents. She had never administered anesthetics to men previously or dealt with war wounds. But if Murray, Anderson, and their junior assistants were woefully unprepared for the challenges of military surgery in 1914, then so, too, was the British Army.

AS IF ALL the logistical problems of transport and evacuation were not enough, doctors were facing medical problems they had never encountered before. Here, too, the army based its practice on experience from the Boer Wars, when rifles made neat holes that allowed bullets to be easily located and extracted, and where the hot, dry conditions of southern Africa kept wound infections at bay. The powerful artillery and high-explosive shells being employed by the German Army in 1914, however, caused large, deep, ragged wounds and complex multiple fractures; shrapnel left dozens of fragments embedded in bone and muscle.[22] Having pompously rejected Florence Stoney's offer of a mobile X-ray unit at the outbreak of war, frontline surgeons had no sure method of locating the metal pieces.

Up until 1915, only the large base hospitals were supplied with X-ray equipment.

At the same time, fighting on the richly manured French and Belgian farmland meant wounds were invariably contaminated by virulent microbes, leading to deadly conditions such as tetanus and gas gangrene. The traditional practice of conservative surgery, in which surgeons cut away as little flesh as possible to cause minimal damage to surrounding tissue, was completely inadequate against rapidly spreading infection. Soldiers frequently had to have limbs amputated to stem infection; even small abdominal wounds were commonly fatal. Blood transfusions were not yet available in front-line medical care, and antibiotics were several decades in the future. There were also unprecedented numbers of head injuries, caused by sniper fire and artillery bombardment, until eventually—in late 1915—it would occur to army chiefs that steel helmets might provide better protection for the men.

The army's surgeons, many of them general practitioners in civilian life, had little or no experience of handling such injuries. They were more used to dealing with minor emergencies such as appendicitis or fractures, and planned operations, such as the removal of tumors. Few had handled devastating war wounds. Now they faced wounds that were "hitherto undreamed of," said one surgeon, in conditions that would "open [the civilian surgeon's] eyes, test his capacity and resources and tend to break his heart as never before."[23] Even veteran surgeons were at a loss. Another surgeon said the septic wounds were "a revelation to the younger surgeons and a shock to the older men."[24]

Likewise, the practice of anesthesia was poorly understood, having changed little since the arrival of ether and chloroform seventy years earlier. The equipment was primitive—usually ether or chloroform was simply dripped onto a mask—and the correct dosage was hard to judge. Few doctors had received any training in anesthesia, so that nurses or even chaplains were often called on to administer anesthetics. Too little chloroform or ether could mean the patient waking or semi-waking and floundering about on the operating table; too much and they never woke up at all. It was not uncommon for frontline surgeons to operate without anesthesia completely, since supplies were frequently inadequate and time often short.

Even if they avoided being wounded by German fire, many soldiers fell sick. As the war continued, filthy trench conditions would lead to the rapid spread of diseases caused by rats, lice, and mosquitos. And then there was shell shock. Even by September 1914, significant numbers of men were exhibiting a cluster of unusual symptoms including tremors, night terrors, mutism, and deafness. Doctors were baffled. Since the outward signs mimicked the symptoms of damage to the brain or nervous system, it was initially assumed the cause was a physical injury to the nerves, although some soldiers were accused of shirking their duties, and therefore risked being executed for "cowardice." The problem would soon assume epidemic proportions, requiring an entire network of hospitals and spawning controversial methods of treatment, ranging from hypnosis and psychotherapy to electric shocks. In time, the challenges thrown up by the war would generate remarkable medical advances—but these were several years down the line.

When Murray and Anderson received their first wounded men in the Claridge's operating theater therefore, they were as ill-prepared as any of their male counterparts. As Murray administered chloroform to the first patient in the converted ladies' lavatory and Anderson took her knife to make the first incision, the two women knew that failure was not an option. This night was a critical test—not only for themselves, but for all women doctors. It was the first opportunity to demonstrate publicly that they were the equals of men. Assisted by their junior colleagues and nurses, they worked late into the night. Claridge's—or L'Hôpital Auxiliare 173, as it was now officially known—was open for business.

WITHIN FIVE DAYS, Claridge's was a fully functioning hospital with one hundred beds in four main wards, plus two small wards for officers. Its operating theater was "in constant use."[25] During that first week, the corps treated casualties brought in by volunteers or begged lifts from friends to collect wounded soldiers themselves.

Hodgson found herself on one such excursion a week after arriving in Paris, being driven to a railway station about eight miles south of the city. On the return journey, she had to sit on the floor of the car cradling one of the men who was thought to have pneumonia. "We are so glad to get out," she wrote home, "but the roads are simply hell! there is no other word to describe them especially when you have a sick man with you & you know that every jolt is agony."[26]

The following day, September 23, on what she described as her first "day off," Anderson drove with a friend to Braisne, a town sixty miles north of Paris and five miles from the front line, which had become a major casualty center. Passing through villages devastated by fighting, she saw smoke rising from German guns firing on Soissons. "I saw more of actual war than I ever expected to see," she told her mother.[27] In Braisne, Anderson found an exhausted young RAMC doctor who almost broke down in tears when she presented him with shirts, socks, and cigarettes for the British troops. He took her to a church packed with injured soldiers lying on straw. As she entered the churchyard, Anderson could smell the foul infected wounds of the men inside. Some were dying, others were already dead. It was a "sight not to be forgotten," she told Alan. The men, who were deposited there daily by horse-drawn ambulances, were "given hunks of cheese & the ones who aren't dying are then carted on again after 12–24–48 hrs delay." She offered to take two of the most severely wounded back to Claridge's and was presented with one man who had been shot through the throat, along with another whose arm was severely fractured. When she hesitated, unsure whether one of them would last the journey, he grasped her arm and pleaded, "Don't leave me behind!" Fortified with brandy and morphine, the two men not only survived the return trip but recovered. Desperate to help more of the wounded stranded within hours of Paris, she sent an urgent appeal to friends in London for some mode of transport.[28]

Her plea was heard: a week or so later, two supporters, a brother and sister, arrived with a lorry as well as an ambulance designed to take four stretchers—"a beautiful motor with springs from which the stretchers are hung."[29] The two siblings even undertook to drive members of the corps to railway stations and medical outposts so they could collect the wounded themselves. Later a second ambulance arrived. Hodgson, who now regarded herself as something of a veteran ambulance aide, volunteered for the first outing on September 26.

SETTING OUT BEFORE dawn in the ambulance and an accompanying car, the convoy—which included Hodgson, Gazdar, and two or three helpers—headed straight for the front line, toward the cathedral city of Rheims, which had been under heavy bombardment from the Germans for a week.[30] It was an eventful journey. As they crossed the battle-scarred countryside, the vehicles suffered two burst tires. The party was stopped repeatedly by police checking their papers, and they were forced to make a detour to avoid bridges that had been blown up. They saw burned-out trees, and telegraph wires that had been cut by shelling. At one point, on hearing shouting in a nearby wood, some of the group thought they were about to be attacked. At this some of the party became "rather upset," which Hodgson thought "so very unofficial." Refusing to be cowed, she and Gazdar nonchalantly ate their lunch on a bridge over the Marne, while the sound of artillery continued relentlessly from the direction of Rheims.

The group was prevented from going farther than Dormans, thirty miles short of Rheims, by police who suspected they were spies—apparently unable to come up with another explanation for the presence of half a dozen British women hurtling toward the front line. Diverted to a field hospital at nearby Château-Thierry, they collected six men—three British soldiers and three French officers—who had been prisoners of war. With four men stashed in the ambulance and two in the car, they returned to Paris at a slow pace so the wounded men could "stand the jolting" and arrived safely though "very exhausted."

There was no letup in the arrival of the wounded as the women at Claridge's took in French and Algerian casualties from the Battle of the Aisne in addition to British and Irish troops. For the French, who lost some hundred thousand men in the first six weeks of the war, these early months were among the deadliest. By the end of September—two weeks after they had set out from Victoria—the women were looking after sixty-eight patients. Anderson was kept busy operating seven or eight hours a day—sometimes for as long as fifteen hours—digging out shrapnel and bullets from ravaged flesh, amputating smashed or septic limbs, and drilling into skulls to relieve pressure from blood clots or embedded bone fragments in head wounds. If she had been inexperienced in military surgery before, she was rapidly gaining experience now. "The shell injuries are dreadful & the men come to us worn out after days in the trenches," she told her mother.[31] "The cases come to us very septic & the wounds are <u>terrible</u>."

Common among the injuries were compound fractures of the thigh, meaning one or both ends of the broken bone emerge through the skin. Since bone and flesh were exposed, these wounds almost invariably became infected. Such cases needed as many as four staff members to dress the wounds—painstakingly peeling and soaking off bandages caked with blood and pus before applying clean ones—and each dressing could take as long as an hour. Since many of the men had been left untreated for days, their wounds were often gangrenous, and many were weak with fever. "We have got several pretty bad fractured femur cases & they are none of them as clean & nice as they might have been," wrote Hodgson.[32] She added, "Oh the stink of some of those gangrenous wounds (How <u>do</u> you spell it). They are so nasty—we got a Frenchman in our ward last night who is dreadful—it is his jaw." In a single day's work, it was rare to see more than two wounds that were not septic, she said. Some patients survived their surgery only to succumb to infection days later. One "very nice Scotchman" died two weeks after successful surgery for a scalp wound when he developed tetanus, said Anderson. She added ominously, "Nearly all those cases die."[33]

Some patients were already showing signs of shell shock. The French and British officers, in particular, were "acutely shocked by the horrors through which they had passed," wrote Murray. Many were young men in their early twenties, barely out of school, who had led older men to their deaths and watched friends die. They could not sleep, she said, and "their nights were haunted by terrible memories and anxious thoughts." Hodgson told her mother at one point that one of the junior doctors had been "up all the night with a man who is off his head & has died since I think."[34]

Most of the men arrived dirty and half-starved; many had not had a change of clothes or socks since leaving England.[35] Although friends of the hospital staff back home sent gifts of clothing, as well as sheets and towels, it was almost impossible to keep up with demand. Hodgson urged her mother to send pajamas, shirts, socks, and handkerchiefs, since many of the wounded arrived wrapped only in a blanket, because their uniforms were "too much torn & dirty to keep near wounds."[36] With heartfelt conviction, she added, "No one in England knows the necessity & misery of the wounded before they get here or [has] the slightest idea of the casualties."

THE DAYS WERE long, the workload relentless, and the scenes harrowing, yet Hodgson's letters fizzed with excitement; she was doing valuable work for the first time in her life—and she was good at it. On a typical day she was up by 7:00 a.m. to make breakfast for the men, then she helped prepare dressings and boil instruments till noon.[37] After dishing out lunch to the patients, she spent the afternoon on errands, such as sending telegrams and shopping for supplies. Back by 6:30 p.m., she helped serve dinner before sitting down to her own. In between times she washed dishes, made soup, wrote letters for the men, and chatted with the officers. If she needed help from one of the few male staff, such as the electrician or hotel manager, "I simply flirt these men into any job," she informed her mother. Her cousin, Olga Campbell, meanwhile, was working mostly on the officers' ward. The men there "take a lot of attention & feeding as 3 of them have to be fed," said Hodgson.

Fraternizing with men, albeit principally with the officers, was a rare freedom. The war brought a dramatic relaxation in the rules of decorum for young middle-class women. Although Campbell and Hodgson had enjoyed comparatively more independence, most young women had previously never been permitted so much as to mix with men unchaperoned or travel alone, much less "flirt." Women who had never seen a man shirtless before were suddenly having to perform intimate tasks for male patients as hospital aides. The experience would bring about a lasting change in attitudes.[38] Yet at the same time that she was experiencing these heady new freedoms, Hodgson was gaining a valuable insight into medicine, encouraged by Anderson and Murray.

In the first few days at Claridge's, Hodgson helped Grace Judge dress the men's wounds, including a serious back wound that she proudly reported managing "fairly satisfactorily."[39] Within two weeks she was assisting Anderson in the operating theater at five operations—"2 very bad jaw wounds 2 amputations (fingers) & 1 bad wrist," she wrote. "They had no effect on me whatever beyond making me frightfully interested. At one of the amputations I had to hold the fingers for Dr Anderson & turn them while she was working," she added. On the wards, Anderson encouraged the orderlies to help with nursing tasks as much as possible. Supported by Anderson, Hodgson was showing a definite knack for nursing, if not necessarily for surgery. When Hodgson cut herself slicing bread and had to be excused from dressing duties in case the cut became infected, Anderson may have had second thoughts about her orderly's abilities in theater.

Although Murray and Anderson could seem austere and imperious, they led by example, working long hours, and commanded enormous respect from their team of women. "Flo is such a darling—and so busy," Hodgson wrote of Murray. "We admire her & Dr G. A. tremendously. They are so quiet & level headed." Yet while praising the two doctors, she was careful to assure her mother she was not turning "suffragetty." Anderson and Murray wore their "Votes for Women" badges all the time, and although most of the doctors sympathized, they "regard[ed] it from the same standpoint as you do," she said. This standpoint was presumably supporting women's suffrage in words but not deeds, at least not to the point of militancy. Hodgson had mixed feelings about the other doctors, however. She was friendly with Gazdar and thought Cuthbert "tall

& good looking." She least liked Judge, who was more brusque. Yet they made "a jolly little party," and all came together at one long table for mealtimes.[40]

AS THE BEDS filled, the corps was reinforced by two more doctors, Majorie Blandy, aged twenty-seven, and Rosalie Jobson, twenty-eight, both LSMW graduates who had just qualified, and ten more nurses, who all arrived by the end of September.[41] Both keen sportswomen, Blandy and Jobson were good friends. Blandy had studied at Cambridge, while Jobson, the daughter of an army surgeon, had attended Oxford before they had both enrolled to study medicine at the LSMW. In addition, the corps was joined, according to one newspaper, by "several Girl Scouts."

Reading about the corps' work in British newspapers, well-wishers sent gifts of cigarettes and hot water bottles for the men as well as money and medical supplies. Friends in Scotland responded enthusiastically to Hodgson's appeal for sacks of oats—since there were "a lot of scotch boys who would love porridge"—as well as tobacco and butterscotch, because the men were "all suggar starved."

Comrades in the suffragette movement took the corps to their hearts. Emmeline Pankhurst led the way, exhorting her supporters to raise £60 for the corps at a WSPU meeting in September where she praised Flora Murray effusively.[42] When she complained about the paucity of the sum, a male sympathizer topped it up to £100. By contrast, the NUWSS, with Aunt Millie at its helm, channeled its energies into raising funds for Elsie Inglis, the Scottish surgeon and suffragist, who—having been spurned by the War Office—was organizing medical units to send to France. Although the campaign for women's votes was officially suspended, Murray and Anderson's unit was clearly identified as the suffragettes' hospital, while the Scottish Women's Hospitals, as Inglis's outfit was named, was closely allied with the suffragists.

The Parisians, too, were generous with their money and time. As news of the corps' work spread, crowds gathered at Claridge's grand entrance to watch the ambulances unloading casualties. Elderly men offered to help carry the stretchers inside, while women showered the wounded with flowers and cigarettes. Local shopkeepers donated sweets and biscuits, the greengrocer added "an extra cauliflower" to their order, and strangers who recognized the women in their distinctive uniforms pressed coins into their hands.[43] The uniform "opened doors and hearts and pockets," said Murray and the Parisians, arbiters of style, pronounced it "chic." Crowds also congregated for the funerals.

Inevitably there were deaths among the men, who arrived not only seriously wounded but desperately ill from blood loss, infection, and shock. According to Murray, the death rate was "lamentably high"—but then the same was true at army medical units too.[44] In fact, the fatalities seemed surprisingly low. Hodgson referred to the "first funeral" at the end of five days; after two weeks, Anderson said there had been two deaths—but both men had been "brought to us almost dying."[45] By the end of September Hodgson said five men had died, but added that "several cases who were supposed to be dying" were actually recovering. Given their lack of experience and the high death rates being recorded by army surgeons elsewhere, it was an impressive record.

Some men were beyond hope by the time they arrived at Claridge's. One officer with a badly fractured thigh had traveled eighty miles on a stretcher lashed to the hood of a car.[46] He was Lieutenant Henry Lowe, who was wounded at the Battle of the Aisne, and he lingered for several weeks before expiring, aged twenty-four. Lowe's older sister Isabel traveled to Paris to sit at his bedside during his last ten days. She was "wonderfully brave," said Hodgson. Another soldier had crawled on his stomach for two hours after his foot was hit by a shell before tumbling into a quarry.[47] He wrote home to say that, apart from his foot, he "couldn't be in better health." Others had already endured hurried operations in medical posts near the front line but needed further surgery on arrival, since gangrene had developed. One "nice boy" had had his foot amputated but developed sepsis in the stump. Anderson amputated his leg higher up and had hopes he would live; his fate went unrecorded.[48]

Whether or not Anderson ever questioned her lack of experience or wavered in confidence, she rarely admitted to doubts. Concerned at one point over some French patients, she wrote: "We try to help them so very hard but I do not feel we have succeeded yet but we have had some desperate cases."[49] Another time she confessed to feeling "tired and sad" after a long night sitting at the bedside of a Frenchman; his arm had been amputated on account of gangrene, but he died. Looking back years later, when understanding of war surgery had advanced significantly, she would confess that in 1914 a case of compound fracture of the femur was "a source of infinite anxiety to the surgeon."[50] This was scarcely surprising, since mortality for such cases at the start of the war was around 80 percent.

Those who died were laid out in a makeshift chapel converted from the hotel grill-room. With its marble pillars and stained-glass ceiling light, the restaurant had been designed for titled guests to linger over steaks and claret. Now decorated with flowers and a plain wooden cross, it provided a serene resting place for British and French soldiers. "It can be flooded with a golden light from its glass roof, and is then really beautiful," Murray and Anderson told supporters.[51] Funeral services were held either in the chapel or at a nearby Catholic church in the early autumn mornings. Onlookers gathered to watch a procession of staff, soldiers, and occasionally relatives as they followed the horse-drawn hearse through the quiet streets. "On the way to church everyone in the street salutes or crosses & women come out & put flowers on the coffin," wrote Anderson. At those times, she said, the Champs-Élysées "was bathed in soft lights; the Arc de Triomphe looked ethereal; the trees were golden and the distances faded into misty blue."

Attending the funerals was regarded as a staff duty. Hodgson followed one cortege for a French soldier who had left a wife and three-month-old baby behind; he had been married only sixteen months. She wrote, "They want us to make a large a show as possible for the poor little wifes sake." The dead were buried in St Pantin Cemetery in northeast Paris, where French and British graves were accumulating. It was a staff duty to write to the families of the dead, too. "One of the best things we can do is to write home to the mothers and wives of those who die," Murray and Anderson wrote. "It does make a difference to know that English women have given help and affection to their sick and reverent care to their dead."[52]

THROUGH IT ALL—the long hours of surgery, the bedside vigils, the slow deaths, the funerals—Murray and Anderson maintained a relentlessly stoical optimism to keep up morale among both the staff and the patients. They found a chaplain to provide Sunday services and some local girls to sing hymns in the courtyard; the men joined in on "Onward Christian Soldiers" from their beds. All the staff took pains to make Claridge's seem homey and cheerful, in contrast to the stark clinical environment of a typical military hospital. "Their minds are full of horrors," wrote Anderson, "& it is a help to them to come into a soothing atmosphere with decent food & soft beds & our gentle merry young orderly girls who pet them with cigarettes & write to their mothers & read to them." Hodgson said, "Everyone says who comes here that the thing which impresses them most is the comfort & friendly spirit, also this is the Hosp. where the men are not longing to be gone."[53]

At the same time that they were proving they could run a hospital with both military precision and cozy domesticity, Murray and Anderson plainly relished the opportunity to use the full range of skills they had gained in their medical training and demonstrate the abilities of women doctors. Despite the challenges and the failures, they took real pleasure in their clinical work. Anderson knew that, of all people, her mother would understand. "It is most awfully nice to have a chance of doing this work," she wrote. "We will get unique surgical experience of every kind. . . . I like that chance v. much but I like still more the opportunity of being a little good to these bruised men."[54] It was quite a turnaround, after years of viewing men as the enemy, to see them now as allies—vulnerable, weakened, and damaged, but jointly fighting a bigger enemy. What was more, after "years of unpopularity" during their suffragette campaign, it was exhilarating to be "on the top of the wave, helped & approved by everyone, except perhaps the English War Office!" Despite the long hours, it felt like "a sort of holiday," she told Alan. "It is so new & so interesting. The difficulties have been & are considerable but I hope we are steering right & will come through!"

It was a novelty for the men to arrive at a hospital run by women. Probably none of them had been in contact with women doctors before, Murray acknowledged. Yet they "trusted the women as they would have trusted men."[55] The fact that those women were well-educated, self-assured, and distinctly middle or upper class was clearly a factor in instilling confidence—and even inspiring a little fear—in the predominantly young working-class men. More accustomed to treating children than grown men, Murray and Anderson seemed to regard their patients as big boys. The French were like "broken children," said Anderson, while Murray wrote, "When they got well and went away, it was like seeing boys go back to school." Transported from the filth, stench, and terror of the battlefield to clean beds and hot meals in the opulent surroundings of a luxury hotel, the men could hardly complain. It was incomparably better than the front.

ALMOST AS TIME-CONSUMING as the sick patients were the hordes of visitors who flocked to see the hospital "run solely by women." As well as relatives, friends, and comrades, who dropped by with gifts, there were French and British journalists, aristocrats and dignitaries, British MPs, and Red Cross officials all eager to see how the women were managing. One French journalist refused to believe the surgery was performed by women until he was shown the surgeons at work. Another French reporter persisted, saying, "Who is it really who operates?" When the attractive Dr. Cuthbert confirmed she wielded a knife, he exclaimed: "<u>Incroyable</u>!" (Unbelievable!).[56]

More believing but no less impressed, British journalists lauded the corps' work with the patriotic zeal characteristic of the early war years. The *Daily Sketch* ran a photo spread showing the doctors at work while noting, "Nursing comes naturally to women, but not all have the calm courage and iron nerve necessary to become a successful operating surgeon."[57] One British journalist described Claridge's as "probably the best equipped hospital in Paris"; another said there was "no hospital more efficient." *The Globe* stressed that these "talented women doctors" were nothing like the "vinegar-faced types" familiar from cartoons; the orderlies, the reporter added, were "educated young English gentlewomen" who conducted their duties with "promptness and lack of fussiness." And the *Daily Mail* noted the "wonderful atmosphere of sympathy and home about the wards." Even the *British Medical Journal*—no friend to suffragette doctors in the past—was effusive. It applauded the corps' "workmanlike order" and said that even if Claridge's was the sole British hospital in Paris, "the medical profession in Great Britain might still continue to regard itself as well represented." Yet for all the efforts at jollity, life for most of the men treated at Claridge's was no party.

One female journalist, who had previously visited Anderson and Murray's children's hospital, arrived at the same time as a convoy of severely wounded men. She was shocked to see their bodies "horribly mutilated and disfigured by shrapnel."[58] Removing the filthy clothing and cleaning the wounds was a "terrible task for nurse and patient," she wrote, so that "one grows sick with the horror of it all as stretcher after stretcher is carried." Despite the distressing scenes, the nurses and doctors worked "quietly and methodically" without wasting a second. She added, "The big sunny wards, and the big men lying smoking and joking at intervals is rather a contrast to the house of toys and children in Harrow Road."

Given the taxing workload, there was little time for rest. But most evenings Murray and Anderson managed to slip away for a quiet stroll together through the empty Parisian streets. "Paris is looking wonderful, especially at night," Anderson told her mother. "There's a little moon & over the town search lights are playing all night from the roof of the Madeleine & the Eiffel Tower. We walked along the river last night—past the Grand Palais & the Chambre des Deputés and came back very refreshed."[59] It was a welcome relief to saunter through romantic Paris at the end of a grueling day in the operating theater. Their confidence was growing; they were doing work they had been trained to do. But that work was about to come under intense scrutiny.

ON SEPTEMBER 27, the crowds parted as Reginald Baliol Brett, the Second Viscount Esher, marched up the steps of Claridge's in his uniform, medals, and spurs.[60] Although he had no official position in the British Army—and wore a uniform of his own design—Lord Esher was a close friend and informal adviser on military matters both to King George V and to Lord Kitchener. Charged with a secret mission to liaise between Kitchener and Sir John French, the commander of British forces in France, he had arrived in Paris the previous night. Having visited medical posts near the front line earlier in the day, Esher had been appalled to find injured soldiers dying from untreated wounds while hospitals stood empty a few hours away in Paris. Equally shocking was the discovery that French Red Cross hospitals in Paris were being run by British doctors because they were unwanted by the army. Now he had come to see one of these hospitals for himself.

Still a handsome man, sporting a vigorous mustache at the age of sixty-two, Esher struck an imposing figure as he strode through the doors of Claridge's and demanded to be shown around. Met by Anderson and Murray in the foyer, he wanted to know who was in charge. When they told him that they were—and furthermore, that the entire staff was female—Esher blurted out, "All women! No proper surgeons?" Stifling their indignation, the women escorted him round the hospital as he fired questions and interrogated the men in their beds. With him, Esher had brought a surgeon, Sir Frederick Treves, who was renowned for serving in the Boer Wars as well as for performing an operation for appendicitis that saved the life of King Edward VII. Now advising the War Office on medical matters, Treves was introduced as being "unconverted to women doctors."

The atmosphere grew increasingly chilly as Esher and his entourage made their progress around the hospital. The French Red Cross representative, Madame Suzanne Pérouse, arrived belatedly on the scene, breathless and flustered. Taken aside by Esher, she was grilled as to whether the women really were "practical surgeons" and asked whether the men "tolerated" them. She assured him that Claridge's was her "best institution" and had "perfect" organization; the men on the wards confirmed her verdict by heaping praise on the staff. Gradually, Esher's attitude altered. By the time he left, he was convinced that Claridge's was a model military hospital and its women doctors equal to any male ones.

Writing excitedly to Alan after the visit, Anderson said, "Lord Esher was mollified when he found absolute hospital discipline in the wards & nothing feminine about them & no one holding anyone's hand." She added, "We thought him hostile & suspicious at first but he melted when we took him round the wards & talked to the men & officers." Hodgson, meanwhile, thought Esher and his party "very haughty & snuffy" on arrival, but after being shown around, she said, they were "frantically interested."

Returning to London, Esher lost no time in apprising Kitchener of the muddle he had witnessed in the army's medical services while lauding the work of the volunteer hospitals in Paris. The RAMC's breakdown in organization was "a horror and a scandal!" he exclaimed, while the "admirable hospitals under Dr Guest and Dr Garrett-Anderson" were "all splendidly manned and equipped, by fully trained nurses and the most eminent surgeons of the day."[61]

Esher's intervention helped bring about rapid and significant improvements in the army's medical care. Over the next few months, the chain of evacuation would be drastically overhauled. More than two hundred motor ambulances were rushed to the front and special hospital trains laid on to transport casualties from the battlefield to the base hospitals on the coast—although the scale and extent of casualties would continue to overwhelm resources. Esher's visit also triggered momentous changes for the women who "manned" Claridge's. Almost overnight, the attitude of the RAMC toward the Women's Hospital Corps was transformed from indifference or hostility to respect and support. And as the fame of Claridge's spread, so army officials and medical men flocked to see the women at work.

Now one of their staunchest supporters, Esher became a regular visitor, often bringing distinguished guests with him to view the novel scene for themselves.[62] One army official refused to believe his colleagues' reports until he saw the evidence with his own eyes. "Well I'm damned!" he announced. "I never expected to see an English Military Hospital run by women." Another asked whether Sir Arthur Sloggett, who commanded army medical services on the Western Front, had paid a visit. Informed that he had not, he mused, "I wonder at that. Great man with the ladies." Wryly, Murray replied, "I expect we are not his kind of ladies." Indeed, they were not.

Keeping her mother up to date with this surprising turn of events, Anderson enthused, "It is quite a new experience to be so popular." She was thrilled to report that one official, the RAMC's inspector of auxiliary hospitals, had placed them first among the units in Paris. Although they had only been in operation a few weeks, she was gaining confidence by the minute. "I wish the whole organisation for the care of the wounded—their transport, the disposition of base & field hospitals & their clothing & feeding cd be put into the hands of women," she declared. "Medical women could do it so much better than it is done—especially if the right med. women were chosen for the job—ahem!!"[63] Determinedly cheerful as ever, she added: "We are having a wonderful time." Hodgson was equally exuberant. One army general, on hearing about their work, had exclaimed, "That is just the sort of show we want to squash."[64] But "he came, he saw, & we conquered." She added, "Don't you think it fine all these old military busters saying that sort of thing, about a woman's hospital too?"

YET FOR ALL the approbation there were still enormous challenges in coping with the casualties, while at the same time the stream of sightseers was becoming tiresome for staff and patients. As well as army officials, there were comrades from the suffragette movement, fellow medical women, aristocracy and royalty—Queen Amelie of Portugal was among the dignitaries—and family members who turned up unexpectedly. Anderson's Aunt Joey—her mother's younger sister Josephine—arrived one day bearing cigarettes and chocolate for the men. One zealous well-wisher brought along a French poet, resplendent with long hair and bow tie, who insisted on giving a recital during the hour assigned for bed baths. Other do-gooders turned up in rest periods determined to stage concert parties. Some of the men grew weary of the tactless questions about their injuries and experiences at the front—as if they were exhibits in a freak show—and asked to have the screens pulled around their beds.

At the same time, the staff faced administrative problems that would have been comical were they not so maddening. The French Red Cross had appointed a Parisian stockbroker, a certain Monsieur Aubry, to supervise the hospital's administration.[65] He spent most of his time chatting and drinking tea. The hotel owners, however, had appointed their own administrative head, referred to only as Monsieur Casanova, who commandeered the best suite and insisted on eating from a special menu. Whenever a convoy of wounded arrived in the night, Casanova lived up to his name by appearing in his pajamas, extravagantly wiping tears from his eyes, and kissing the hands of the doctors, while a train of "strange ladies" wrapped in blankets followed in his wake. Periodically erupting into rages, he would issue wholesale dismissals to the Belgian kitchen staff, and Murray had to employ all her diplomatic skills to charm him into backing down. When the two managers fell out over some trifling disagreement, Murray had to negotiate a truce.

These rows between the two rival managers at Claridge's were emblematic of the wider arguments that erupted between the director of the French Red Cross in Paris and the governor of French army medical services in the city. When the former criticized the latter, the governor retaliated by blocking the transportation of wounded men to Red Cross hospitals. At one point, when the corps was refused documentation for its ambulances to travel out of Paris, Murray stomped along to see the governor in his lavishly appointed office. She refused to leave until he produced the requisite forms. Hardened by her suffragette experiences, she was implacable when occasion demanded.

Throughout September and the first half of October, most of the patients treated at Claridge's were British. But as the army hastily reformed its medical services, so British casualties were increasingly transported to base hospitals near the coast. Anxious to keep their beds filled and continue the work they had come to do, the women sent their ambulance to forage for French casualties from the battlefield near Soissons. On October 2, wounded French soldiers arrived in relays. After performing five operations without a break, Anderson dashed down a hurried dinner before scrubbing up for a sixth—a trepanning, the delicate procedure of drilling into the skull to relieve pressure on the brain. Men from every region of France—from Brittany to the Pyrenees—as well as from the French colonies of Algeria and Morocco, now occupied the beds in the marbled halls. Just as they had cooked porridge for the Scottish troops, so the staff provided special dishes, local wines, and herbal tisanes to make their patients feel at home.

One Algerian soldier had to have both feet amputated owing to frostbite caused by the harsh conditions when sleeping outside.[66] Visitors brought him and his compatriots baskets of fruit to remind them of home, but it was little compensation for such disability. Two patients brought in with the French casualties were actually English brothers who had joined the French Foreign Legion when war broke out. The first arrived at Claridge's after insisting on being taken to an English hospital; his brother had been struck deaf and mute with shell shock and was sent to a French unit. Eventually, after much searching and paperwork, they were reunited at Claridge's. Puzzled by the man's unexplained condition, the other patients hollered in chorus behind him until finally, one evening, he turned around and smiled. Soon after, he recovered his speech, too.

Despite the efforts marauding for French casualties, mid-October brought a lull in arrivals at Claridge's. As the Allies and Germans attempted to outflank each other by maneuvering northward in the so-called race to the sea, British troops rushed to defend Flanders, and the wounded were now directed to Boulogne and neighboring ports. Although this was clearly a welcome improvement for the casualties, Murray and Anderson knew the shift threatened their very existence. "As the fighting line recedes, it becomes increasingly difficult to get patients in to Paris," Anderson told her brother. Murray had spent a day driving around the Chantilly area north of Paris looking for casualties in vain, she said. Toward the end of October, Hodgson told her mother the workload was "getting very slack" and complained that it was "most dismal having not very much to do & all the empty beds about."[67]

By now, the X-ray apparatus that Anderson had appealed for had arrived. Set up in the hotel basement with an adjoining darkroom, it proved an essential tool in locating bullets and shrapnel. Although the glass plates were cumbersome and the images grainy, the women were ahead of most army medical units in using X-rays. Yet since the equipment was primitive, emitting X-rays in all directions and needing several minutes for each exposure, the process was highly unsafe both for patients and staff—although nobody realized it at the time. A photograph in a British newspaper showed two RAMC surgeons watching with fascination as the doctors at Claridge's used the X-ray equipment for the first time—to locate a bullet in the arm of a soldier wounded at the Battle of the Aisne.[68] Hodgson was keen to see what all the fuss was about. She watched Judge take X-rays of two wounded men and pronounced the experience "very interesting" but "not exciting."

DESPITE THE CONTINUING challenges in tackling wounds and handling officialdom, the women of the WHC were hitting their stride. They were enjoying the opportunity to put their skills to good use while gaining vital experience in saving lives and pioneering new techniques. It would have been devastating to have to pack up and go home now. If they couldn't find patients by scavenging around Paris, Murray and Anderson decided, then they would have to look farther afield.

3

Sunshine and Sweetness

Boulogne, October 31, 1914

Louisa Garrett Anderson and Flora Murray stepped onto the platform at Boulogne in the late afternoon.[1] After the deserted streets of Paris, the scene that greeted them was like a vision from hell. Every street in the Channel port was choked with army trucks, Red Cross ambulances, and marching troops, all vying for passage. The sea appeared to be just as congested as the land. Hospital ships, hastily converted from cross-Channel steamers, jostled for mooring in the docks with passenger ferries and fishing boats. On the quayside, stretcher-bearers attempted to lift wounded men from the ambulance trains at the same time that passengers flooded down the gangplanks from the ferries. Crowds clustered to gawk at the commotion.

Having taken up quarters in Boulogne in mid-October, the Royal Army Medical Corps had commandeered every major hotel and sizable building to establish its new medical base and evacuation port. Two weeks later, when Murray and Anderson arrived, ambulance trains were bringing up to 1,200 wounded soldiers into Boulogne every day from the front line near the Belgian border. One army nurse, who had reached Boulogne at the end of October, said the town was "a seething mass of ambulances, wounded men, doctors and nurses." Another visitor described Boulogne as a "city of hospitals."[2]

Murray and Anderson had arrived in this maelstrom of chaos and confusion at the height of the First Battle of Ypres. As British, French, and Belgian forces raced to head off the Germans in their push toward the coast, the armies had clashed in a series of battles along a forty-mile front through Belgium and northern France. British soldiers, diverted to the region from the battlefields of the Aisne and reinforced by more troops from Britain and India, were engaged in constant battle from October 21 onward. The heaviest fighting was concentrated around the Belgian town of Ypres, where hand-to-hand battles led to record numbers of casualties. The seven-week Flanders conflict would claim the lives of some 8,000 British soldiers with nearly 30,000 wounded—effectively wiping out the core of the original British Expeditionary Force—while French casualties would number more than 50,000 killed or wounded.[3] Many of the British wounded were now streaming into Boulogne. Just like the frontline medical posts, however, the doctors and nurses in Boulogne were now hopelessly overwhelmed.

The fresh medical mayhem came as no surprise to Anderson and Murray. Eager to find a new source of patients, because of the decline in casualties coming to Paris, they had already sent three staff members—assistant surgeons Rosalie Jobson, Majorie Blandy, and Gertrude Gazdar—on a reconnaissance mission to Boulogne the previous week. The young women had traveled as part of a mercy mission of British surgeons and nurses from voluntary hospitals in Paris. When they offered assistance to army medical chiefs, however, they were told they were not needed—even barred from visiting the military hospitals. Using the ingenuity that had become the corps' trademark, the three women from Claridge's persuaded a friendly matron to let them into one of the hospitals under the guise of nurses. They were shocked by what they found.

The three women had bluffed their way into the largest of the army's Boulogne hospitals, set up a few days earlier in a collection of sugar warehouses on the quayside. Officially named No. 13 Stationary Hospital—but better known as the Sugar Store Hospital—this depot had become the main reception and distribution point for casualties. The makeshift facility was so crowded that orderlies had to climb over the wounded on stretchers to distribute food and water. The lack of staff meant that many of the men had not had their dressings changed since being picked up from the battlefield days earlier.[4] In one huge shed designated for the "walking wounded," the men lay on straw or sat on empty barrels, their clothes still caked in mud and their wounds covered by bloodstained bandages. Dressings, medicine, and water were in short supply, and there was only one stove on which to boil water, making it almost impossible to perform aseptic surgery. The following day, when the three women returned and sheepishly revealed their medical qualifications, the doctor in charge was so desperate he asked them to help.

Jobson, Blandy, and Gazdar spent the next few days helping at the Sugar Store Hospital. When Gazdar returned to report back to Claridge's, Jobson and Blandy remained behind. Released from their duties with the Women's Hospital Corps, they would spend most of the next six months at the Sugar Store Hospital. Jobson and Blandy were officially accepted as surgeons under the auspices of the RAMC—thereby becoming the first women doctors attached to the British Army. A volunteer nurse working alongside them said, "The lady doctors have been invaluable, their zeal unflagging. They are splendid operators, and in the midst of the worst rushes never careless."[5] Whatever army officials had told Jobson and Blandy, it was plain more medical aid was urgently needed.

Learning of the chaos in Boulogne, Murray and Anderson had determined to set up a new hospital right in the heart of the army's medical colossus. Since every suitable building there had already been taken over by the army, they had sent Grace Judge to search the surrounding area. She had returned with news of an empty hotel in Wimereux, a seaside resort about two miles north of Boulogne. Now Anderson and Murray had come to inspect the building to see if it would be suitable for their needs.

BUILT AT THE END of the nineteenth century as a luxury seaside villa, the Château Mauricien had since been converted into a hotel catering to the hordes of well-to-do British tourists who flocked to

Wimereux every summer.[6] Known as the "Nice du Nord," Wimereux had become a fashionable retreat for the idle rich. In recent months, however, the resort had been transformed from a seaside idyll into a satellite of the army's vast medical machine.

The town's two biggest hotels, the Hôtel Splendid and the Hôtel Grand, where tourists had until recently lounged and partied, had been hastily converted into military hospitals; a ward in the Hôtel Splendid's casino was labeled the "Baccarat Room," alluding to a popular card game. The resort's wide golden sands, where tourists had strolled a few months earlier, were now dotted with convalescing soldiers in "bedraggled khaki."[7] Even the striped bathing huts on the beach had been put to use: they were now isolation units for patients with contagious diseases. Whereas most of the town's hotels and chalets were usually boarded up for the winter, the resort now bustled with military vehicles and army personnel.

Murray and Anderson found the Château Mauricien in a street behind the esplanade the morning after their arrival and quickly discovered that the hotel had seen better days. With its tall windows and sunny verandas offering views of the English Channel, the picturesque villa was surrounded by pretty gardens featuring stables, garages, and greenhouses. Inside the château, rooms were ornately decorated with painted ceilings, marble pillars, and heavy curtains. The building had been shut up since the outbreak of war, however, and its maintenance had been neglected. The roof now leaked, the chimneys were blocked, the boiler was broken, and the drains overflowed. The owner, the town's mayor, was nevertheless determined to extract a high price from two obviously well-off British women. Murray and Anderson spent the best part of Sunday morning haggling with the mayor's agent, a man with the "appearance and manners of a bluff sea captain," but were forced to agree to an extortionate rent. Convinced the mayor was "on the make," Anderson told Alan, "It is not ideal but it is the only thing." Murray, ever optimistic, and in spite of the November chill, described the hotel as "full of sunshine and sweetness."[8]

Moving into the Château Mauricien the same day, Murray and Anderson, with their customary resourcefulness, set about transforming it into a "passable hospital."[9] They contracted with French workmen (who all happened to be employed by the mayor) to sweep the chimneys, fix the drains, and repair the heating. They procured furniture, mattresses, and a kitchen range—also through the mayor—which arrived at the hotel in two rickety carts along with cutlery, which came, rather alarmingly, from a former typhoid ward. As the hospital took shape over the next few days, the hotel pantry was converted into an operating theater, one of the greenhouses became a linens storeroom, and a three-story cottage on the grounds was turned into accommodations for staff. Meanwhile, Murray and Anderson wired Paris with an urgent request for staff and supplies.

BACK AT CLARIDGE'S, Mardie Hodgson had been packing medical equipment and vital supplies in anticipation of the move. She had also ordered two hundred more blankets to be shipped over from Barker's in Kensington.[10] Since it was possible they might need to evacuate the new hospital at a moment's notice, should the Germans breach Allied lines, she had pared supplies to a minimum. Two days later, on November 2, Hodgson and a crew of volunteer drivers left Paris in a convoy of four cars and one ambulance, with a skeleton crew staying behind at Claridge's to tend the few remaining patients. Pulling up outside the Château Mauricien that evening, they unloaded fifty canvas beds along with bales of blankets and medical supplies. More baggage had been sent on by train.

As soon as she arrived, Hodgson dashed off a note to her mother with an urgent appeal for hot water bottles and bed linens. Taking in her new staff quarters, she reported: "Our room is very nice but there is no furniture 1 double matrass on the floor & 2 chairs is all we have 1 wash basin between 3 & we carry our own water across the yard." Since they were unwilling to pay the mayor further exorbitant fees, Anderson and Murray had drawn the line at renting bedsteads for the staff. Although the château was built with a walled garden and "endless green houses," Hodgson thought the kitchen "rather small" for a projected hospital of seventy to eighty beds. She

was still delighted at the change of scene, since she and Olga Campbell had grown "sick of fooling around & doing nothing" in Paris.[11]

As the beds were being made up and the operating theater
equipped, Hazel Cuthbert arrived from Claridge's with a team of
eleven nurses.[12] Meanwhile, Anderson's own cook, Eliza Fenn, and
her housemaid, Annie Goodwin, came over from London to take
command of the kitchens. Quickly establishing order, they recruited
twenty women, all Belgian refugees, as kitchen staff and supervised
the catering, with the aid of a checklist of French-English transla-
tions pinned to the wall. The return to English cooking after months
of French cuisine was a popular change with the staff, who tended
to prefer everything British.

Another welcome arrival was Arthur Campbell, Olga's father
and Mardie Hodgson's uncle, who had turned up in Paris in October to help with carpentry jobs at Claridge's and now decamped
to Wimereux to lend a hand there. "I am sort of general utility orderly," he wrote home. "Any odd job is turned over to me—such as
taking to pieces the balustrade of the staircase to enable stretchers
to be taken up—Putting up clothes lines—Making shelves etc for
a disinfecting chamber—Making splints—repairing door locks and
any odd job that may be needed—not a very glorious occupation
but still it all helps."[13] An energetic and practical man, Arthur had
worked in diamond mines in South Africa and trekked through the
Transvaal with Cecil Rhodes in his youth before establishing his tea
plantations in Ceylon. Now aged sixty-four, he was one of only a
handful of men who would find a long-term place within the corps.

Another arrival in the party from Paris was Chester Fentress. He
was an American tenor living in Paris who had initially volunteered
at the American Hospital before offering his services as an orderly
at Claridge's. Fondly adopted by the corps, Fentress enlivened Claridge's by throwing impromptu parties in his room, dressed in a
black silk kimono. He introduced the staff to his close friend Hu-
bert Henry Davies, a British playwright, who likewise helped with
hospital chores. Having appropriated his elderly aunt's decrepit old
car—and its chauffeur—Fentress was now helping with the move.[14]

Thanks to the corps' efficiency, just four days after Murray and Anderson took possession of the château they were ready to accept sixty patients. There was just one problem. To receive British casualties flooding into Boulogne, the corps needed the army's approval. The initial response of army officials had not been promising. Since then, however, Jobson and Blandy had proved their worth at the Sugar Store Hospital, and Gazdar had been warmly received at the RAMC's Boulogne headquarters. At the same time, Murray and Anderson knew that positive reports of their work at Claridge's had filtered through to Boulogne from army medics who had visited them in Paris. But most crucially, they had calculated that once they had a functioning hospital fully prepared with empty beds, willing staff, and an ambulance at their disposal, the army could not say no.

ON NOVEMBER 5, Murray and Anderson called on the two highest-ranking RAMC officers in Boulogne in their makeshift headquarters in a dingy hotel room. In Murray's words, it had "hideous French wallpaper on the walls."[15] The two men were probably Sir Arthur Sloggett, who had arrived in Boulogne at the end of October after being appointed commander of medical services on the Western Front, and his deputy, Lieutenant Colonel Charles Burtchaell.[16] A dapper, mustached man in his fifties who lived up to his reputation as a "ladies' man," Sloggett was described by one contemporary as resembling "Mr Punch," with a "breezy manner and a crimson nose."[17] To Murray and Anderson's amazement, Sloggett not only confirmed that the army was willing to use the Château Mauricien to "the fullest extent," but agreed to grant the unit official status as an auxiliary military hospital. It was an unprecedented move. Attached to No. 14 Stationary Hospital in Wimereux's Hôtel Grand, the Women's Hospital Corps would work directly under military command. Their food, coal, and gasoline rations would be provided by the army—although the staff would still be unpaid volunteers. An official contract was signed on the spot to certify that the hospital was recognized by the War Office. The Château Mauricien auxiliary hospital, as it was now officially titled, had become the first British army hospital to be run by women.

Elsewhere in France and Belgium, British women doctors, nurses, and other volunteers had established other hospitals and ambulance units that were now providing medical aid to the front line.[18] Among them was the Millicent Sutherland Ambulance, a unit set up by the Duchess of Sutherland, which had spent six weeks behind enemy lines in Belgium before relocating to slightly safer premises in Dunkirk. Likewise, Dr. Hector Munro's Flying Ambulance Corps—whose members included motorcycle enthusiasts Elsie Knocker and Mairi Chisholm—had run a field hospital in Ghent before being forced to evacuate by advancing Germans. Similarly, Mabel St Clair Stobart, who had previously run a medical unit in the Balkan Wars, had set up an emergency hospital in Antwerp before staff there had been forced to flee. Stobart's unit would later take over a sixteenth-century château near Cherbourg. Meanwhile, Elsie Inglis was still busy organizing her Scottish Women's Hospitals. She would establish its first base in the medieval abbey of Royaumont, near Paris, in December.

But Louisa Garrett Anderson and Flora Murray had become the first women doctors to be formally sanctioned to run a military hospital for the British Army. It was a remarkable turnaround. In the three short months since the onset of war, they had gone from being suffragette militants working against the British government in the cause of the women's war—effectively enemies of the state—to becoming medical officers attached to the British Army.

Being absorbed into the army naturally meant being subject to army bureaucracy. When Sloggett asked whether the corps had a quartermaster to take charge of supplies and administration, Anderson quickly confirmed that they did—while silently appointing Olga Campbell to the post. Having arrived from Claridge's to help Mardie Hodgson with the preparations, Campbell was taken under the wing of the quartermaster from the Hôtel Grand and escorted to the army supply depot. She returned with her car packed with vast quantities of cold meats, fruit, cheese, tea, and sugar as her fellow quartermaster shook his head in bafflement at the depot's unaccustomed generosity. The army even installed a telephone.

Gleefully reporting the news to Alan, Anderson wrote, "It makes all the difference having been taken over by the War Office. The army rations strike me as excellent in quality & amt & they require very little supplementing so that our expenses are reduced tremendously."[19] Murray was just as jubilant. Their "hearts leapt" at the army's acceptance of the corps, she said, since it had always been their ambition to see women doctors working as army surgeons under the British War Office.[20] A proud Hodgson wrote home with news of her cousin's unexpected promotion. Campbell, she said, had been "hobnobbing" with the quartermaster from the "big hotel" and now had "endless books" in which to record supplies. Poor Olga, her cousin wrote, was already "fair dazed with calculating so many men at so many oz per day—as it has to be worked out for every condiment not only for the wounded but for us also." She added, "There are hundreds of wounded here & we hope to be very useful."[21] Despite Hodgson's gross underestimate of the casualties, the corps would certainly prove useful.

THAT SAME EVENING, November 5, the corps's ambulance waited in the line of vehicles at the Boulogne quayside, ready to load its first patients.[22] Within two days, twenty-three patients had been admitted into the sumptuous ground-floor ward of the Château Mauricien, and another ten were expected that night. Unfortunately, Hodgson was also on the casualty list—again—having cut open her head when leaning out of the tram that ran between Wimereux and Boulogne and hitting a telegraph post. Breaking from her busy operating list, Anderson had put a stitch in the cut. Within two weeks, the first patients were sufficiently recovered to be sent back to England for convalescence, and a few days later the hospital was full again.

The addition of the Château Mauricien brought the number of army and voluntary hospitals in the Boulogne area to ten, with a total of three thousand beds. The number of hospitals soon expanded to eleven with the arrival of an Indian medical unit, which moved into the Jesuits' college. As the Battle of Ypres ground on with little gain on either side, wounded men arrived daily in the ambulance trains plying their way between Boulogne and the front. At times the bombardment was so intense the shelling could be heard in Boulogne. In total, some twenty-five thousand wounded men would be admitted into the area's hospitals during the Battle of Ypres; many more were either patched up and sent straight back to the battlefield or transferred by hospital ships to Britain.[23] Throughout November and into December, the corps' ambulances—a second arrived at some point—shuttled along the coast road between Boulogne and Wimereux.

One British volunteer working in Wimereux at the time described the eerie scene in Boulogne that occurred daily. Red Cross and private ambulances backed up to the platform every morning and evening to await the arrival of the trains. When a train pulled in, one expected "noise, bustle and the bursting open of every carriage door," she said. Instead, there was such silence that "one wonders, is it an empty train or a train of dead?"[24] Then, slowly and quietly, the nurses descended, the walking wounded emerged, and the stretcher cases were lifted down. Having raced to the quay, the ambulances then crawled back to Wimereux with their fragile loads. Rough seas sometimes washed over the coastal road, making it impassable, and the ambulances had to wait for the tide to ebb before they could reach the resort.

At the end of their second week in Boulogne, Anderson wrote to Alan—the first time she had had time to put pen to paper since arriving—to update him on their progress. "We are quite busy here & rather nicely placed although not luxuriously," she said.[25] The first convalescent patients had just left for home "in great spirits at going but quite sad to leave." There were "a great many handshakings & good wishes all round." That day, Sunday, November 15, she had brought in an army chaplain to lead a service on the ground-floor ward. There was no piano or other accompaniment, but the men "sang well & liked it." She added, referring to her maid and cook, respectively, "Annie & Eliza are a tremendous help & are working very hard. I think they are quite interested but it is a great change for them to run an institution with 60 beds & a staff of 20 with Belgian refugees under them."

Grateful as she was that at last she was able to do such work with the official stamp of the War Office, Anderson was beginning to betray a weariness at the relentless onslaught. Aware that family and friends back home were volunteering for active service or were already in training for the front, she confided to her brother, "It is so bad that one feels it can't go on much longer & yet neither side can afford to stop."[26] Having seen the brutal effects of battle at close range for nearly two months, she felt sickened by "the great horror of this war." The thought that her brother might volunteer was alarming. Writing to Alan's wife, Ivy, who was expecting their fourth baby, she said, "It makes one's heart stop—but he & you must decide."[27] Like so many others involved in the war effort at home or abroad, she felt the only way to cope was to carry on and try to alleviate the suffering. "The thing has to be fought out," she said, "& nothing matters except that we shd each of us do our best."

Yet despite the nightmare continuing less than sixty miles away, there were some compensating factors. "The sea is perfectly lovely here," Anderson told her sister-in-law. "Wimereux stands rather high & there is a sweep of coast. The sea has been quite rough lately & at night the search lights over it are beautiful." Hodgson agreed. Her head wound mended and the stitch removed, she sent her mother a postcard with a picture of the Château Mauricien in calmer times, with a hotel guest in a straw boater hat enjoying afternoon tea under a striped sunshade on the lawn. "Just had a lovely walk down the shore," she wrote. "It is blowing hard but the search lights look lovely over the waves."[28]

NOW THAT THE Château Mauricien was fully operational, Murray returned to Paris to supervise Claridge's with Hodgson at her side while Anderson remained in Wimereux with Campbell as her capable deputy. Despite the lack of new admissions in Paris, there were still convalescent patients who needed attention. In Wimereux,

Anderson worked long hours in the operating theater, with Gazdar and Cuthbert as her assistants and the team of eleven nurses on the wards. Although the hospital was smaller than Claridge's, the amount of work and pace of arrivals was significantly heavier, with "a great deal of major surgery."[29]

Just as at Claridge's, the injuries at Wimereux included smashed limbs, multiple gunshot and shrapnel wounds, plus horrific mutilations of the body and face. According to one nurse who worked at the Sugar Store Hospital, men arrived with fingerless hands and sightless eyes, with their "mouths swollen beyond all recognition" and "ugly scalp wounds." The stench of gas gangrene—akin to the smell of a dead mouse—filled the nostrils. Most of the men arrived in shock, devastated by what they had seen and done, traumatized by witnessing the deaths of friends and enemies alike. "There is a look of weariness in their eyes that appals one," said the nurse. "They all have it—the trench-haunted look."[30]

As well as contending with battle injuries and shell shock, the men suffered deteriorating health from long periods in the foul trench conditions. Diseases such as trench fever, dysentery, meningitis, diphtheria, measles, and influenza thrived in the squalor. Infectious cases were routinely sent to No. 14 Stationary Hospital, in Wimereux's Hôtel Grand, where they were isolated in the bathing huts.[31] Most of the men were infested with lice—which in turn often infested those caring for them. The lice, along with the growing population of rats—engorging themselves on rotting bodies—spread diseases such as typhus. As autumn advanced, heavy rains turned the trenches and surrounding land into quagmires, which brought new problems. Trench foot, a painful condition caused by wearing permanently wet socks and boots, resulted in more gangrene cases, and the battlefield downpours hampered the stretcher-bearers, who had to wade through mud up to their knees to collect the wounded.

With the onset of winter and plummeting temperatures—the first snow fell in mid-November—men arrived with frostbitten fingers and toes, which also led to gangrene. At that point the only feasible course was amputation. The evacuation process had improved with the arrival of the first motorized ambulances in October and specially fitted ambulance trains by mid-November, but horse-drawn ambulances still formed the mainstay of the RAMC's transport at the front.[32]

Most surgeons, however, still practiced the traditional conservative approach to wounds, so that tetanus, septicemia, and gas gangrene spread, often with lethal results. In November 1914, a Scottish surgeon, Henry Gray, based in an army hospital in Rouen, began to pioneer a radical new approach. He cut away all dead and damaged tissue to leave a large gaping wound, which he left open and regularly cleaned for several days while checking for infection—with good results. But Gray did not publish his research until 1915, and the practice only became standard two years later. "Very few of the surgeons had previously been familiar with wounds such as those caused by shell-fire," wrote one Boulogne-based army surgeon, and the cases of gas gangrene and trench foot were "entirely novel" to all.[33]

Anderson had, by this point, performed hundreds of operations at Claridge's, and therefore had at least as much experience of military surgery as her army colleagues. She rarely described the visceral reality or complexity of the surgery she was undertaking in letters home, although she told Alan there "is plenty for us to do," with "ambulances running in & out of the courtyard night & day."[34] She was so busy she had little time even to keep up with the war news: whenever she was not in the operating theater, she was writing letters on behalf of the wounded. Whenever possible, she wrote personally to the families of every man when he was admitted. Yet for all the medical challenges and appalling losses, she relished the task she had taken on. By November 17, Anderson could tell Ivy that the hospital was "running nicely now." They had sixty beds full and were set to expand to seventy. She added, "I am <u>thankful</u> we came out. It was quite the right thing to do."[35]

It was exhilarating to feel that the corps was being taken seriously at last by both the army hierarchy and fellow male doctors. It was novel, too, to feel empathy and respect for men, after so many years engaged in the bitter suffrage campaign. "The men are really <u>very</u> nice," Anderson told Ivy. "We get so fond of them. They love having fires in their rooms & English food & comfortable beds & having letters written to their wives etc etc & a girl quarter master who is very attractive as well as efficient." Although she was generally disapproving about marriage, especially for women doctors, she knew the value of a pretty face to an ailing man. She added, "My admiration for men has gone up so tremendously I feel <u>quite</u> different about them now & it is such a blessing to do so. For years at home I had seen only their worst side & now I am seeing a splendid side of courage & self sacrifice for an ideal, that no woman would better." The sentiment was apparently mutual. One Scottish patient, asked by a visitor where the male doctors were, retorted, "What for should we be wanting male doctors here?"[36]

As well serving as a bridge between men and women, working within the corps spanned other divides. It was the first time that most of the women staff—who had previously mixed almost exclusively in middle- or upper-class society—had experienced any close relationships with working-class men. Anderson wrote, "The Tommies are wonderfully articulate & sweet to us & grateful <u>in words</u> for the little that we are able to do for them." Murray expressed similar views. Compared to the grand and lofty rooms at Claridge's, the Château Mauricien was much smaller and more intimate, so the relationship between staff and men was particularly close, she said.[37] Getting to know the soldiers in their care, the women learned about the men's pasts—and the recent terrors they had suffered. "The women felt strangely near the Front," she wrote, "for the men came down from the lines in a few hours, and their tales of the mud and wet in which they were standing almost up to their waists, the agony of frostbite, the terrible shortage of ammunition and the superiority of the German guns made pitiful hearing." Yet even as she felt empathy for the soldiers, Murray still held the male establishment responsible for the war. Some of the men had signed up before the war with no expectation of ever being called to fight in a foreign land, she said. Then, finding themselves caught up in the slaughter, they were warned they would be shot for desertion if they left.

It was no surprise that the men felt grateful for being transported from the misery and horror of the trenches to the comfortable and airy villa overlooking the sea. As soon as they were unloaded from the ambulances in the château's courtyard, they were greeted with cups of steaming cocoa or soup before being helped or carried to a reception room supplied with hot water, clean towels, and soap.[38] As well as a comfort, the hot drinks and warm baths served a practical purpose. Understanding of resuscitation techniques was in its infancy at the beginning of the war. As the war advanced, surgeons would realize that men in hypovolemic shock—where excessive bleeding led to lowered blood pressure—needed intravenous fluid replacement and blood transfusions. But hot drinks to replace fluids and raise temperature, and warming patients with blankets, hot baths, and hot water bottles, offered some of the same benefits.

For many of the men, this reception provided the first warm drink and hot food that had passed their lips since being wounded. For some, it was their first encounter with soap and water since arriving at the front. Warmed, washed, and nourished, and changed into clean pajamas, the men were settled in their beds with freshly laundered sheets and colorful blankets, like children in a nursery, before having their wounds dressed or being prepared for surgery. The largest ward had been set up in the villa's "grand salon," an elegant ground-floor drawing room with neoclassical columns and elaborately decorated ceilings, while other wards had been created in the bedrooms and billiard room. Some of these rooms were "veritable sun traps," according to one observer, providing a haven of rest.[39]

Just as at Claridge's, the women at Château Mauricien went out of their way to provide their patients with domestic comforts and morale-boosting diversions. In addition to the English cooking supervised by Eliza and Annie, there were religious services and concert parties. Friends kept up a supply of bed linens and warm clothing shipped over from Britain; some even crossed the Channel, their cars packed with gifts, including rubber rings to help cushion painful wounds and board games to keep the patients amused. One friend presented the corps with a gramophone—an instant hit with the men. It was played "incessantly," Anderson told Alan, with breaks only for the daily round of dressings and post-lunch naps.[40] The men found the "pleasure of cigarettes & cakes & chestnuts is incomplete without it," she said. "For these reasons I like it better than any other present I ever had."

Hodgson meanwhile kept her mother busy with appeals for blankets and clothing. In a typical letter she asked for "grey flannel dayshirts also flannel bed jackets preferably scarlet, because they do brighten the place up," as well as "20 or 30 bedsocks" to be given as presents to the men when they left.[41] At one point, Alan himself arrived, bringing with him a carload of pheasants—"the last word in luxury," said Murray.[42]

NOT SURPRISINGLY, MANY of the men were sorry when the time came to leave—either for hospitals in Britain if their injuries were too serious to return them to active service, or back to the front if they were deemed fit enough. The continuing flood of fresh casualties and the demand for more men to replace them in the battlefield meant the military hospitals were under constant pressure to discharge patients and free up beds. The RAMC officers were "zealous" about turnover, said Murray, and visited weekly to check that patients were not malingering. In the brief time they tended them, the women grew fond of their charges—and grimly aware of what awaited those heading back to the front. "As the day came nearer," said Murray, "their eyes would follow the Chief Surgeon around the ward, apprehensive of discharge."[43] For those returning to the front, the women assembled a parcel of gifts—including the bedsocks sent by Mardie Hodgson's mother—and all the staff turned out to wave them off. Yet there was "no getting over the horror of going back," said Murray.

Some of the men treated at the Château Mauricien sent letters thanking the women for their care after they returned to Britain or to active service. "We get lots," Anderson told Alan. "Some very sweet ones."[44] One soldier, Private Jack Canham, who had been shipped home to recuperate in Manchester, wrote, "I have not forgotten your kindness to wards me," and sent his love to all the staff. He added, "I must say you all done your best to make me as happy as you possabe could." Others wrote from their hospital beds to tell their families about their experiences in this novel hospital run by women. Corporal David Watt, who had been a railway porter before joining the Scots Guards, had already been wounded once and recovered at home before returning to the front near Ypres, where he was hit by a bullet in the leg. He had sheltered in a trench for twenty-four hours as shells fell around him before being picked up and brought by ambulance train to Boulogne. From there he was admitted to the Château Mauricien in November. "We are very well treated and cared for here; they do anything for us," he wrote. "You see the place is run by the Women's Hospital Corps and they are very good to us." Another, Lance Corporal Frank Reynolds of the Oxfordshire and Buckinghamshire Light Infantry, had been wounded in the face, neck, and shoulder by fragments from a bursting shell. His brother George had pulled him out from a mound of debris, but the four men with them had all been killed. "I am in one of the very best hospitals—a ladies' hospital," he wrote home. "Lady doctors do all the work—no men at all, so you can guess I am all right."[45]

One patient, however, felt rather less comfortable when he found himself surrounded by women. Anderson recognized him as the police officer who had arrested her during the "Black Friday" demonstration in Whitehall four years earlier. Embarrassed, the poor man said, "I wouldn't have mentioned it, Miss. We'll let byegones be byegones."[46] The incident was later depicted in a cartoon in *Punch* showing a stern and bespectacled Anderson quizzing a bashful soldier while nurses giggle in the background.

Letters came from widows and bereaved mothers, too, thanking the staff for caring for their loved ones. Whenever a patient died, Anderson made a point of writing to his next-of-kin, providing details of his last days and—in accordance with army custom—praising his heroism. One widow, whose letter Anderson preserved, wrote her to say, "I must thank you from the bottom of my heart for the careful and devoted attention which you gave to my Husband and the attempts made to alleviate his sufferings." Although Anderson rarely referred to the deaths of patients in her letters home, she admitted to Alan, "We get letters like this all the time—they are so touching."[47] The dead were buried in the nearby military cemetery on a hill overlooking the sea. During the ceremony, the Lord's Prayer was read in French and the "Last Post" played by a "boy bugler."[48]

The specter of death was impossible to avoid. Only a few months had passed since the outbreak of war, but already bereavement had become a familiar experience to many. With the hospital's proximity to the cross-Channel steamers, it was often visited by soldiers and civilians desperately searching for missing friends and relatives. One was a retired colonel who was trying to trace his son. "We have such a lot of people here who have lost a beloved son—or brother," Anderson told Alan. She was probably thinking of his own position, but one of the corps' nurses, who worked at Claridge's, lost a brother near Ypres in November.[49] "It is a terrible business for everyone," wrote Anderson, "but far the worst—as it always is—for the people left behind."

BY LATE NOVEMBER, when the First Battle of Ypres ground to a stalemate, the armies on both sides exhausted, depleted, and entrenched in freezing mud, there was a slowdown of casualty arrivals in Boulogne. Yet the hospitals remained full of sick and convalescing soldiers, while the ambulances were kept busy transferring patients to the hospital ships or back to their camps. Now that the pace of surgery had eased, Rosalie Jobson and Majorie Blandy took a break from duties at the Sugar Store Hospital and came to help at the Château Mauricien—although Jobson, at least, had good reason to linger in Boulogne. At the Sugar Store Hospital, Jobson had met her future husband, Gordon Morgan Holmes, a brilliant neurologist who had worked at the renowned National Hospital in Queen Square, London, before enrolling with the British Red Cross at the outbreak of war.[50] He would become one of the army's foremost experts on shell shock. Both aged twenty-eight, the pair found a shared love of medicine and mutual respect through working together in the grueling conditions. They would marry in 1918, after Gordon proposed to Rosalie while rowing on the Thames during leave.

The comparative relaxation in workload gave Olga Campbell a chance for a well-deserved break from her quartermaster duties. She went to London with her father, Arthur, before returning laden with gifts, including a soccer ball for the men, and brimming with fresh enthusiasm for her work.[51] Like many caught up in the horror of war, whether they were soldiers or volunteers, she felt restless and impotent when away from active service. War was traumatic and monstrous, but Campbell felt it was better to throw herself into working than to submit to the false banality of home life. Her return was warmly appreciated: Anderson had been "lost without her & inundated with all kinds of difficult things . . . which I didn't understand."[52]

Back at the Château Mauricien, by November Campbell wrote an exuberant letter to her younger brother Keir. "I am simply bursting with health—this is an extraordinarily healthy spot," she wrote. "We all eat like tigers & as you know army rations are very liberal & also very good."[53] She was proud of her organizational skills—"I wish you could see my store room," she bragged to Keir—and delighted with the new gramophone, which was being kept hard at work on the top floor, where the convalescent men had been moved. "The men simply love it, its raucous but cheery cries pervade the house of an evening," she said. "It is a wonder-fully cheery place. I love to hear the gusts of laughter that descend every now & again."

The jaunty air was no doubt also an attempt by Campbell to boost her brother's spirits, since he was training to be sent to the front in the New Year. "There is one merciful thing," she counseled. "You will find that everything as it comes seems the natural & in-evitable thing to be doing—A man told me who had lain for hours badly wounded with apparently no chance of being picked up that he had never felt the least bit worried or sorry . . . as the signs of haemorrhage & weakness came on he had just watched them with interest and felt that it was all perfectly natural and fitting." She told

Keir she had resolved to study medicine when the war was over. "I shall probably fail to get there—but I'm going to have a try."

Even as the beds slowly emptied during the lull in fighting, the hospital wards had a constant stream of visitors. Passenger ferries were still crossing the Channel—despite the lurking German U-boats—so Boulogne and the surrounding area had become a magnet for relatives visiting the wounded, as well as sightseers eager to catch a glimpse of the war machine. One welcome visitor, who arrived on November 27, was Henry Nevinson, the journalist who had read the roll call of staff when the corps left Victoria in September. So much had happened in the intervening ten weeks.

As a seasoned reporter of many past conflicts, Nevinson had been frustrated by the War Office's refusal to let journalists near the front—not to mention the press corps' meek acceptance of government censorship. So in October, he had traveled independently to France in the hope of seeing the fighting at first hand. Since then he had been visiting volunteer-run field hospitals and ambulance units, and—as a man of action as much as words—been helping to ferry the wounded from the front line to medical aid.

Despite his long experience of war, Nevinson had been shocked by the condition of the casualties he encountered, including one "boy" of twenty-three with his intestines "dashed out, & the far-off look of death upon him."[54] His account, titled "Realities of War," had been deemed too horrific to publish in the *Daily News*, though it would later appear in the American journal *New Republic*. Nevinson met Anderson at the quayside in Boulogne and walked with her along the coast road to Wimereux to visit the Château Mauricien. He was no doubt relieved to find that Flora Murray, with her fierce manner, was absent.

Touring the wards, Nevinson met one man who was speechless from shell shock and another who had undergone a "wonderful new operation" to mend his fractured thigh with steel pins. Although he did not reveal whether this operation was Anderson's handiwork or that of a surgeon earlier in the evacuation chain, it was a technique that Anderson later employed. After taking tea with staff, he walked along the esplanade under a "stormy moon" before meeting Anderson for dinner. Back in London two days later, Nevinson devoted an afternoon to "trying to get things out for Dr G. A."

Evelyn Sharp, the suffragette journalist who was Nevinson's companion, and had once been an intimate friend of Anderson's, visited Wimereux at around the same time—most probably with Nevinson. Observing the compassionate care that Anderson and her corps provided, Sharp noted the "bitter irony of our civilization, which first compels men to tear one another to pieces like wild beasts for no personal reason, and then applies all its arts to patching them up in order to let them do it all over again." When the "patching is done by women," she wrote, "the ironic tragedy of the whole thing seems more evident."[55]

Just a day or two later, another familiar face appeared unexpectedly. It was Lord Esher, back in France to review the changes in medical care. Anderson was in the middle of operating when Esher arrived, but he waited patiently for her to finish, and then they sat together in front of the fire, "talking things over quite friendly."[56] Anderson later told Alan, "Considering his desperate hostility a few weeks ago it is really funny. He even made friends with Eliza and Annie." A few weeks later, Esher sent her a scrawled note to say he had spoken with Sir Alfred Keogh, who was now in overall charge of British army medical services, impressing upon him "very strongly" that "no one has done more splendid work" than the Women's Hospital Corps. He added, poignantly, "Were I wounded, I would prefer your hospital to any I have seen—and I have seen most!" Anderson sent the letter to her brother so he could share it with their mother. Although Elizabeth Garrett Anderson was now "very wandery," Louisa reasoned that her mother "probably likes me doing this work and knowing, if she knows, that it has gained recognition for Women's Work."[57]

A further seal of approval came a few weeks later when Sir Frederick Treves, the surgeon Esher had once introduced to Anderson and Murray as "unconverted to women doctors," returned to France to report on medical care for the British Red Cross. He pronounced the wards in the Château Mauricien "cheerful, tidy and well placed" and declared that the work was "carried on with great earnestness and enthusiasm."[58]

JUST AS THE PACE in the Boulogne hospitals was slackening, so work in Paris suddenly picked up. With no hope of advance near Ypres, the Allies had shifted their attention south again, to the region of Champagne, in the hope of breaking through German lines. Attacks by the French, with British support, from early December led to high numbers of casualties without significant gains. At Claridge's, at the behest of the army, the corps had set up an extra thirty beds at the end of November to cope with an expected influx of 150 wounded. Army medical chiefs had come to regard Claridge's effectively as an auxiliary army hospital, much like the Château Mauricien, even though it was technically still supervised by the French Red Cross. "We are again prepairing for more wounded," Hodgson wrote home. The central courtyard had been enclosed to provide an extra ward, which was "all ready even to the night shirts & jackets on the beds & the towels & soap," she said.[59]

A few days later, on December 4, the first British wounded arrived on ambulance trains diverted to Paris. Anderson dispatched some of the staff from Wimereux to help in the capital, while Hodgson was fully employed fetching casualties from the station. One convoy brought ninety-six wounded in a single afternoon.[60] Hodgson was so busy that, she said, "I only occasionally have time to think of anything outside my immediate job."[61] Her work was not helped by the continuing organizational obstacles. They had trouble obtaining sufficient coal through the French authorities to heat the cavernous building, which meant there was no hot water for baths on the day the huge convoy arrived. Staff had to heat up gallons of water on gas burners. At times, the wards at Claridge's were so cold that the men had to be kept in bed with blankets and hot water bottles. "We are near perished with cold here," Hodgson exclaimed.[62] She obtained some coke-burning braziers to help heat the wards;

even if they were only partially effective, the men enjoyed cooking chestnuts on them.

The difficulties were exacerbated by the fact that one of the orderlies, Cuthbert's sister Galantha, had been sent home at the end of November as "incapable." According to Hodgson, she was "so forgetful & cannot be trusted to see anything through."[63] Her place was taken by Isabel Lowe, the elder sister of Lieutenant Lowe, who had died at Claridge's in October from wounds sustained in the Battle of the Aisne. Having watched the corps at work during the ten days she had spent at her brother's bedside, she now wanted to show her gratitude.[64] Like Vera Brittain, the writer whose memoir, *Testament of Youth*, encapsulated the experience of a generation— and many more women who lost brothers, friends, and lovers in the war—Isabel Lowe found some solace in contributing to the war effort while grieving for her brother. Despite being nicknamed "Slow" by Hodgson, Lowe, who was twenty-eight, proved a loyal worker who would remain with the corps for years to come. She and Hodgson became firm friends.

As well as the British wounded, there were more French and French colonial patients to fill the beds at Claridge's. One Frenchman with a severely fractured thigh had spent the previous two months in hopelessly overcrowded French military hospitals, and was surprised when Murray slowly and painstakingly eased the gauze from his gaping wound.[65] He had been used to French doctors ripping the dressing away in haste. Another patient was a "Turco"—an Algerian—with severely frostbitten feet, who was likely to require amputation of one or both.

Hodgson not only kept up with the colossal task of organizing transport and supplies, but was also gaining experience in the operating theater. Together with Lowe, she was charged with preparing the surgical instruments. "We got everything ready & only forgot a sling of all the necessary things," she wrote home after one session.[66] Despite the gruesome sights, Hodgson enjoyed working in theater, although she hoped that someone else would take charge when the time came for the Algerian man's amputation—an especially unpleasant operation. If she was charged with the task, she wrote, "I shall take it as an enormous complement because that will mean they think me competent to manage my share & hand all the necessary things & prepare it all."

Hodgson plainly took enormous pride in her work. "I do long to tell you how very happy I am to be here & <u>know</u> I am useful," she told her mother. "Sometimes our jobs seem trifling, but I know that they help."[67] She was even starting to sound a bit "suffragetty" in her letters home. "We have made a pretty big splash, & all about so little I mean the women here are doing no more & no better than they have done for years in London & elsewhere."[68] She longed for her mother to see the new ward with its thirty brass beds covered in blue-and-red striped blankets and its glowing coke brazier in the center. "At this moment," she wrote, "there is a crowd around the piano at the far end & the men are all singing & having a lovely time, they are so happy & it sounds so nice."[69] Hodgson had grown enormously in maturity. Writing to her stepfather, she briskly explained that she could not accept one young woman, a family friend, who was keen to volunteer, since it was "quite impossible" to fit in another girl at Boulogne—"especially one who like Elsie cannot bear the sight of blood."[70] She was intensely proud of her cousin Olga, too, and thrilled to report that "Flo"—that is, Murray—had insisted "she could not do without us."

Both Anderson and Murray were well aware of the vital contribution that the cousins made to their two hospitals. "I can't tell you what a happiness it has been to me to have Mardie here these last weeks," Murray told Hodgson's mother. "She is so sweet & helpful & her gaiety & buoyancy are very comforting & pleasant."[71] In a similar vein, Anderson wrote, "I do not know what Dr. Murray & I wd have done without Olga & Mardie. . . . They are dear girls & they promise to make remarkable women." Echoing Murray's appeal to keep them a little longer, she added, "The separations which are entailed are the price we pay for our great position."

SEPARATION WAS A TRIAL for both Murray and Anderson too. It took more than a week for letters to travel the 160 miles between Paris and Boulogne in wartime conditions, and the train journey was at least eight hours. Anderson told her sister-in-law, Ivy, "We hate being apart—& I miss her help very much here where there is a great deal of organising & business in addition to a lot of surgery."[72] While Murray was a quietly efficient administrator who kept calm under pressure, Anderson knew her own strength lay in the hands-on work of the operating theater. When Ivy sent her a bundle of warm clothes, Anderson asked her to order duplicates "for Flo," to fight the Claridge's chill. She wanted gloves with long fingers, mouse-colored puttees (leggings to wear over ankle boots), and a "leather waistcoat like mine only if possible mouse colored or brown rather than yellow & slender size."[73] She even provided little sketches to indicate the ideal shape for Murray's boyish figure. In early December, the pace in Wimereux slowed sufficiently for Anderson to visit Paris for a day; the following week, she made the visit again "for a glimpse of La Directrice without whom I get on badly."[74]

By now—in mid-December—the Château Mauricien was emptying fast. Since hostilities had more or less ceased on the Flanders front line, patients were being discharged daily and dispatched to Boulogne for the hospital ships returning to Britain. As ambulances filled the yard to take the men home, patients and staff shook hands, Anderson told her brother, and some of the men made "shy & nice remarks," telling them "that if it weren't for their wives & babies they wd have liked to stay on."[75]

Yet, just as the British were leaving, a new patient arrived: their first German prisoner of war. Murray and Anderson had been horrified on their first train journey to Boulogne to overhear a French nurse discussing a German patient who had lost the use of his hands, and was deliberately fed last by the staff. They believed the Hippocratic Oath bound them to treat everyone equally. As Anderson wrote, "I hope we will make him like the English if he feels nasty about them now, but he doesn't look as if he did."[76] When the

German recovered and was told he was being transferred to England, he looked puzzled and insisted, "But I am in England now."

AS CHRISTMAS APPROACHED, Murray and Anderson knew they would have to spend the holiday apart, but they were determined to make the time as cheerful as possible for the staff and patients at their respective hospitals. They generously packed Hodgson and Campbell back home to Scotland for a ten-day break; after three months away from their families, they were both thrilled to return—though all too aware of the additional strain they left in their wake. Hodgson felt "quite a deserter," she wrote to her mother as she waited in Boulogne to cross. But, she told her, "<u>Home</u> seems to be the eternal refrain of this letter—it is such a good place."[77]

In Wimereux, the kitchen staff peeled carrots and made plum puddings in the run-up to the festivities, and the doctors had decided to wear "funny noses" for the day. "We are going to make an effort at real gaiety here for Xmas day," Anderson reported to Alan.[78] "It has a sad side to it but I expect it is best to do it." She had little appetite for celebrating; the strain of the long hours, the separation from her family and *La Directrice*, and the return of the men to the trenches took its toll. "It is difficult to know what to do this year—but I expect it is best to go right on," she said. For the first time, however, she spoke of disbanding the corps, because "Dr Murray & I must come home & take up the old threads." Murray said the same, telling Hodgson's mother they would probably close the venture in March. "Six months away from one's practice is as much as it will stand, & as more hospitals come out every week we shall probably feel that we can be replaced."[79]

In Paris, where every bed at Claridge's was now full, the hospital was turned into a veritable Christmas grotto—but with a peculiarly martial emphasis. Most of the decorations were created by the convalescing men, so that in addition to paper chains crisscrossing the ceilings, the walls were festooned with decorations featuring "aeroplanes, long guns, rising suns, [and] statues to liberty and victory."[80] One effort, which featured three battleships and the Union Jack beneath the motto "The Flag of Freedom," went a step too far for Murray's liking. When she objected that there was "no freedom for women under that flag," the men slunk away and changed the last word to the more accurate "England."

On Christmas Eve, choirboys from a local church bearing colored lanterns sang carols in the wards, and the nurses hung stockings at the end of each bed. Like excited children, the men woke at 5:00 a.m. to open their gifts in a scene "reminiscent of nursery life." After getting the dressings round over early, staff pushed all the beds and tables into the largest ward to serve Christmas dinner—roast turkey with sausages and all the trimmings—for eighty-six men. Then Murray and six nurses brought in flaming plum puddings in a procession cheered by the patients. There was beer and port to toast the king's health and Christmas crackers for the men to pull.

Dinner was followed by a packed evening of entertainment, beginning with a pantomime based—very loosely—on Little Red Riding Hood, written by Dr. Cuthbert. Staff took various parts, including a cow that required several prompts before it appeared. According to Murray, "the men said that they had never known such a Christmas: it was something to tell in the trenches, something to write home—a memory treasured by patients and staff alike."

FOR ALL THE forced frivolity, the New Year brought no hope for an end to the war. Lord Kitchener had been right. When some of his cabinet colleagues had suggested the war would be over by Christmas, he had grimly forecast it might very well continue for years to come. The soldiers who had dug in for the winter on the Western Front were already desperate for an end to the carnage. The doctors and nurses were exhausted by the task of patching up wounded men only to send them back to the slaughter. Friends and families back in Britain were sick with the perpetual anxiety of waiting for telegrams and letters. And after more than three months of relentless toil, Louisa Garrett Anderson and Flora Murray were ready to disband their corps, return home, and pick up their "old threads."

Making a brief visit to London and Suffolk to see family and friends after Christmas, Anderson met her pal Nevinson at London's Liverpool Street Station and told him her plans. "She was very charming again," he wrote in his diary. "Thinks of returning from the French hospitals soon." This would be welcome news, he knew, to Evelyn Sharp, Anderson's friend, though he added, darkly, "but Dr. F. M. comes with her & so trouble is renewed."[81]

Back in Boulogne by January 6, 1915, Anderson took up the reins at the Château Mauricien for the time remaining. Although they would keep the château going until spring, she and Murray had decided to close Claridge's early, owing to the obstacles they continued to encounter with French officials. Both the French Red Cross and the British Army voiced regrets about the closure. Red Cross officials insisted that Claridge's was their "best installation," while army officers told the corps they had "set a standard which is quite unknown even among auxiliary hospitals."[82]

Hodgson, who had returned from Scotland with Campbell with her enthusiasm undiminished, was immediately thrown into a frantic week in Paris. She worked tirelessly evacuating patients and packing supplies, which were sent on to Boulogne in fifty-eight bales and boxes. On January 8, Hodgson gathered with Murray, Anderson, and a handful of staff members and friends for a farewell dinner in a Parisian restaurant. It was a "great success," but there was more than a tinge of sadness to the celebrations: Claridge's, said Hodgson, was now a "thing of the past." Anderson glumly sent the news to Alan. "We closed Claridge last week—much to our regret—& some of the Corps went home & some are taking short leave holidays."[83] All who had worked in Paris and Wimereux—doctors, nurses, and orderlies—would later receive the 1914 Star medal, known as the "Mons Star," for their contributions in France.[84] Murray and Anderson also had a special medal struck for all those who had worked in the Women's Hospital Corps.

While some of the staff returned to their families for a well-earned rest, Hodgson and others transferred to the Château Mauricien to help in Wimereux. There was scarcely enough work to keep them occupied, however. By February, the incessant rain had transformed the Ypres region into a sea of mud. Any hope of advance from either side was out of the question, and all fighting had ground to a halt. The stream of sick and wounded arriving in Boulogne had dwindled to a trickle, and the beds in the Château Mauricien were emptying fast. A lull had fallen over the trenches, over the medical centers in Boulogne, and over the little château beside the sea at Wimereux. It would not be long before the members of the corps would have to pack up their bags and head home. Their big adventure, they thought, was over.

4

Good God! Women!

War Office, Whitehall, London, February 1915

Flora Murray and Louisa Garrett Anderson entered the War Office on the corner of Whitehall and Horse Guards Avenue with a mixture of anticipation and trepidation.[1] In the five months since they had last been living in London, the city had changed beyond all recognition. By day, the streets were thronged with women driving cars and delivery vans, riding motorcycles as telegram messengers, and patrolling as police volunteers. By night, the city was empty, dark, and hushed. Street lamps were extinguished, clocks were muffled, and searchlights raked the sky for the air raids, which were expected at any moment. As the two women climbed the marble staircase in the palatial War Office, which had opened nine years earlier, they saw a building bustling with activity. Since most of the permanent staff had been deployed to France, the offices were mainly run by reservists; boy scouts scuttled up and down the corridors bearing messages, and "lady clerks"—another novelty—clattered away at typewriters. Anderson and Murray were shown into the office of Sir Alfred Keogh, the most senior doctor in the British Army.

A seasoned army surgeon who had seen action in the Boer Wars, Keogh, now fifty-seven and sporting a bristling mustache, had retired from service in 1910 only to be called back as director general of army medical services soon after the outbreak of war in 1914.[2]

Born and educated in Ireland, Keogh was renowned for his superlative organizational skills and contempt for red tape. He had transformed the army's medical services before the war and brought in further sweeping changes in late 1914—including the introduction of motor ambulances and ambulance trains—to address the challenges at the front.

The winter lull in fighting in France had enabled both sides to reinforce and extend their trenches, so that now these earthworks stretched four hundred miles from the North Sea to Switzerland. This new front line, which would remain largely static for the next four years, meant that medical centers could be established much closer to the field of battle, with hugely improved evacuation chains. Casualty clearing stations, in particular, were being rapidly expanded so they could perform swifter and more complex surgeries, saving many lives. Yet Keogh knew he still faced serious problems. It was clear, despite these improvements, that the army's medical provision could not cope with the scale of casualties that German firepower could inflict. With a new "push" set to begin on the Western Front as soon as weather permitted, and more battle zones opening up farther afield, Keogh urgently needed an extra fifty thousand beds in Britain—and more doctors—to treat the inevitable casualties.

Encouraged by the friends and supporters they had made among the army's medical chiefs in France, Anderson and Murray were eager to continue the work they had started. Although they had been ready to disband the Women's Hospital Corps at the end of 1914, army officials in Boulogne had urged them not to give up their military work. They needed little more persuasion. Glowing reports of their hospitals in Paris and Wimereux had been forwarded to the War Office by the most senior RAMC officers in France, including Keogh's deputy, Sir Arthur Sloggett, the "ladies' man" who was now one of their staunchest allies. Lord Esher had also relayed praise of their work "in the highest terms."[3] It was through Sloggett and other army chiefs in France that they had secured this critical meeting with Keogh. Four years earlier, Anderson had been arrested in Whitehall, only yards from the War Office, for her part in the Black Friday demonstration. Six months ago, the War Office had sent women doctors away with a stinging rebuff. Now it was asking Murray and Anderson for their help.

Keogh began by telling them he had heard "nothing but good" of their work but wanted to know who was really running their unit. Conscious that many voluntary hospitals were being financed by wealthy aristocratic patrons (many of them women), he was evidently wary of interference from benefactors. When the two women confirmed that they alone were in charge of the Women's Hospital Corps, Keogh replied, "Then we can talk."

To their astonishment, he invited them to run a military hospital in the heart of London with up to one thousand beds. Like the Château Mauricien, it would be supplied by the army with War Office funds. But unlike any other British army hospital ever, it would be run solely by women, with an almost entirely female staff. Indeed, Keogh promised Anderson and Murray complete freedom to appoint whichever staff they pleased. It was, as Anderson immediately recognized, "a great opportunity."[4]

The two women dashed, jubilant, back to France the following day and immediately began closing the Château Mauricien. When they called on Sloggett to tell him that Keogh was going to put them in charge of a hospital in London, he spluttered, "Good God! He isn't?"[5] Quickly recovering himself, he added, "Well, when I think of it, I expect you'll be able to do it." A few days later, on February 19, the women of the WHC crossed the Channel with their cargo of equipment and arrived in Dover.

News of their new challenge, however, had preceded them. Keogh had announced his offer to them the previous day at an event to raise funds for an extension of the London School of Medicine for Women. Applauding the achievements of the LSMW, Keogh revealed that he had received "numbers of unsolicited letters from Paris and Boulogne" declaring that the work of the women doctors in France was "beyond all praise" and "an example of how such work ought to be done." So impressed had he been, he said, that he had invited Murray and Anderson to take charge of a five-hundred-bed hospital in the center of London—"and, if they pleased, of a hospital of 1,000 beds."[6]

It was a huge gamble, as Keogh well knew. Writing to thank one colleague for backing his "revolutionary proposal," he said, "I hope they won't let me down!" Many within the War Office, however, were vehemently opposed to female doctors muscling into their ranks. Keogh would later admit that he was pressed to abandon his plan, and he was well aware he would meet "scorn and ridicule" if the venture failed.[7]

For all his sincere and encouraging words, Keogh was motivated as much by necessity as liberalism. In the first five months of the war, forty-six doctors had already lost their lives.[8] Desperate not only to fill these gaps but boost medical provision at the front, Keogh was about to issue an appeal for two thousand more British doctors, as well as doctors in the British Commonwealth, to volunteer their services. Yet the stream of medical men and students enlisting in the army had already left hospitals and practices at home dangerously understaffed, while medical schools were emptying fast. In London, only three surgeons were left at St Mary's Hospital, and almost none at St Bartholomew's, while thirteen out of fifteen junior doctor posts at St George's were vacant.[9] Indeed, the drain on medical schools was so severe that the president of the General Medical Council, Sir Donald MacAlister, had asked the army to send back the students it had only recently recruited so they could finish their studies.[10] There were serious concerns that the civilian population would soon be left without adequate medical care.

Former hardline opponents of women in medicine were suddenly forced to change tack. Faced with empty benches in the medical school at Cambridge University, professor of surgery Frederick Howard Marsh urged hospitals to appoint women doctors to vacant posts and declared "another epoch for women is at hand."[11] Leading government figures, members of the medical establishment, and even royalty threw their weight behind the appeal to expand the LSMW in order to train more women doctors. *The Times* added its voice to the call for more medical women to address the "serious and increasing dearth of medical men."[12] Even Prime Minister Herbert Asquith, who had fought against women's demands for so long, gave his backing to the appeal, admitting that the war had instigated a "turning-point" for medical women.[13]

For Murray and Anderson, Keogh's gamble represented the opportunity they had been waiting for. It was a decision born of both "courage and wisdom" that would produce sweeping changes in "magnitude and importance," said Murray.[14] Not only did it give medical women their first official chance to serve their country as part of the war effort, but it was a testament to the value of women doctors and a message from the country's top medical military authority.

RETURNING TO LONDON, Murray and Anderson moved back into their house in Kensington. After their months of separation in France, they would never live apart again. They began preparations for their new hospital immediately. Yet despite the support of the most senior medical figure in the War Office, it was not going to be easy. In early March, they were told they had been allocated a former workhouse near Covent Garden in central London. Peering warily through the entrance on their way to a meeting at the War Office, they were shocked to see the site piled high with rubbish and filth before being turned away by an officious gatekeeper as "unauthorized persons upon government premises."[15] Once they gained official entry to the building, the obstacles—and the antagonism—only increased.

The St Giles's and St George's Workhouse in Endell Street, in the heart of London's Theatreland, was a forbidding five-story hulk of four blocks arranged around a dingy courtyard. The only entrance was a narrow lane off the upper end of Endell Street, squeezed between a public washhouse and a church. When they emerged from this dark tunnel, Murray and Anderson discovered that the courtyard was divided by iron railings into sections, much like animal pens, where the workhouse inmates had until recently exercised. The labels, denoting categories such as "Old Males" and "Young Females," were still attached to the padlocked gates. First erected in 1727 and rebuilt in the late 1800s, the workhouse was reputed to have been the inspiration for Charles Dickens's *Oliver Twist*; the oldest block contained a long room that was believed to be the setting for Oliver's interview with the Poor Law guardians.[16] The old workhouse mortuary, with slate "pigeon holes" to store coffins, still survived, and stairs led down into "ancient and grimy" cellars. The workhouse had closed in 1914, and the rooms had then been used to house Belgian refugees. Not finding it the most promising location, Murray pronounced the building "grey and sombre-looking"; another observer called it a "sad and gloomy place."[17] It was a world away from Claridge's.

Major alterations were needed to convert the grim Victorian institution into a smooth-running military hospital. The exercise pens, padded cells, and iron chains once used to restrain workhouse inmates all had to be removed. Electric lighting, modern cooking facilities, and lifts capable of taking stretchers had to be installed. And the entire site needed to be cleared, cleaned, and painted. Stacked to the ceilings with a jumble of old furniture and littered with junk outside, the place was "indescribable chaos," said Murray.[18] Now that they had the support of the army's surgeon-general, the might of the military machine behind them, and four hundred workmen on the job, the renovation should have been straightforward. Yet the women met barriers and hostility at every turn.

Medical chiefs in the War Office did as little as possible to help, while other officials were deliberately obstructive. Most army officers seemed to regard the Women's Hospital Corps with a mixture of incredulity, humor, and distaste. When Murray and Anderson called at Endell Street one day to check on progress, the RAMC colonel in charge of the conversion greeted them with the words, "Good God! Women!"[19] Convinced that the idea of women running a military hospital was both ridiculous and dangerous, he attempted to persuade them to abandon their plans before storming off in disgust. He was swiftly followed by his deputy. Another RAMC officer refused to take them on a tour of the building with the excuse that he did not know his way around. Undaunted, the women clambered over the rubble to make their own inspections.

After weeks of little or no progress on the site, Murray and Anderson finally took matters into their own hands. They directly petitioned Keogh, insisting that the renovations be put under their command, and Endell Street Military Hospital was formally handed over on March 22. Using their customary brand of "mild militancy" that had worked such miracles in Paris and Wimereux, the two women then charmed, cajoled, and threatened the workmen so that the alterations that had proved so troublesome could be completed in a more timely manner. Within a few weeks, the job was done. Under the pretense that Kitchener himself was taking a personal interest in the project, they even persuaded the men to give up their bank holiday to complete the task.[20] At one point, desperate to clear the laundry room of hundreds of damp and filthy mattresses, the two women tracked down the official responsible for their removal and refused to let him leave his office for the weekend until he telephoned through the required order.

Meanwhile, Keogh arranged for Anderson, Murray, and Campbell to attend a course in military administration at the Queen Alexandra Military Hospital in Millbank beside the River Thames. There, in contrast to the general hostility they were battling on the site, they were surprised to be treated with "much kindness" and gained valuable insights into how to run a military hospital.[21] Finally, at the end of March, Murray and Anderson moved into rooms on the second floor of Endell Street that constituted the old workhouse Master's House. They would live together there for the next four years along with their pair of black and white Scottish terriers, Garrett and William.[22]

BY THE BEGINNING of May, the hospital was taking shape. There were 520 beds lined up in seventeen wards, two operating theaters, an X-ray room, a pathology laboratory, a dispensary, and, of course, a mortuary. The wards were all named alphabetically, in accordance with military custom, but—in a strike for feminism—instead of being denoted simply by letters, Murray and Anderson named them after female saints, ranging from St Anne to St Veronica. In fact, the War Office had initially assumed the hospital would be called "St George's and St Giles'," after its former workhouse setting, but the two women were adamant it would not be named after male saints. Thus it became, and would remain, the Endell Street Military Hospital.[23] An additional room in the basement, where drunks were put to cool off, was dubbed the "Johnnie Walker Ward"—the only place within the entire hospital bearing a male name.

Just as in France, Murray and Anderson were determined the wards should be homey, bright, and cheerful—in contrast to the "chilly whitewashed walls and gloomy brown blankets" of typical army hospitals.[24] Cleaned of their workhouse grime, the wards were painted in fresh green, and the high ceilings and tall windows gave the rooms a light and airy aspect. The beds, lined up in two neat rows, were covered with colorful quilts—striped blue and red in one ward, salmon pink in another—and fresh flowers were arranged daily by volunteers, who were supervised by Anderson's sister-in-law, Ivy. Designed to resemble cozy sitting rooms rather than hospital settings, the wards were hung with pictures, patterned screens shielded the open fires, and easy chairs were dotted around. Since the electric lighting installed by the army provided only dim pools of light, the women appealed to Anderson's old school, St Leonard's, which sent 180 reading lamps so the men could read and play cards in bed.

On the ground floor, a large room was set aside for recreation, with a library and billiard table at one end and a stage at the other. A remnant from the workhouse, the stage was transformed by pretty blue curtains embroidered with the W.H.C. initials and the suffragettes' motto, "Deeds not Words," emblazoned above. The courtyard outside was converted from a barren, utilitarian exercise yard into a verdant and fragrant haven scattered with planted tubs, window boxes, and sunshades. Staff accommodations were arranged on three floors in one of the blocks.

As the work progressed, Anderson and Murray set about recruiting some 180 staff members, to include 14 doctors, 29 trained nurses, and more than 80 orderlies. Those women who had served with the corps in France formed the nucleus of the workforce, and 1,000 interviews were conducted to find the rest.[25] As in France, Murray was appointed chief physician (or "doctor in charge"), while Anderson was chief surgeon. To find the rest of their medical team, they drew on their connections in the LSMW and the suffrage movement, ensuring that all the women doctors would be not only professionally trained but also loyal to the cause.

First in line among the new doctors was Louisa Woodcock, who had supervised the corps' fundraising work in London and was now appointed second physician. Reserved and kindly with a deep social conscience, Woodcock had studied at Oxford before taking up medicine and had cowritten a report on medical care for the poor with the social reformer Beatrice Webb. She would become one of the most hard-working and best-loved members of the corps. To help Anderson in the operating theater there were six assistant surgeons, including Gertrude Gazdar and Rosalie Jobson, who had served in France. Gazdar and Jobson now had a few months of experience treating battlefield wounds, but none of the others had previously dealt with major trauma. The youngest two of the new recruits, Gertrude Dearnley and Winifred Buckley, aged thirty and thirty-one, respectively, had only qualified in the past three years. Buckley, who was born in Calcutta, where her father had worked as a civil engineer, had served only one year in a junior post at Anderson and Murray's Harrow Road children's hospital and six months as a house surgeon in Hull. Fun-loving and gregarious, if sometimes slightly odd—she once downed six raw eggs mixed in milk to save time eating—she would come to regard her work at Endell Street as "perhaps the happiest time in her life."[26] In addition, Anderson and Murray recruited several women specialists, including a pathologist, an ophthalmologist, a radiologist, and a dental surgeon, to act as consultants.

Without exception, the Endell Street doctors were all graduates of the LSMW—since no mainstream medical school, in London at least, was yet open to women—and the vast majority of them had never previously treated men. The radiographer, Eva White—who, at twenty-eight, was the youngest—had only just graduated. Amy Sheppard, the ophthalmologist, who was fifty, had qualified more than twenty years previously; she had spent her entire career at the New Hospital for Women. Helen Chambers, the pathologist, who was thirty-five, was the only one who had ever worked in a large general hospital, the Middlesex in London. Modest and reserved, she had distinguished herself as an expert in cancer research and cowritten a number of research papers. Several of the doctors had been active suffragettes—although none had been imprisoned— and all but one were single. Only Eva Handley-Read, one of a handful of female dental surgeons in Britain, was married. Sheppard, in fact, lived with a fellow woman doctor, Frances Ede, with whom she enjoyed a loving relationship in the manner of Murray and Anderson.

As with the original corps in France, the nurses had significantly more experience in looking after male patients and providing general medical care than the doctors. Although Murray would make little mention of them in the book she later wrote about Endell Street, it was the nurses—the twenty-nine qualified "sisters," as they are called in Britain, a number that later increased to thirty-six— who would spend the most time with the patients and assume day-to-day responsibility for their care. While the doctors worked long hours in the operating theater and provided clinical advice on the wards, it was the nurses who prepared patients for surgery and cared for them postoperatively, dressed their wounds and alleviated their pain, helped ease their minds, and oversaw vital daily tasks, including washing, eating, and exercise.[27]

Six of the sisters appointed at Endell Street had worked with the corps in France. One of them, Evelyn "Evy" Clemow, came from a prosperous Cornish family that owned a string of hotels and wine merchants—including the only company allowed to import Veuve Clicquot champagne into Britain. Educated in private schools in France and Germany, she was fluent in both languages. Clemow had wanted to study medicine but was dissuaded by her father; instead, she trained as a nurse at Guy's Hospital in London. Her work at Wimereux won high praise from Anderson, who described her as "a very good nurse" who was "most assiduous & careful & reliable & very kind to her patients."[28] Many of the other nurses were the daughters of doctors, vicars, and other professional men from similarly well-to-do backgrounds and had been educated at private girls' schools.

They were all expertly supervised by Grace Hale, who would work as matron at Endell Street throughout its lifetime. Formerly matron at the New Hospital for Women, she had been transferred at the outbreak of war to a military hospital in south London.[29] Murray had secured Hale's move to Endell Street by pulling a few strings with Keogh. A War Office memo agreeing to her release noted that although the New Hospital was keen to have her back, the staff there was also anxious to support Endell Street, since it would be a "difficult hospital to run." The daughter of a grocer, Hale, aged forty-three, had trained at the prestigious St Bartholomew's Hospital in London and was highly experienced. One colleague described her as "a capable, conscientious and efficient organiser." She was popular with all the staff.

It was the eighty or so women orderlies, however, who performed most of the daily drudgery of basic nursing as well as cooking, cleaning, and running errands—all under the watchful eye of the ward sisters. Although the orderlies were termed "nurses"—and addressed by doctors and patients alike as "nurse"—most had little, if any, training in nursing skills. Some had already volunteered for war work as "VADs"—members of Voluntary Aid Detachments run by the British Red Cross—while others were recruited directly by Murray and Anderson. A large number of these untrained, or largely untrained, women had been recruited to perform traditional nursing duties in military hospitals at home and overseas, and the influx was already triggering concerns. Professional nurses and the nursing press were worried about eroding standards and differing approaches—especially given the social divide between working nurses and the mainly middle- or upper-class volunteers.[30] Commenting on the arrangement at Endell Street, the *British Journal of Nursing* warned that supervising such a large number of willing but inexperienced women would likely prove a "heavy and anxious" task for the ward sisters, even if the orderlies were "carefully selected from the cultured class from which probationers should always be drawn."[31]

This small army of nursing orderlies was indeed drawn from the "cultured class." They were more used to being waited on—their clothes laundered, meals cooked, and shoes polished by servants— than to tending to somebody else. Some were debutantes from titled families; one was even believed—probably apocryphally—to be a niece of Winston Churchill.[32] It was a common sight, one patient would relate, to see "luxurious motor-cars" dropping off the orderlies outside the hospital in the morning and collecting them at the end of the day. But Flora Murray would defend them vigorously for "laying aside their habits of ease and pleasure" in order to shoulder the burden of hospital work.[33] It was the orderlies, she stressed, who were largely responsible for the "distinctive character" and "fine spirit" at Endell Street. "They brought laughter into the wards," she said. That was a commodity that would be sorely needed.

Well aware of the mammoth challenge ahead, Murray and Anderson were determined to hold onto the key members of the corps who had proved their worth in France. Olga Campbell was appointed quartermaster, assuming the vital role of organizing all stores and medical supplies as she had in France—although now she was responsible for managing a hospital five times the size of Claridge's. Mardie Hodgson was appointed transport officer, with three assistants, in charge of preparing for the arrival of the wounded as well as organizing outings, greeting visitors, and maintaining a strict watch on the gate; Isabel Lowe worked closely with her as one of the chief orderlies.

Campbell's father, Arthur, was still determined to do his bit. Having moved with his wife, Ethel, into Murray and Anderson's house in Bedford Gardens, he continued his sterling work as general handyman and would become adept at crafting artificial limbs. To help with the heavier labor, which it was believed the women orderlies could not manage, the RAMC supplied an officer and twenty men. These included the three male orderlies, Privates Bishop, Price, and Hedges, who had accompanied the corps to Paris, and who were now transferred into the RAMC detachment at Endell Street. There was one more addition to the corps. Hodgson had smuggled an Alsatian puppy back from France, hiding it in her bra, according to family lore. The dog, which she named Eepie after Ypres, would take prime position in staff photographs along with Garrett and William.[34]

Now that they were all officially in the army, the women were given nominal military ranks. Although they would never be granted official commissions or be entitled to wear military uniforms and insignia, they were all awarded army pay and allowances. Murray and Anderson were paid according to the level of a major—Murray would later be promoted to the equivalent of lieutenant colonel—while the other doctors were paid as lieutenants or captains. They were the first women to be regarded effectively as army officers, and upon her promotion Murray would become, nominally at least, the highest-ranking woman in the British Army. The distinctions were not just symbolic. Their military rank was a significant factor in helping the women maintain discipline among the thousands of soldiers who would soon come under their care.

Like officers in the army, the women at Endell Street would refer to each other by their surnames—although they also used nicknames to subvert the army's masculine culture. Amy Sheppard, for example, was known as "Sheppie." Nobody, however, would dare to refer to their two leaders by any nickname. They were always Dr. Murray and "Dr. G. A.," or "the COs," short for "commanding officers." Although technically only Murray was commanding officer, it was understood that the job was shared. The women orderlies were considered ordinary enlisted soldiers—just like Tommies, one patient noted—and they received standard army pay of 1s 2d (one shilling and two pence) a day—"whether they want it or not," he added pertinently.

Denied official army uniforms, the women at Endell Street wore the same practical grayish-brown skirts and jackets they had designed for France, with red shoulder straps to denote the doctors—blue for the orderlies—and the WHC initials in cloth shoulder titles. Later the cloth badges were replaced by metal ones emblazoned with the words "Endell St." The staff made a point of proudly wearing their uniforms in public, albeit with their heads chastely covered by a cap with a trailing veil, and they soon became a familiar sight on

London's streets. One newspaper applauded their outfit as "a great relief from the drab khaki and blue serges that many women are wearing for their war work."[35] On the wards, the orderlies exchanged their jackets for white overalls, while the nurses adopted more traditional bluish-gray tunics covered by white aprons and headdresses.

It was enormously time-consuming and challenging work to sort through the one thousand women who applied while negotiating the bewildering army paperwork and regulations—especially since Murray and Anderson were still running their Harrow Road children's hospital. But determined to make a success of the extraordinary opportunity they had been granted, they rallied family, friends, and suffragette comrades to support their enterprise by volunteering their money and talents. One member of the staff, making an appeal for donations through the press in March, urged: "We want pianos, gramophones, pictures, and motor-cars—and we have not the slightest doubt we shall get them." The hospital, she pledged, would be a "home from home for Tommy." She added, "We are going to show the men how these things should be done."[36]

ARRIVING AT ENDELL Street amid the mayhem, as the builders worked overtime to finish their tasks and orderlies scurried around with furniture and bedding, the American actress and author Elizabeth Robins was among the first to respond to the appeal for help. Born in Louisville, Kentucky, but mostly raised by her grandmother in Ohio, Robins had married a fellow actor in Boston when she was twenty-three.[37] After her husband drowned himself in the Charles River in a fit of depression and jealousy, Robins had made her home in England and her name on the London stage playing formidable female characters from Henrik Ibsen. With her pretty, impish face, striking blue eyes, and profusion of coppery hair, Robins had drawn numerous admirers of both sexes. She would never remarry but had a long-term love affair with William Archer, her Ibsen translator, and was close friends with the poet John Masefield and the author Henry James, as well as the Liberal politician Sir Edward Grey.

Breezily rejecting advances from suitors, she once pushed George Bernard Shaw out of a taxi into the gutter.

Having retired from the stage in 1902 at the age of forty, Robins had turned to writing—she published fourteen novels—and thrown herself into the suffrage movement. Her play *Votes for Women!* made a powerful case for the women's cause, and she put her stage presence to good use by giving rousing public speeches. Her passion had inspired Evelyn Sharp, Anderson's formerly intimate friend, to join the movement, as well as captivating Sharp's admirer Henry Nevinson. Robins had helped to found both the Women Writers' Suffrage League and the Actresses' Franchise League.

Now fifty-two, Robins had largely retreated from London life to a farmhouse in Sussex. She spent much of her leisure time with her close companion Octavia Wilberforce, who had just begun training in medicine at the LSMW. Although Wilberforce was more than twenty years her junior—Robins said she was "more my child than my 'friend'"—the pair would have an intense and sometimes claustrophobic relationship for the rest of Robins's life. Now, however, Robins ventured out of her semi-seclusion in response to an appeal from her friend and fellow novelist Beatrice Harraden, also a committed suffragette, to help set up a library for the wounded men soon to be arriving at Endell Street.

Catching the early train to Victoria, Robins arrived in Endell Street around 10:00 a.m. on May 10. She knew the area well, having trodden the boards at many of the local theaters in her heyday. Entering the old workhouse courtyard for her first day's duty, she was regaled by the clamor of workmen's hammers and drills. Despite the noise and dust, it was clear—as she wrote in the diary she had kept meticulously since the age of thirteen—that the hospital "slowly approaches readiness."[38] Working companionably with Harraden, Robins sorted, stamped, and shelved books in the new recreation room until early afternoon. It was a laborious, dirty job, but Robins felt exhilarated. She was part of this thrilling new adventure—one led by women she loved and admired, and with whom she shared suffragette ideals.

Robins and Harraden had met up some weeks earlier to discuss their plans for the hospital library. Both were already friendly with Anderson and Murray through their suffragette work and had been enthusiastic supporters of their medical mission in France, as well as their children's hospital. When the two doctors asked them to volunteer at Endell Street as "honorary librarians," Harraden and Robins did not hesitate. At their first meeting, Murray told Robins that the corps' experience in France had taught them that many soldiers were "more wounded in their minds than in their bodies."[39] Providing patients with books as a diversion from the physical pain of their wounds and the emotional trauma of their war experiences was entirely in keeping with Murray and Anderson's nurturing approach to treating the war wounded. The two doctors may also have been inspired by the War Library in London, which had been set up by a literary enthusiast, Helen Mary ("May") Gaskell. Gaskell had rallied the public at the beginning of the war to donate books and magazines to send to British troops in hospitals at home and abroad.[40] Immediately embracing their challenge, Harraden and Robins sent appeals to friends, publishers, and fellow authors asking for donations. They were overwhelmed by the response. Publisher friends sent huge consignments of fiction, biography, and travel books, while authors presented signed copies of their own works. Others donated thousands of popular magazines, such as the *Tatler* and the *Illustrated London News*. Some were rather too generous in their response, contributing "shoals" of tatty paperbacks and dated magazines that the librarians shoveled into sacks to be pulped. Harraden would later say she had never been "so dirty and so indignant."[41] Ultimately the Endell Street library would boast more than five thousand books and would be described as the "finest" hospital library in London. Working hard to organize and catalog their stock as the hospital took shape around them, Robins described those first few weeks as "unforgettable."[42]

TWO DAYS AFTER Robins's first shift in the library, on May 12, 1915, the first patients arrived at Endell Street. Although the beds were ready and staff in place, the patients turned up two weeks earlier than the War Office had promised. Workmen were still laboring onsite, and cutlery had to be hired at short notice. Much to Flora Murray's chagrin, however, these first patients were all convalescent cases, 100 men transferred from other military hospitals in London—no doubt to clear beds. Many of them, Murray complained, were "the troublesome, the idle, the grousing, or those who were unsatisfactory for some reason," whom staff elsewhere were evidently keen to get rid of.[43] But then that same night, the first convoys of wounded men arrived, straight from the battlefields of France. Within two days the staff members were nursing 246 men. By the end of the first week, all 520 beds were full.[44]

Robins and Harraden were flustered by the sudden rush. "War Office have sent soldiers to Endell street before the workmen have finished," Robins exclaimed in her diary. "They've made hay of our library. Harraden in despair."[45] Postponing her return home so she could help out, Robins found the recreation room full of convalescent patients rifling through the neatly ordered books, hammering on the piano, and even, eventually, breaking the new gramophone. Despite the disorder, it was all "v. cheerful & good natured," she said, and many of the men wanted most to talk about their experiences at the front. One soldier gave Robins a poem written by a friend who had been killed. Others were wheeling themselves about in invalid chairs.

After rescuing the scattered books and firmly locking the bookcase, Robins went to seek out Murray "in her sanctum" to complain about the chaos. Life in a military hospital was a "different world," she said—and it most certainly was. She added, "Poor fellows. All that needless suffering. A never to be forgotten afternoon." Murray did her best to placate Harraden and Robins, but she had rather more to worry about than a few displaced books and a broken gramophone.

Endell Street had opened just three days after the Allies had launched their joint spring offensives against the German Army on the Western Front.[46] The winter stalemate had ended on March 10 with a surprise attack by the British, bolstered by Kitchener's new recruits and troops from elsewhere in the empire, which had succeeded in capturing the village of Neuve Chapelle but at the cost of heavy losses. Then both sides had battled from their entrenched positions for more than five weeks through April and May in what would become known as the Second Battle of Ypres.

On top of the horrific mutilations still being caused by heavy artillery, the Germans had a new weapon. They first released chlorine gas on April 22. French, British, and Canadian forces—newly arrived in France—were terrified by the enveloping gas clouds, which burned the eyes, mouth, and nose and then attacked the lungs, causing choking and suffocation. One nurse, who helped treat more than two hundred gassed men in a single night in France, described the experience as the "most distressing" she had ever known.[47] Gas would continue to be used as a deadly weapon—by both sides—in various forms throughout the war.

Despite this horrifying new threat, on May 9 French and British troops launched their spring offensives in a renewed effort to break through German lines and seize the Vimy and Aubers Ridges. The attempt proved an unmitigated disaster since the preparatory bombardments failed to destroy German defenses, so that thousands of men were mown down by gunfire as they sought in vain to reach enemy trenches. In one of the most disastrous days of the war, more than eleven thousand British soldiers were killed or wounded. Despite the setback, the Allied assault would continue into June, with some of the worst fighting taking place from May 15 to 27 at the Battle of Festubert.

Meanwhile, in March, British naval forces had launched a disastrous attempt to wrest the Dardanelles strait from Turkish control, leading to significant shipping losses. This was followed, on April 25, by an ill-judged landing on the European side of Gallipoli, the peninsula guarding the strait, by British and French troops, along with substantial reinforcements from the Australian and New Zealand Army Corps (ANZAC) and a sizable Indian contingent. The fighting at Gallipoli would result in some three hundred thousand casualties.

As the wounded, sick, and gassed troops were shipped over in rising numbers from France and the eastern Mediterranean, they were met at British south coast ports by Red Cross ambulance trains, which transported them to London terminals. From these stations, volunteers in private cars and motor ambulances, organized by the new London Ambulance Column, set up through public donations, ferried the injured to military hospitals in the capital. The spectacle brought crowds of sightseers, who gathered at railway stations to watch the stretchers being unloaded and cheer the wounded men.

The increasingly common sight of wounded men arriving with the mud of the trenches on their bloodstained clothes brought the war right into the heart of London. One observer, visiting London in early May, noted "more soldiers, more bandages and limps, and more nurses" wherever she went. The sight of wounded soldiers eating in restaurants had become so commonplace by that point, according to another diary writer, that one man sat at a table with his head entirely bound in a bandage, yet "no one even glanced at him."[48] In May alone—the month Endell Street opened—more than forty-three thousand sick and wounded troops arrived in the United Kingdom from France, plus more than two thousand British, Australian, and New Zealand casualties from the Mediterranean.[49] It was the highest monthly total since the start of the war. Many of these wounded were recent recruits—Kitchener's New Army, as they were dubbed—who had enlisted in a rush of patriotic enthusiasm just months earlier.

These unprecedented casualty figures had brought the army hospital system close to the breaking point. On May 17, in the same week Endell Street opened, the War Office issued an urgent appeal for beds to the London Hospital, in the city's East End, since there were some fifteen thousand wounded waiting to be shipped from Boulogne.[50] All the beds there, however, were already full. Because it was close to several of the railway terminals that were receiving casualties, including Charing Cross, Waterloo, and Victoria, Endell Street was now in the front line of the capital's medical care. Ultimately, more than three hundred hospitals would be designated to receive the war wounded in London, ranging from the big five general hospitals to convalescent homes in converted townhouses. In terms of beds, though, Endell Street was one of the capital's twenty largest units. Within central London, it was one of the ten biggest hospitals, and its proximity to Charing Cross meant it would frequently receive the most serious cases.[51]

The imminent arrival of a convoy at Endell Street—often in the middle of the night—was announced by two blows on a large bell in the hospital courtyard. As soon as they heard the sound, the duty doctors, nurses, and orderlies hurriedly dressed and assembled outside. When the ambulances rumbled into the courtyard, the RAMC men slid out the stretchers and placed them on the ground. At times, according to one ambulance nurse, the smell of chlorine gas still clung to the men's uniforms mixed with the ever-present stench of gangrene.[52] The doctors, usually supervised by Murray and Anderson, assessed the patients' conditions and assigned them to a ward, and then Olga Campbell or one of her staff members logged their names, regiments, numbers, ranks, and medical details in the army-issue Admission and Discharge Book. While the paperwork was being filled out, the men were given hot cocoa and cigarettes. Then women orderlies took up the stretchers and carried them to the lifts and up to the wards.

One orderly would later remember the panic that ensued when the bell struck in the middle of the night. "We were up in a second and incredibly quickly stuffed our nightdresses into our dark blue bloomers, popped on our uniform, caught up our hair in our bonnets and reported down in the yard."[53] Electric lights were blacked out, to avoid offering German airships targets for a raid, and the only illumination came from a "dark"—covered—lantern. Then the ambulance "rolled quietly in, the stretchers slid out, those willing to take the head and shoulders stood by Dr Murray, the others stood a little further away." One young surgeon, who dozed momentarily after being woken by the tolling bell at 4:30 a.m. one night, rushed down in a fluster to find the orderlies already lined up on one side of the yard and the night sister with her lantern on the other. "Then came the ambulances," she said. "Silently the stretchers were lifted down from the motors which held four and a nurse."[54] Although the convoys most often arrived between midnight and 3:00 a.m., sometimes the bell would ring in the daytime, and the orderlies would run out of the offices and stores and line up ready to help.

The most complete description of the convoys arriving at Endell Street, however, comes from Beatrice Harraden, who watched the scene from her perch in the library. Harraden would use her experience at Endell Street to write a novel, published in Britain in 1918 as *Where Your Treasure Is* and in America as *Where Your Heart Is*. Her story follows a jewelry shop owner, Tamar, whose friend works as an orderly at St Ursula's Military Hospital, which was closely based on Endell Street.[55] Trying her best to ignore the war and the wounded, since she is "rather frightened by sick people," Tamar visits the hospital reluctantly, then finds, to her horror, that a convoy is on its way. Surveying the scene from a discreet corner, she sees young women running "from all quarters" to line up in front of the (male) sergeant major as two women doctors—the CO and chief surgeon—emerge from an office. "Then in glided four large grey ambulances marked *Red Cross*. Out of them in succession were lifted the stretchers, with their wounded freight, and laid on the ground. At once, at a sign from the Sergeant-Major, two girls stepped out from the line, and with an ease and agility which astonished Tamar, bore the soldier to the lift, directions as to his destination being given by the C.O. from her list. This process was repeated with four more ambulances, and yet another four, until all the wounded had disappeared and all the orderlies." Some of the wounded men, Tamar observed, were "clasping the flowers which had been showered on them at the station." Then the orderlies returned with their empty stretchers and the ambulances dashed away. The doctors vanished, the sergeant major dismissed the stretcher-bearers, and people began crossing the courtyard again.

As many as eighty men might arrive at Endell Street in a single convoy, many of them needing immediate surgery. Although some of the wounded would have received emergency aid at the newly expanded casualty clearing stations near the front line, or on hospital ships heading back across the Channel or through the

Mediterranean, many still arrived directly from the battlefield, especially at times of a big military "push," when the field hospitals were quickly overwhelmed. During the Battle of Neuve Chapelle in March, for example, some of the casualties reached London hospitals within twenty-four hours of being injured.[56] Since Endell Street received a high proportion of stretcher cases bearing the most seriously injured men, many needed urgent attention. Often twenty to thirty operations would have to be performed in a single day, and as soon as beds were emptied they filled again that same night.[57] At the heaviest times, the staff would be woken every night for a week to admit fresh casualties. From its opening day, the hospital would admit between four hundred and eight hundred cases every month.

If the arrival of the convoys at Endell Street presented an eerie sight for the women, it was all the more strange for the men arriving from the front. After traveling for hours or days from France or the Mediterranean, some of them slipping in and out of consciousness, many of them in shock, they must have thought they were dreaming—or worse—when they emerged from their ambulances into a dimly lit courtyard populated almost entirely by women. Often the wounded men were "speechless with astonishment" when they realized their stretcher was being carried by two "flappers," said Murray.[58] Yet within an hour or so of arrival they had not only grown accustomed to the idea of the "flappers' hospital"—they were singing its praises. Far from being alarmed when they found out they were going to be treated by women, they developed "amazing confidence" in their particular doctor, she claimed, while their faith in the chief surgeon, Anderson, was "unbounded." Murray wrote, "Each man thought his ward the best ward in the hospital, and his doctor the best doctor on the staff." Indeed, the men were so fascinated by the rare sight of a female dental surgeon that they pointed Eva Handley-Read out to visitors. Amy Sheppard, the ophthalmic surgeon, was regarded with awe, since it was believed—falsely, Murray insisted—that she had broken more windows than any other suffragette. Only one patient would ever ask to be transferred elsewhere because he did not wish to be treated by a woman doctor, Murray said, but he just as quickly changed his mind and begged his mother to plead for his return. On occasion, patients were asked whether they would prefer to be treated by a male doctor elsewhere—since some of them had wounds in intimate places, and many were suffering from venereal disease—but this offer was invariably refused.

Many of the men arrived with horribly septic wounds. Although gangrene was relatively rare among the convoys, the vast majority of wounds were infected to some extent. From the start, Anderson was keenly interested in finding ways to combat these infections. She worked closely with her pathologist, Helen Chambers, in testing various methods and logging their results. In a joint research paper published in *The Lancet*, charting their efforts to tackle septic wounds in one thousand patients in the first six months at Endell Street, they concluded that standard antiseptics were virtually useless.[59] They had slightly more success with three new approaches: Eusol (Edinburgh University Solution of Lime, a combination of bleach powder and boric acid first trialed in 1915), salicylic acid paste (a derivative of aspirin), and washing the wound with a salt solution. But most wounds healed in time if they were left open, drained, and regularly dressed, they noted.

Among their cases was a nineteen-year-old soldier with a bullet still lodged in his knee whose wound had turned "very septic." Anderson performed an operation to clean out the wound, and once the infection receded, she removed the bullet in a second operation. The youth made a full recovery. Another soldier had already had a "guillotine" amputation of his thigh—an emergency procedure cutting straight through the limb like a slice of bread—which had left the bone protruding from an "extremely septic" wound. After treating the infection, she amputated the limb higher up using the standard procedure, making flaps of skin and muscle to cover the stump.

The hospital also treated soldiers with general ailments ranging from rheumatism and heart conditions to psychological problems. Two men with acute mental disturbance arrived at Endell Street just a few weeks after it opened.[60] One was described as "blasphemous and homicidal," while the other was "deeply religious and suicidal"—a potentially explosive combination—and both were violent and noisy. Since there were no special secure facilities, the men were detained together in a tiny room, guarded by some of the male RAMC officers, while the women frantically telephoned local army barracks for help. After four days of anxious telephone appeals, an elderly colonel arrived on the scene, obviously under the impression that the women were unduly alarmed because they were unaccustomed to psychiatric cases. Glibly remarking that these were "not nice cases for ladies," he offered to calm the patients. Murray, who had—of course—previously worked in an asylum, showed the colonel into the patients' room. But as the colonel attempted in vain to "soothe" one of the men, the other seized him from behind. He was rescued by several of the female orderlies after a "regular scrimmage." Orders were promptly given to have the two patients transferred to more suitable accommodations. The incident left the women doctors "almost helpless with laughter," Murray said, though it could not have been especially funny for the two poor patients.

Despite the nightly arrival of convoys, the grousing convalescents, and occasionally violent patients, Anderson was passionately enthusiastic about the hospital's progress in those first few weeks. Speaking at a fund-raising tea for the LSMW on May 17—just five days after the arrival of her first patients—she joked that running a 550-bed military hospital (she plainly had ambitions for expansion) was like treating "550 large babies." She said, "If you have found out the way to treat children—what toys they like, what they like for tea, and what frightens them when going to an operation—you have gone a great way to find out how to run a military hospital."[61]

The press, too, was eager to talk up the fighting spirit that Endell Street exemplified. At one of the lowest points of the war—when headlines were reporting one defeat after another, columns were filled with notices of casualties, and news of the sinking of the *Lusitania* by a German U-boat on May 7, with the loss of 1,195 lives, was spreading shockwaves through Britain and America—journalists were desperate to report any piece of good news. Although much of the coverage focused on the novelty of women doctors treating male patients, often with a jocular or incredulous tone, the press seized on the story of the military hospital "manned by women." National newspapers ran regular features extolling the work at Endell Street, with photographs depicting cheerful patients being treated by its "lady doctors." Pictures of its "exceptionally pretty" orderlies in their "beguiling" uniforms adorned the pages of newspapers and magazines. A typical article in the *Daily Chronicle*, headlined "The All-Woman Hospital," described Endell Street as "a model institution," declaring, "The Endell-street hospital is a triumph not only for women in medicine, but for women in administration." The *Pall Mall Gazette* asserted that "the Endell-street Military Hospital proves what women can do when the opportunity is afforded them." And *The Suffragette*—which now filled its columns with examples of women's war efforts, rather than their militant actions—congratulated Murray and Anderson on the "splendid work" they were doing in the "National Crisis."[62] Taking a similarly feminist tone, the *British Journal of Nursing* remarked on the "subtle difference" between Endell Street and other military hospitals, which it attributed to the fact that it was "woman's kingdom."

The article in the *British Journal of Nursing* echoed a theme, picked up by other journals, that Murray and Anderson were always at pains to emphasize. Endell Street, they argued, was not just equal to male-run military hospitals in its professional care of the wounded; it was superior, because of its feminine attention to domestic detail. Escorted around Endell Street by the matron, Grace Hale, just a few weeks after the hospital opened, the *BJN* reporter declared the building "spick and span, cheerful, comfortable and efficient." The writer noted examples of the feminine touch and enthused about the "wide and bright" wards with their vividly colored quilts and screens, the "nutritious and appetisingly served food," and even the mortuary with its purple hangings, which "bears evidence of women's care." In particular, the writer added, there were flowers everywhere—on the wards as well as in the courtyard, where convalescing patients lay on couches, sat on chairs, or strolled about amid the "scent of heliotrope and other sweet-smelling flowers." Murray pasted the newspaper cuttings into a scrapbook that survives to this day.

In the wider world just as much as in suffragette circles, the opening of Endell Street was regarded as the harbinger of a new wave of freedom and equal opportunity for women doctors and for women in general. Leading the way, Keogh urged, "The idea that the medical education of women is an experiment must pass away. It has proved its worth, and nobody can doubt that it has come to stay—and to stay for the public good."[63] Taking Keogh's advice to heart, hospitals were now falling over themselves to recruit female doctors to posts left vacant by men who had gone to the front. An article devoted to the contribution of women doctors to the war effort in *The Times History of the War*, published soon after Endell Street opened, not only applauded Murray and Anderson's work—and featured a photograph of Murray in uniform at her desk—but reported the first appointments of women doctors to jobs at Great Ormond Street Hospital for Children, the Chelsea Hospital for Women, and the Female Lock Hospital (for women with venereal disease)—albeit in junior posts.[64] Meanwhile, it said, people who had been forced to visit women doctors in private practice as a "war-sacrifice," since their usual doctors had gone to the front, had discovered "that skill had nothing to do with sex."

At the same time, medical schools attached to major hospitals opened their doors to women students for the first time. The *Girls' Own Paper* ran a feature extolling the virtues of a career in medicine for young women, with an illustration showing a hopeful candidate practicing first aid on her "docile small brother."[65] One "lady doctor" interviewed by the *Manchester Courier* expressed the hope that the war might remove the prejudice against women doctors.[66] She added, however, a warning note: "But are these women to be deprived of their posts when the men return from the front?" *The Hospital* magazine preferred to believe the doors that had opened would not close when the war ended. Even *The Lancet*, previously a lukewarm supporter of medical women, at best, welcomed the rush of women doctors supporting the war effort, predicting that after the war the scope of women's medical work would be "immensely widened."[67] Some newspapers went further and argued that the example of Endell Street would not only bring equality for women doctors but might even help win women the vote.

It was all very well to garner plaudits from the press for the novelty of "lady doctors" treating war heroes in a homey new hospital, seen through the rose-tinted lens of early war jingoism. But the women also had to deliver the best possible care for a relentless flood of seriously wounded soldiers in the face of continuing obstruction within the War Office and the hostility of much of the male medical profession. With a significantly bigger hospital than before, a much larger workforce whose members were mostly new and untrained, along with the bureaucracy of army regulations to negotiate, the early days were a make-or-break trial.

"The first month was a difficult one," Murray later admitted. "The work poured into the hospital, making new and heavy demands upon every one. Equipment was short, and the women had everything to learn and no one to advise or help them." Since many of the army officials designated to assist them were singularly unhelpful or positively obstructive, the women had to find out for themselves how the labyrinthine military system worked—and would later have to waste precious time correcting the registers and returns they had previously filled in. Only later did they realize that the War Office officials "did as little as possible" to help them, Murray wrote. "Having thus made it as difficult as possible," she remarked, "the authorities left the women to sink or swim." Winifred Buckley, one of the new assistant surgeons, said army officials deliberately avoided helping Endell Street for fear they would be held responsible for its demise, which they all considered inevitable, writing, "It was thought that the life of the hospital could not possibly be longer than 6 months." The male corporal in charge of the RAMC detachment at Endell Street later said he had been assured by his colleagues that the hospital would be a "failure and disaster."[68] Even Keogh would later admit that his colleagues subjected him to "great pressure" not to go ahead with the Endell Street experiment, since it would surely fail.[69]

But perhaps the most disturbing signal was picked up by Robins. As she made her rounds of the wards to deliver books in those first few weeks, she chatted with the men and wrote letters for them.

A familiar face from her days on the stage and still an attractive and vivacious woman, she was a popular visitor for the men. She became particularly friendly with one patient, Dawes, and fretted over another, a blind Canadian—possibly blinded by the gas attack at Ypres—whom she described as "pitiful."[70] In those early "unforgettable days," some of the patients took her into their confidence, and as a "lay-onlooker" she saw the "same little drama" enacted again and again. This drama differed rather from the scene Murray painted of cheerful men expressing unbounded confidence in their women doctors. Although none of the patients Robins spoke to asked to be transferred elsewhere, several confessed that they believed they had been sent to a women-run hospital primarily because the military authorities deemed them to be hopeless cases. "When us chaps found they'd sent us here, we thought we hadn't a dog's chance. We ain't worth botherin' about," said one, in a typical comment. They had been sent to Endell Street, they thought, to die.

If Endell Street failed, it would be a highly visible disaster—for women doctors and for the women's movement in general. The staff bore a "double responsibility," Beatrice Harraden said, as doctors who had to safeguard the welfare of the soldiers entrusted to their care and as women who wanted to vindicate the confidence that had been placed in their abilities.[71] Without a doubt Endell Street's opening marked a milestone in medical women's achievements. Anderson, Murray, and their staff had proved that women were capable of handling both the complexity and the horror of modern war surgery. Others, including Mabel St Clair Stobart in Antwerp and Cherbourg, and Elsie Inglis, who was leading the Scottish Women's Hospitals, were already following in their footsteps.[72] Yet Endell Street was, and would remain, the only military hospital under the auspices of the British Army to be staffed solely by women doctors and run entirely by women. It was a shining beacon of the potential of women and a tribute to suffragette ideals. Anderson would always insist that the success of the corps' work in Paris and Wimereux was due in large part to the impeccable organizational skills they had learned in the Women's Social and Political Union.[73]

But everyone knew there was a long way to go before Endell Street could be pronounced a success too.

MURRAY AND ANDERSON were well aware that the success of their project was imperative. But it was also an act of love. Proving they could run an efficient and professional military hospital together was the clearest demonstration of their mutual devotion. The coming months were going to prove tough, as the simmering tensions were about to bubble over.

The Laughing Cure Theory

Endell Street, London, June 24, 1915

Elizabeth Robins crossed the hospital courtyard and entered the recreation room ready for a busy day in the library.[1] In the six weeks since the hospital had opened she had established a routine, staying with friends in London from Monday to Friday when she helped at Endell Street, and resting in her Sussex home on the weekends with her faithful companion Octavia Wilberforce. Fortunately, she could draw on a long list of well-heeled friends with whom to stay. At present, she was lodging with Jean Hamilton, wife of Major General Sir Ian Hamilton, who was at this moment in command of the doomed attempt to wrest the Dardanelles from Turkish control. Jean had dropped Robins off at the Endell Street gates that morning.

Life in the library had also settled into a comfortable routine. As well as sourcing and sorting the books, Robins and Beatrice Harraden spent their time touring the wards with notebooks at the ready to ascertain the men's reading tastes. This was easier said than done. Some of the patients at Endell Street had no interest in reading, while others had never learned to read at all; some, too traumatized by their battle experiences, simply refused to look at a book. The "very idea was a sort of terror to them," Harraden later said.[2] But by first tempting the men with illustrated magazines or picture books, the two women gradually encouraged them to move on to popular novels, and some, occasionally inspired by films they had seen, even became absorbed in classics by Shakespeare or Dumas. Some men wanted books on hobbies they had enjoyed in their civilian days—one requested a book on horse-breaking and another on growing roses—while others consumed detective thrillers by the dozen. Most were no doubt eager for distraction from their memories of the trenches, although one man, at least, requested a book on high explosives. It was a hospital rule that any book requested on any subject in any language should be provided, and so the book was duly obtained.

Far and away the most favored author was Nat Gould, a former sports journalist who had turned his hand to writing adventure novels, mainly centered on horse racing, which he churned out at a rate of five a year. Whenever a parcel of Gould's books arrived on a ward they were seized on by the men and then passed from hand to hand in "a sacred, secret, underground way."[3] Harraden believed a Gould book was "as valuable as a pigeon's blood ruby"—one of the world's rarest gems—although both she and Robins were pleased to note that their own novels were in high demand as well. They never attempted to influence the patients to read "literary" books or educate their tastes, said Harraden, on the principle that "it's no good forcing caviar on people who are hankering for cockles."[4] As well as distributing favorite books, Robins and Harraden dispensed cigarettes and matches, wrote letters for the men to their families and sweethearts, and listened sympathetically to their tales of heroic acts and hellish ordeals. All in all, Robins felt, her unpaid shifts at Endell Street were both rewarding and appreciated.

But when she walked into the library on June 24, she found discord and turmoil. One of the library assistants, a medical student at LSMW, had quarreled with Flora Murray, Robins learned, and Murray now insisted she be dismissed.[5] It was not the first time arguments had erupted between these two. Robins had returned from a weekend break a few weeks earlier to discover that the student had lost her temper with Murray, and it was only when she was made to apologize that the air had cleared. Whatever the student had done to upset Murray would remain obscure. But as Robins gleaned in a hasty debriefing from Harraden and Bessie Hatton, a suffragette novelist and playwright who oversaw the hospital's recreation department, Murray was adamant she must go. Gamely, Robins volunteered to break the news. After dismissing the student later that day, she breathed a sigh of relief: she had resolved a difficult situation. In reality, the problems—in the library and on the wards—were just beginning.

Over the next few months, tensions would flare between Flora Murray and the librarians, the entertainment organizers, the ward visitors, and even the nurses—as Robins would faithfully record in her diary. Although Robins herself would always seem to float above these troubles, retreating to friends or to her Sussex home when it all got too much, she often bore the brunt of the complaints, especially from Hatton and Harraden. Indeed, soothing Harraden's anxieties would prove to be an almost daily labor.

An intelligent and scholarly woman who had gained a first in her arts degree from London University, Beatrice Harraden had published her first book, a children's story, in 1889.[6] Her first adult novel, *Ships That Pass in the Night*, published four years later, was an instant best seller, but since she had sold the copyright for a paltry sum, she had seen none of the profits. She would struggle financially for most of her life. A committed suffragette, she had had her belongings seized after refusing to pay income tax. Like Anderson, she had resigned from the WSPU over the autocratic conduct of the Pankhursts. Now fifty-one, Harraden was short and bespectacled, with cropped gray hair and a perpetual frown. She was a kindly and earnest person but highly strung, and she took her responsibilities— and her friendships—extremely seriously. One doctor at Endell Street described her as "very quiet and retiring, and intensely sensitive and sympathetic."[7] She often went to "endless trouble" to discover which reading material each man preferred and helped those whose reading had been neglected. A suffragette comrade said, "To know Miss Beatrice Harraden is to love her."[8] Robins's companion Octavia Wilberforce would take a rather more jaundiced view, later branding Harraden a "parchment faced serpent."[9] Wilberforce was patently spurred by jealousy—and with some reason, as Harraden, who never married, was plainly besotted with her blue-eyed, flame-haired colleague at Endell Street.

Just a few days before the debacle over the library assistant, Harraden herself had suddenly threatened to resign from Endell Street, under the conviction that Murray disliked her.[10] She felt "slighted," she told Robins, and convinced her work in the library was unwanted. Yet when Robins questioned Murray, Murray was surprised that Harraden had that impression, and immediately took pains to mollify her. Only a day after the library assistant had received her marching orders, however, Robins found Harraden "nervous & inclined to tears." A few days later Harraden was ruffled again—apparently over the lack of space and help allotted to the library—so that Robins had to troop into Murray's office once more and attempt to build bridges between the pair. Murray, said Robins, was "most forbearing," and even offered to give up her and Anderson's own sitting room to accommodate the library. The library remained in its small corner of the recreation room, but Murray assigned one of her orderlies, whom she could scarcely afford to spare, to help with the book rounds.

By July, Robins was growing understandably "weary of so much complaint" from Harraden. After a long talk together—one of many about the perceived difficulties—she concluded that her fellow writer was a "strange little being." Harraden's gripes and anxieties would continue—although she would remain the chief organizer of the Endell Street library, unpaid and often underregarded, throughout the hospital's lifetime. Harraden was evidently overly sensitive, and Murray perhaps not sufficiently appreciative of her efforts, but the novelist was not the only one to complain during the course of 1915 about the exacting Endell Street regime.

The nurses protested next. When she turned up at Endell Street on July 22, Robins was shocked to hear that nine nursing sisters—nearly a third of them—had risen in "revolt" the previous week. "They dislike Murray's manners & they love G. Anderson acc. to BH," she confided to her diary.[11] Murray had "treated them like dirt," she wrote, adding, "Great ructions but the nurses are ultimately smoothed more or less." Quite what had triggered the nurses' revolt and what form it took was left unsaid, although it is possible that Murray's tendency to take the sisters' work for granted while lauding the orderlies was related to the struggle.

A month later, as summer temperatures soared, tensions in the recreation department were rising. Robins had taken leave for the whole of August to stay with friends in Yorkshire, and Harraden and her new assistant complained of feeling exhausted from their long hours in the library. Harraden was desperate for a break so she could recuperate and get time to work on her latest novel, and her assistant, Di Forbes, was unwell and would not be able to "hold out much longer without a change."[12] Yet neither could take time off without someone to cover their work. "I have told Dr Murray many times that I am going away but even now the assistant is not to hand," Harraden lamented to Robins while gently inquiring when her friend was thinking of returning to London. "I've been so 'called upon' in many directions. . . . I need a spell of rest from ordinary life."

Meanwhile, Bessie Hatton felt equally worn out from organizing the relentless round of entertainments and activities demanded by Murray to maintain the men's morale—"Miss Hatton thinks too many," said Harraden. Hatton, a novelist and playwright who had cofounded the Women Writers' Suffrage League, was likewise unable to take leave until cover was found. Robins would eventually return to Endell Street in early September, but the tensions would continue.

IT MAY BE HARD to sympathize with the petty grumbles and perceived slights being raised by Robins and Harraden at a time when the doctors and other staff members were working tirelessly to save the lives of desperately injured men. Harraden and Robins were both plainly overanxious women with no prior experience of hospital or military life. But they were not alone in bridling at the authoritarian command at Endell Street. There's no doubt that Anderson, and especially Murray, were hard taskmasters and strict disciplinarians. They needed to be. Running a military hospital required military order. Like their male army colleagues, they had to command respect and maintain control among their nearly two hundred staff members—as well as more than five hundred patients—while ensuring that the complex hospital machinery ran as smoothly as possible. They set high standards both for their staff and for volunteers because they had to. For Murray and Anderson, as for other military surgeons, the first priority was patient care. Even Robins would later admit that Murray's unswerving demand for perfection stemmed from her determination to do her best for the patients, whether she was coercing a volunteer into lending a car for motor trips or begging a friend to promise a job to a "maimed man who wanted to die."[13] After years of demanding rights for women, it was men's needs that came first now—although she and Anderson never forgot what was at stake for women, too.

Murray and Anderson had to demonstrate that their hospital was at least as good as any run by their male counterparts. Indeed, Murray would always insist that the work of her staff should not just equal but exceed that expected of men. "We had this drilled into us," one orderly would say. "You not only have got to do a good job but you have got to do a superior job."[14] In order to prove that women could run a military hospital, Murray and Anderson had to act like men.

Not surprisingly, many at Endell Street regarded their two commanders with a mixture of wonder and terror. Winifred Buckley, the assistant surgeon, admired both women immensely and was said to "worship" one of them—though which of the two she worshiped was not disclosed.[15] Other staff members described being petrified when called to Murray's office for a reprimand over some small misdemeanor. Murray, in particular, could seem austere and imperious, but she bore chief responsibility as doctor in charge for ensuring the success of the hospital. As such, it fell to her to smooth out trivial difficulties (not least in the library) and she became the most visible wielder of staff discipline. Anderson, by contrast, spent much of her time ensconced in the operating theater, protected from minor irritations and army red tape. Whereas Murray had to maintain a constant aura of authority, Anderson was more likely to erupt in a fit of anger, and then regain her composure moments later. Anderson was "small, quick and energetic in her movements," with a "quick fussiness" over the right way to wheel a trolley, according to one Endell Street doctor; Murray was "tall, calm and unhurried," yet could issue a reprimand with a "quietly beckoning finger."[16] One of the orderlies said Murray's presence was so powerful that staff members were aware she was walking down a passage behind them before they saw her. "She cast a spell over all the hospital," the orderly said.[17] There were tensions and arguments at other war hospitals, too, of course, not least the Scottish Women's Hospitals unit at Royaumont Abbey near Paris, where one doctor resigned in 1915 in a row over surgical practices, and other staff complained of overwork.[18]

Nerves were on edge on the home front everywhere in 1915. The stresses and strains at Endell Street in its first months were emblematic of the deepening anxieties across the country as the war approached its first anniversary with no end in sight. What had seemed a just and honorable decision to go to war twelve months earlier, when victory was thought to be within easy reach, now felt like a mad and unstoppable descent into a bottomless abyss. The early rush to volunteer for active service in a tide of patriotism had given way to accusations of widespread incompetence and futile slaughter. As defeat followed defeat, Asquith's Liberal government had fallen, partly over revelations about a shortage of shells at the front, combined with accusations over the naval disaster in the Dardanelles; it was replaced by a national coalition government at the end of May. Although Winston Churchill, First Lord of the Admiralty, was one casualty in the political shakeup, for the moment Asquith clung to power. The continuing crisis in Gallipoli, where soldiers were now entrenched in stalemate just as solidly as those in France, had undermined confidence in British military strategy and leadership. Britain itself was even coming under enemy fire by naval bombardment, both on the east coast and from the air. And if people thought the Americans might rush to their aid by joining forces with the Allies, this hope was fading fast.

The national mood was graphically captured in a novel by H. G. Wells, *Mr. Britling Sees It Through*, set during the first eighteen months of the war. The semiautobiographical story begins when an American guest arrives for a weekend of innocent fun and frolics at the house of his friend, the author Mr. Britling, in the tranquil English countryside of July 1914. A year later, Britling's son has been killed in the trenches, his male secretary is missing, believed dead, and his American friend is consumed by guilt at his failure to play an active role in the conflict. The war, says Britling, no longer has the "simple greatness" that initially made sacrifice seem worthwhile. Ideas about fighting for freedom have been replaced by "dark questionings" about "carelessness and incapacity." Faced with the sight of so many women in mourning and the growing multitude of disabled men, the war has become "a monstrous absurdity."[19]

Something of this same desperation tinged the atmosphere at Endell Street. Those first few months, straddling the first anniversary of the war, were difficult days for the entire staff. Battling to come to grips with their new building, new regime, and new demands, as the casualties arrived in a relentless tide, it surely was a case of "sink or swim." As the bell announcing fresh convoys continued to toll night after night, the hospital's beds were increased to 573, and these were full most of the time. Brief lulls in the arrival of convoys were quickly followed by new rushes of work, when all the patients deemed fit enough to be transferred to convalescent beds elsewhere were hurriedly discharged to make way for new admissions. Anderson and her assistant surgeons were kept busy in the operating theater often for seven hours at a stretch.

As in France, the surgeons were tackling severe and complex injuries, including fractured spines, thighs, and arms; shattered knees and elbows; general wounds caused by gunshot or shrapnel; and nerve damage.[20] During 1915, head injuries were still numerous—before steel helmets were finally introduced—although many recovered well. One young soldier had been shot by a bullet that penetrated 1¼ inches into his brain, but four days after surgery he was sitting up in bed sewing. The flow of compound fractures, especially thighs, kept Olga Campbell's father, Arthur, busy crafting wooden limbs and surgical apparatus. The radiographer, Eva White, was fully occupied too, using her X-ray machine to locate bullets and shrapnel as well as imaging shattered bones and joints. One man's upper arm was found to be smashed into a hundred pieces, but by stabilizing the bone the fragments united. He left the hospital able to use his arm again—with an X-ray picture as a souvenir.

The X-ray machine was a popular novelty. The men referred to "going to the pictures" when they were sent for an X-ray, and the staff enjoyed posing for photographs on the X-ray table. Although the scale and nature of the men's injuries were often horrific, not just for the patients, but for staff, too, the range of experience staff gained was invaluable. As Murray put it, from a professional point of view the work was "excellent" and gave women "an exceptional opportunity in the field of surgery." In addition to the surgical wards under Anderson's command, there were two wards containing sixty beds for less "military" medical cases—including appendicitis, pneumonia, and other diseases—overseen by Murray and Louisa Woodcock. The hospital ran a busy casualty room, too, where soldiers who fell sick or were injured in accidents while on leave were brought in day and night. The demands were seemingly endless.

As chief surgeon, Anderson was determined to use the experience to the fullest extent, but she also made a point of introducing her own distinctive and pioneering approach both in terms of bedside manner and fostering teamwork.[21] Every morning she met with her assistant surgeons, the physicians, and the pathologist to discuss the cases admitted overnight as well as any patients of particular concern. These early morning conferences were highly unusual for the time and presaged modern surgical team management. The surgeons spent the rest of the morning on ward rounds assessing patients' progress and their afternoons in theater. Then every evening, from 5:00 to 7:00 p.m., Anderson visited the wards herself to consult with the patients with the most serious injuries and discuss her proposed approach. She would encourage the men to talk about their experiences before explaining their options and offering her professional opinion, presented as advice about the best way forward. "She never hurried a man in his decision, unless it were urgent," said Murray. Anderson's gentle and empathetic manner echoed the emphasis on listening to patients that she had observed under William Osler in Baltimore, although it may well have also stemmed from her training at the LSMW. But it was certainly an unfamiliar approach in Britain, where the "doctor knows best" attitude would prevail for decades to come.

Most of the men unloaded from the ambulances in the Endell Street courtyard were ordinary British soldiers—privates rather than officers—who had been injured or who had fallen sick in the continuing devastation on the Western Front. Wounded officers were generally treated in smaller and significantly more comfortable hospitals converted from luxury hotels and private mansions, where they could choose meals and wine from gourmet menus.[22] Since the bulk of the original British Expeditionary Force, the professional standing army, had been annihilated by the end of 1914, most of the men were recent volunteers. They had been recruited in the rush to enlist during the autumn and winter and then trained in British camps before being packed off to France in early 1915.

One soldier arrived at Endell Street blind, deaf, and mute after being wounded in the Battle of Hill 60, part of the Second Battle of Ypres during April and May. Although he soon recovered his sight and hearing, he remained unable to utter a word, despite the efforts of his fellow patients to rouse him. On one occasion they splashed water on his face; on another—rather rashly—they pulled his chair out from under him. But laughter, rather than frights, proved to be the best medicine. Taken on an outing to a local theater in July, he burst out laughing at one of the comedy acts and then issued a "torrent of fluent speech."[23] The story, which made a welcome change from the daily casualty lists, raced around the world, even making headlines in the *New Zealand Herald*. There was a smattering of officers, too, at the hospital. Flora Murray made a rare appearance in the library at one point, seeking some books on Admiral Horatio Nelson for a young officer; she evidently felt he needed uplifting by a heroic example.[24]

Though mostly working class, the soldiers filling the beds came from every walk of life and every corner of Britain. In their former lives they had worked as miners, dockworkers, carpenters, actors, salesmen, and factory workers. Regional newspapers were peppered with mentions of local sons who lay wounded or had died in Endell Street. One man, Private William Glen, had worked for a boiler-maker near Glasgow before signing up in September 1914. He died of his wounds at Endell Street in June, aged thirty-three, leaving a widow and five children. Another, John Noel Pinnington, who came from the Scottish borders, was one of three brothers who had been wounded and sent to different hospitals at the same time. Admitted to Endell Street in July, he recovered only to die on the Western Front two years later. One young lad, Thomas Miller, an apprentice boilermaker from Sunderland who had signed up as a private despite being underage, died at the hospital in June after being wounded near Ypres, aged eighteen.[25]

By mid-August the hospital was full to bursting. According to Harraden, the workload had never been so heavy. A week later, however, it was ominously "very slack," with only 250 patients, and most of these convalescent.[26] There was a reason half the beds at Endell Street had been hurriedly emptied. At dawn one morning at the end of August, the first convoys of wounded Australian and New Zealand troops began to pour in from Gallipoli.[27]

AFTER INVASION FORCES had first landed on the Gallipoli peninsula in April, the Allied troops—including soldiers from Australia, New Zealand, and India—had endured some of the worst conditions of the war. Under constant bombardment and repeated charges from the Turkish forces, the men were battling for survival on narrow strips of land in searing heat. Food and water were scarce, while parasites feasted on the corpses and spread lethal diseases. "Anything you opened, like a tin of bully [corned beef], would be swarming with flies," said one soldier. "They were all around your mouth and on any cuts or sores that you'd got, which then turned septic."[28] With no fresh water on the peninsula, dysentery was rife. Half of the men who fell ill, as opposed to being wounded, were brought down by dysentery. Under such conditions medical personnel onsite struggled in vain to maintain the men's health and provide adequate sanitation. One soldier who was laid low by dysentery fell into a latrine and drowned in his own excrement. Evacuating the sick and wounded proved to be a formidable challenge. The number of casualties far exceeded expectations so that there was a shortage of stretchers and evacuation vessels; the small boats used to ferry the wounded to outlying hospital ships came under constant fire. A final desperate attempt to seize victory in August with renewed assaults at Cape Helles and what had become known as Anzac Cove, along with a new landing at Suvla Bay, went predictably awry.

The Gallipoli campaign, which would limp on until troops were finally evacuated in January 1916, ultimately cost more than thirty thousand Allied lives, with seventy-six thousand wounded. Among the casualties was Henry Nevinson, Anderson's journalist friend, who had gone to the Dardanelles as a war correspondent for the *Manchester Guardian*. He was hit in the head at Suvla Bay, but his pith helmet saved him.[29] Two of Olga Campbell's brothers, Keir and Bruce, were likewise wounded during the Suvla Bay assault.[30] Both recovered to fight again, but others were not so lucky. Sir John Milbanke, a cousin of Octavia Wilberforce, was killed at Suvla. Evacuated first to Egypt and from there to Britain, the casualties arrived in London at the end of August, and before long they occupied two hundred beds at Endell Street.

Ordinarily strong and healthy by comparison with the British men, the Australians and New Zealanders arrived at Endell Street wasted by disease and weakened by poor nutrition. They looked "gaunt and grey" from their ordeal, said Murray.[31] Many had lost forty pounds or more during their months of deprivation, and they lay "silent and apathetic" in their beds. The few who were capable of walking wandered off to investigate their surroundings "like grey ghosts in the dim morning light." Those who were sick, rather than wounded, were isolated in special wards to reduce the spread of infection. The pathologist, Helen Chambers, worked overtime investigating foreign parasites and unfamiliar diseases. Before long she had identified a number of parasites and other organisms, which she exhibited on slides for staff to see with accompanying lectures. There was little that Chambers could do without antibiotics or other medicines to combat the microbes, but with bed rest and good food, most of the men soon began to regain weight and recover their spirits.

When Elizabeth Robins finally returned to Endell Street at the beginning of September after her month-long break, she found the beds were filled with Australians and New Zealanders. As she made her ward rounds distributing Australian newspapers and taking requests for books—the Australians were eager for bushranger stories to remind them of home—she quizzed the men for news of Ian Hamilton. After two days back she grumbled that her sense of well-being had faded and she felt "tired as of old."[32] Taking tea with Murray and Anderson she found them, not surprisingly, stiff and on edge. They gave little encouragement to Robins's latest hobby horse, her mission to persuade the army to send women to the front as stretcher-bearers.

Robins had published an article making her argument in the *Daily Mail* in August, and had even secured an interview with Keogh to push her case. Murray and Anderson, however, said they had come to sympathize with the War Office view that untrained women would be a hindrance in active service. They staunchly believed women could do the same jobs as men, but only if they received adequate training.

News of the latest patients in Endell Street, and the unique hospital in which they were being cared for, filtered across the globe. Newspapers in New Zealand and Australia began publishing details of men being treated in the women-only hospital as early as September. Fascinated by the novelty of women doctors, the *Sydney Daily Telegraph* reprinted a jaunty letter from one patient to his father in Randwick, a suburb of Sydney. "The only men in the hospital are the patients, two or three orderlies from the Royal Army Medical Corps, and the big policeman at the gate," he wrote. Certain that on the basis of his experience nobody after the war could begrudge women the vote, the soldier declared, "The whole hospital is a triumph for women, and incidentally it is a triumph for suffragettes." It is hard to resist the suspicion that Robins or Harraden had dictated his letter for him. The news cutting found its way back to Britain and was duly pasted into Murray's scrapbook.

Once they began to recover, the ANZAC troops appeared to be both better educated and more enlightened than their British counterparts, at least according to Murray. Since women in Australia and New Zealand had enjoyed the vote for several years, the men could not understand why it was denied to women in Britain. Indeed, the New Zealanders would become so converted to the idea of women doctors that when their commission ordered at the end of 1915 that all New Zealand patients be transferred to a single designated hospital, they begged to be allowed to remain in Endell Street.[33] The Australian troops were also known for their independent minds and reluctance to kowtow to authority. Initially, the Endell Street staff were puzzled by the frequent visits from anxious-looking officers from ANZAC headquarters, until they were told that the Australian men had a reputation for being "very wild" and had caused outbreaks of rebellion in other military hospitals. There were no such problems in Endell Street, however, despite predictions.

War Office skeptics had forecast that the women at Endell Street would be beset by difficulties keeping control of their male patients. But with her military-style uniform, her quietly authoritarian manner, and the confidence gained from her privileged background, Murray held sway over her patients just as she did over her staff with seemingly little effort. Although army rules were strictly enforced, so that patients were not allowed out unaccompanied, at least during the first two years of the war, Murray rarely had to issue a reprimand. On those few occasions when a patient stepped out of line, she would ask the RAMC sergeant major to leave her alone with the offender and then appeal to his better nature. Almost invariably, the man was reduced to tears. One fellow, thus chastised, returned to his bed and pulled his blanket over his head. When he was finally persuaded to reemerge, he told his comrades: "I've been up before men and up before women . . . and God save us from the women!"[34] The fact that Murray and Anderson were old enough to be the mothers of many of these young men no doubt helped. The *Tatler* magazine declared there was "not a better disciplined place in the three kingdoms," and attributed the secret to the women's gentle guiding approach. Like good horsewomen, the hospital's commanders had the "gift of 'hands,'" it argued, on the basis that "if you can't control him with a strong pull, try a weak one." One newspaper remarked that Endell Street "knows no vexatious rules" and added, "Patients, placed on their honour, render willing obedience to ministering angels, who anticipate their every want."[35]

Hard on the heels of the Gallipoli fiasco came news of the Battle of Loos on the Western Front when British forces, in their biggest push of the war so far, used gas for the first time as they attempted to storm German defenses on September 25. Early reports were triumphal—Elizabeth Robins hailed the "victory" in her diary—but the celebrations were premature.[36] Although the British captured Loos, they could not breach the Germans' second trench system and the casualties reached more than fifty thousand. The wounded began arriving at Endell Street within days, the taint of chlorine gas still clinging to their uniforms. Visiting her wards, Robins talked to the men about their experiences of the "great battle." One young Scotsman wept as he described the devastation. It was all "thrilling—terrible," said Robins.

On top of the anguish generated by the latest battle disasters, German airships were now raining down destruction on British civilians. The first Zeppelin had appeared over London at the end of May. Awed by the spectacle of the airship lumbering in the night sky, Londoners rushed into the streets to watch rather than take cover. One observer hung out of his bedroom window, the better to see "the wicked Zeppelin in the sky, like a long grey lighted train."[37] Another was transfixed by the sight of an airship "floating like a huge silvery electric blue cigar." The first to reach London dropped eighty-nine bombs and thirty grenades on the East End and northeastern suburbs, killing seven people. Four more air raids followed over the course of 1915, each one more destructive than the last. In the fourth raid, on the night of September 8–9, a single Zeppelin dropped several bombs on Bloomsbury, only a few streets north of Endell Street, before heading toward "the City," the capital's central business district and historical core. Hundreds of windows were smashed in nearby St Bartholomew's Hospital, and an omnibus was blown to pieces near Liverpool Street Station, killing nine passengers outright and fatally injuring its driver. Robins, staying with a friend in Chelsea that night, heard a "great rushing sound" outside and then "Bang. Bang!" Having sent the servants to take cover below, she and her friend ran to open an attic window and watched, entranced, as the "oblong grey cloud" hovered backward and forward, emitting a "large bright star falling to darkness" as it released its deadly load. There were no air raid warnings—for fear of unduly alarming people—and virtually no aerial defenses. The handful of antiaircraft guns firing shrapnel caused more damage on the ground than in the air.

The fifth attack, on October 13–14, brought the trail of destruction almost to Endell Street's doorstep. That night, three Zeppelins spread terror across the defenseless city. One of the airships cruised lazily over the Strand before releasing bombs into the heart of Theatreland. Watching as it moved toward Covent Garden, dropping incendiary bombs as it went, one Londoner said, "It was beautiful, but awful too." One of the biggest bombs fell on Wellington Street, a few hundred yards from the hospital gates, fracturing a gas main and killing seventeen people, who had been buying refreshments from street vendors during a theater intermission. A total of 71 people were killed and 128 injured. Since details of the Zeppelins' damage were censored from the newspapers, the women at Endell Street swapped gossip. The Zeppelins would not return until 1916, by which time they would be even bigger and more destructive.

AGAINST THIS BACKGROUND, Anderson and Murray attempted to keep spirits up with a relentless succession of entertainments and diversions. Their approach to maintaining order was always a case of carrot as much as stick. Indeed, it seemed that the more the war misery increased during 1915, the more the two COs demanded a dizzying round of recreations to compensate. Although other war hospitals also endeavored to keep their patients occupied and entertained as part of a nurturing approach, Endell Street excelled in this respect. It was Anderson's philosophy that "the men can never suffer from too much amusement."[38] Bessie Hatton was worn to a frazzle, arranging two or three events every week. The pace amounted to more than a thousand artistes visiting each year, as well as a variety of daily occupations to keep the men busy.

Under this tireless schedule, the men were regaled by variety shows on the wards, theatrical dramas on the hospital stage, and concert parties in the courtyard. Murray and Anderson drew on all their connections to bring in fresh distractions, while Hatton recruited her friends in the theater world to form an entertainment committee dedicated to ensuring that whatever the war unleashed, the show must go on. Musician friends joined forces with musically talented staff members to create the "Endell Street Orchestra." This ensemble played regular concerts in the courtyard where they could be heard by all: patients who could limp there on crutches, those who could be wheeled there in their beds or invalid chairs, and those confined to the wards, who listened through the open windows. Patients were encouraged to invite their friends and families to join the fun, and on summer afternoons and bank holidays the square was packed to capacity. With red and blue sunshades positioned over patients' beds, fruit and ices on sale in the canteen, and children skipping around the flower tubs, the scene took on the air of a seaside pier.

The undisputed stars of the hospital stage were the "Endell Street Follies," a troupe of female actors, singers, and dancers who performed uplifting variety shows. Bandaged men in their beds, in wheelchairs, and on crutches were helped or carried down in the lifts to enjoy the shows in the packed hall. Festooned in colorful and exotic costumes, the performers played music hall hits, cracked topical jokes, and played the piano or violin while encouraging the audience to join in with rousing choruses. The Follies soon gained a reputation beyond Endell Street. Newspapers described them as the "most welcome prescription in the hospital" and "a fine vindication of the laughing cure theory."[39]

There was no escape from the fun and frolics. In between this endless program of entertainments, there were visits to the wards from other assorted performers, including a conjuror, a fortune teller, and a boxer.[40] Another visitor, who arrived unannounced one day in the autumn of 1915, was a lone Scottish pipe-major in his kilt and full regalia, who marched into the hospital courtyard and began to play his bagpipes. The visit had been arranged as a surprise for the men from Highland regiments. When they heard the strains of their regimental tunes, the men crept from their beds and crowded at the windows like "children enchanted by the Pied Piper." Some of them, said one of the doctors, had not left their beds until that moment.[41]

In the gaps between the visiting entertainers the men were treated to outings. Wearing their distinctive "hospital blue" flannelette suits and red ties, which marked them as wounded heroes rather than shirking civilians, the men were taken to the theater, on boating excursions along the Thames, and to watch cricket at Lords. Society hostesses invited the patients to their grand London townhouses for afternoon tea. The Endell Street Tommies were always popular with the moneyed and titled guests, who enjoyed grilling them on their frontline ordeals.

Those men who were too ill—or too despondent—to be enticed out of the hospital were visited in their sickbeds by a seemingly endless tide of well-wishers, although Murray imposed strict visiting hours. These rules did little to deter the stream of celebrities, politicians, relatives, and acquaintances who arrived at the gates at all hours, eager to do their bit for the war effort by comforting a wounded soldier or, sometimes, to edge a little closer to the thrill of war. Even if some of the visitors were a little ghoulish, most were clearly appreciated by the men; some of them would keep in touch for years after the war.

Among the visitors who were never turned away were the royal family. George V and Queen Mary toured Endell Street at least once—in February 1916—and Queen Alexandra, the king's mother, was a regular visitor to the wards, often bringing gifts for the men.[42] Patients would treasure the engraved walking sticks and embroidered handkerchiefs she dispensed for years to come.

One visitor was treated with even more deference than the king and queen—at least by Flora Murray. Emmeline Pankhurst—suffragette royalty—came in November, and Murray personally escorted her around the hospital.[43] Now working closely with David

Lloyd George, the newly appointed minister of munitions, Pankhurst had organized a women's march in July for the right to work, countering opposition from trade unions against women taking men's jobs.

When not being entertained by rousing wartime songs, knockabout comedy, or visiting celebrities, the men were encouraged to keep their hands and minds busy with diverting hobbies. As well as being plied with books and magazines by Harraden and Robins, they were taught knitting, basket-weaving, and needlework by volunteers led by Anderson's sister-in-law, Ivy. Many produced excellent work, including some seven thousand embroidered regimental badges, as well as soft toys, tea cozies, and framed pictures depicting idyllic English gardens and country scenes, which were sold at annual sales to raise funds. Some became so absorbed in their work that they picked up their sewing frames as soon as daylight dawned and only laid them down when darkness fell. One patient, a coalminer in civilian life, stitched a picture depicting a basket of fruit; another skilled needleworker was a former butcher. A few of the works still survive. One soldier made a cloth bag embroidered with a picture of a doctor—probably Anderson—in the distinctive Endell Street uniform, with her cap pushed back to reveal a glimpse of coppery hair; the figure is walking two dogs resembling Garrett and William.[44] Another, a former nightwatchman named Walter Elmy, who had enlisted as a gunner, stitched a romantic picture of a dovecote in pastel shades—with only one arm. His left arm had been amputated after a gunshot wound. The sight of burly butchers and miners working at their stitching frames with all the dexterity of Jane Austen characters naturally caught the attention of the newspapers. One reported how proud the women felt of "their soldier needle-workers." Delighted by this graphic example of gender reversal, Murray said, "We have proved that men, too, can sit at home and sew."

IF THE MEN stayed cheerful despite the desperate times, some of the staff felt closer to tears as 1915 drew to an end. In a determined effort to banish all thoughts of war during the holiday season, staff, volunteers, and patients alike were recruited to transform Endell Street into a merry winter wonderland and play their parts in a flurry of celebrations. The men were pressed into action making decorations to adorn their wards. Competing for a prize for the best-dressed ward, they entwined holly around bed frames, suspended Chinese lanterns from the ceilings, and crafted their own displays from scraps.[45]

Bessie Hatton and her recreation department worked day and night planning a glut of festive entertainments. The twin highlights of this program were a pantomime based—loosely—on Aladdin and a "Pageant of Saints" that paraded through all seventeen wards. Hatton cajoled leading actors to take part, while Harraden and Robins devised the pageant procession, which entailed volunteers dressing up as the saints whose names were represented in the hospital wards.[46]

As the pre-Christmas panic intensified, so the strains among staff increased. When Murray paid a rare visit to the library, Harraden challenged her, saying, "I believe you think we do nothing."[47] Hatton, meanwhile, was convinced that Murray was taking "no interest" in the theatrical preparations, so that participants felt "hurt & disheartened." No doubt Murray had rather more important matters to contend with than soothing disgruntled volunteers. Despite Murray's lack, or perceived lack, of attention, both the pantomime and the pageant proved to be resounding triumphs that garnered glowing press reviews. *The Queen*, a high-society magazine, declared that out of all the Christmas entertainments staged in hospitals across London, the Endell Street pageant took the "palm."[48]

The pantomime, two days later, won even more plaudits. As a bevy of stars from the London stage assumed the roles of Aladdin, Widow Twankey, and the Magician, the men in the audience were transported to a fanciful land of the Arabian Nights with a curious Endell Street twist. One scene involved a line of orderlies being drilled by their special constable in front of the hospital gates; another featured Murray and Anderson, skillfully taken off by actresses, performing an operation to install a heart in the previously heartless Magician. The men loved it, applauding the Endell Street references and joining in the songs. *The Times* pronounced the event a "great success."[49]

Behind the scenes, however, the bubbling cauldron of discontent had reached a boiling point. Relating details of the pageant's success to Robins, who was recuperating from a cold at home, Harraden was beside herself. Harraden, convinced that the orderlies were still enjoying preferential treatment, accused Murray of upsetting the volunteers, the recreation department, and the nurses. "Anything like Dr M's attitude towards the Recreation Department I've never seen," she complained to Robins. "She and the others are mad on the subject of the orderlies—it seems a positive obsession." Murray, she said, regarded Hatton and the entertainment committee as "mere serfs & slaves," and the nursing sisters were upset because instructions for the pageant day had been given to the orderlies rather than to them. Harraden was peeved, too, at the pecking order devised for members of staff to meet the royal family—Queen Alexandra and her daughters, the Princess Royal and Princess Victoria, and granddaughter Princess Maud—who were guests of honor at the pageant. "The orderlies were all marshalled up to greet the Royalties with the Drs, the Matron following like a meek rabbit & the Sisters non-existent," she said.[50] Imploring her friend Robins to return soon, Harraden was eager for an urgent conference.

Robins had heard enough. Complaining of lumbago, a rotten tooth, and general exhaustion, she resigned from the library post and promptly took up an invitation to visit her brother in Florida. Harraden was devastated. The news came as a "bomb," she told Robins—not a word to use lightly in the circumstances—and she coolly declined meeting with Robins before she left, saying the decision had "left me sort of stranded."[51] After shopping for clothes for her trip, Robins called at Endell Street to say goodbye to Anderson, who stressed how upset Harraden was at her departure. "It is evident I'm a monster for being ill," Robins raged in her diary. "I resign—very thankfully. It's too much."

Although Robins's abrupt exit did little to reduce the friction in the entertainment department, it perhaps had some surprising influence overseas. When she sailed for New York a few weeks later on the SS *Rotterdam*, she bumped into Edward House, President Woodrow Wilson's closest friend and confidant, who was returning to America to advise Wilson on the United States' policy toward the war.[52] Wilson had been reelected on a platform of maintaining American neutrality, but House—nicknamed "Colonel" House, although he had no military rank—wanted to support Britain and France by mediating a peace treaty with Germany. Becoming friendly with House and his wife during the ten-day voyage, Robins made a passionate appeal to the Colonel to push the case for America to enter the war behind the Allies. She used her experience at Endell Street to bolster her argument.

At Endell Street, said Robins, she had witnessed the voluntary contribution and cooperative spirit of both the women staff and the fighting men. She believed that spirit was typical of the English—she meant British—war effort. She told House: "If I had never known any English but those I had known in the Endell Street Military Hospital, I should know where my sympathies in the war must be." Evidently moved by her words, House urged her to write about her views—as she subsequently did in a piece for the *New York Times*, published a few weeks later. In her article Robins recounted the transformation she had seen in England since the start of the war. Men and women had put aside their own needs to join the army and help on the home front in a "spirit of voluntary co-operation" that had produced a "civilising effect" on the entire country. She was convinced that Britain would not accept a peace deal that failed to guarantee freedom for its allies, and she called on her compatriots not to let England "bleed to death" for its beliefs. There is no evidence that Robins's arguments changed House's views, but it is tempting to think that the values demonstrated at Endell Street had a small impact in eventually persuading America to enter the war.

FOR ALL THE gripes and grumbles, it was clear as 1915 turned into 1916 that the women at Endell Street had defeated the cynics in the War Office. They had not only survived for more than six months, but had proved publicly and defiantly that women were just as capable of running a military hospital as their male counterparts. As matron Grace Hale put it, faced with the struggle to sink or swim, "the Corps swam and is still swimming." But the trials were far from over.

6

Almost Manless

Endell Street, London, February 1916

Nina Last was shown to her dormitory in the staff quarters known as "the Barracks." A dismal room with eight narrow beds and one tiny window, it was filled with the stench of the postmortem room below, as well as an incinerator nearby where amputated limbs were burnt.[1] With typical wartime irony, the room was nicknamed "The Murray." Ever since she had heard about the plans to open Endell Street Military Hospital, twenty-year-old Last had been determined to work there. Her younger sister, Barbara, who was eighteen, had already been recruited straight from school as a nursing orderly. The fact that Last invariably fainted at the sight of blood had done nothing to deter her from applying, and neither had her sister's reports that the work was "pretty grim." Yet as she now surveyed her spartan living quarters, permeated with the smell of death and decay, her nerve nearly failed.

Brought up in Buckinghamshire, the daughter of a vicar and eldest of four children, Last had enjoyed a comfortable middle-class childhood. Along with her sister and two younger brothers, she had been looked after by a nanny and then taught at home by governesses. To round off her education—and perhaps to rein her in—at sixteen she had been sent to a finishing school for five terms. Sporty and headstrong, Last had a keen sense of adventure and was popular with the young men she met, while her sister was more reserved. Last had been at a tennis party in August 1914 when news came through that war had been declared. She would never see the young men from that party again: all of them—she would later say—were killed in the early years of the war.

As her male friends rushed to enlist, Last had been determined to play her part in the war effort too. As soon as she was old enough, in early 1915, she had enrolled as a VAD, or member of a Voluntary Aid Detachment, working as an assistant cook at a country mansion in Hertfordshire, where a wing had been converted into a hospital for forty convalescent soldiers. The move was prompted by necessity as much as anything else. Her parents' investments had declined in value during the war, so she needed to pay her own way. When Barbara was accepted as a nursing orderly at Endell Street soon after it opened, Nina had fixed her sights on following her there. Yet while Barbara was "a born nurse," Nina would freely admit she had neither talent nor desire for nursing. She had applied, while working her twelve-month stint as a VAD, with the hope of obtaining a clerical job.

When a vacancy finally arose, Nina Last had rushed excitedly to London. The contrast, after the tranquillity of the Buckinghamshire countryside, was stark. After eighteen months of war, the capital's streets were thronged with soldiers, and every available building had been converted to military purposes. Even the lake in St James's Park had been drained to provide land for temporary War Office buildings. London, according to one observer, was "contracting to a War Camp."[2] Finding her way to Endell Street, Nina had entered the black iron gates with misgivings.

The job interview had proved an "alarming" experience, since the two commanding officers—Anderson and Murray—struck Last with terror. "Dr Murray was a dour Scot," she later recalled, and Dr Anderson "severe." She was impressed, however, by the fact that both women had been active suffragettes; although she had been too young to take part in the suffrage protests herself, Last had admired the marching, chanting women from afar. Noting their pale, thin faces, no doubt made all the more gaunt by the strain of running Endell Street, she was convinced the two women bore the marks of hunger strikes. Despite her anxieties, Last had made it through the interview and been accepted for a month's trial as an orderly.

Now, as she unpacked her belongings on her bed, the one farthest from the window, she knew she faced "a severe test" if she stayed at Endell Street; but at least she was now "really in the thick of things." She took possession of her uniform and would look after it with pride. A photograph taken soon afterward shows her looking thoughtful but resolute in her buttoned-up jacket and bonnet cap with its long gauze veil. As she had suspected, the next few weeks were going to be a tough test indeed.

NINA LAST WAS one of more than 120,000 volunteers—most of them women—who worked in hospitals and convalescent homes in Britain and overseas during the First World War. The vast majority were members of the VAD scheme. Although the women appointed to nurse, clean, cook, carry stretchers, and run the offices at Endell Street were recruited directly by Murray and Anderson, many arrived there after serving as VADs. There, they were employed on much the same principles to do much the same work. They also brought many of the same problems.

Founded in 1909, the VAD scheme had originally been set up to train men and women in first aid and other skills in order to supplement army medical services on the home front in readiness for war. By 1914, there were roughly eighty thousand members of Voluntary Aid Detachments up and down the country, overseen by the British Red Cross Society and the St John Ambulance brigade.[3] Roughly two-thirds of them were women, and most—though not all—came from middle- or upper-class backgrounds with little or no experience of physical labor or military discipline. While some earned certificates in first aid, hygiene, and cooking, and a few were qualified nurses, most had limited or no medical knowhow. What they lacked in practical abilities, though, they often made up for in gusto. One VAD, Katharine Furse, entered her women's unit in a stretcher-bearing competition run by the War Office only for her team to drop both stretcher and patient, bringing disgrace on the entire detachment.[4]

When war broke out, thousands of VAD members deluged the War Office with appeals to help at the front, while thousands more applied to join VAD units at home. At first, Lord Esher, who had been instrumental in forming the scheme, was said to have wished he had never bothered, since its members were "so tiresome in their clamouring."[5] Despite her stretcher-carrying disaster, however, Katharine Furse was grudgingly permitted to take twenty women VADs to Boulogne—the first VADs to go overseas—in October 1914. Like Murray and Anderson, she found the army's medical chiefs both hostile and bewildered. "They could not make us out—women were such a nuisance in war time," she said. Undaunted, Furse and her team set up a "rest station" in some disused railway carriages, brightened up with tubs of sweet peas and nasturtiums, and provided hot drinks and first aid to thirty thousand wounded men as they arrived on ambulance trains over the next five weeks.

Now that these pioneer VADs had proved their worth, it was the War Office that was clamoring for their help. From February 1915 the War Office appealed for VADs to work as assistants under trained nurses in the extensive network of military hospitals being set up at home and overseas. Hurriedly trained in basic nursing skills, this army of VADs, most of them women, were paid £20 a year plus board and lodging to provide the bulk of hospital care for Britain's wounded men. That autumn the scheme was expanded, and VADs were recruited to take over jobs as clerks, cooks, cleaners, and pharmacy dispensers to free up men to serve. This unprecedented invasion of well-intentioned volunteers descending on the nation's hospitals brought inevitable problems. Titled ladies of leisure in jewels and furs flocked to VAD headquarters in London, now ably run by Furse, demanding to do their bit. Many were society figures, daughters of peers and politicians, who worked an hour or two in a hospital between social engagements. Some sent their unflattering blue uniforms to be retailored by their favorite couturiers, while others wore pearl necklaces under their shirt collars.[6] Their arrival created widespread friction among the professional nurses.

Qualified nursing sisters, who had learned their clinical skills and codes of practice during three years of training on hospital wards, were understandably concerned that these partially trained women would be wholly unsuitable, and unsuited to nursing desperately sick men. Many worried that these "ignorant amateurs"— who were generally addressed as "nurse" or even "sister" by doctors and patients alike—would seriously dilute professional standards. Worse, since nurses, unlike doctors, had no system of registration, they feared that VADs might muscle in on the profession after the war—rather as male doctors suspected their female counterparts might do.[7] Leading the backlash, the *British Journal of Nursing* complained that the sight of Red Cross nurses in hospitals in France wearing white silk stockings and high-heeled shoes "shocks one's sense of propriety."[8] But the VADs did not always help matters themselves.

Many VADs plainly resented being ordered to perform menial tasks by professional nurses, whom they regarded as their social inferiors because they had to work for a living. Some evidently saw themselves as serving out of some higher ideal of patriotism and self-sacrifice simply because they were volunteers. Some even pointed out that while professional nurses were paid a proper wage to do their jobs, it was the nursing assistants who carried out most of the work in military hospitals. Murray patently shared this view, as did Furse. A popular ditty making the rounds of military hospitals—a variation on a familiar army song—quipped, "The V.A.D.s do all the work; The Sisters get the money!" Furse agreed that although it was a "nonsense verse," there was "a glimmer of truth in it."[9] In one sense it was inarguable: by their sheer weight of numbers, the VADs did provide the bulk of the labor, and for little reward.

Other volunteers—notably the writer Vera Brittain—would characterize the sisters and matrons they worked for as callous and bullying harridans, toward both the VADs and the patients, while depicting themselves as almost saintly.[10] Brittain, who started work as a VAD at a London war hospital in October 1915, saw herself as tackling the work with a "sacred glamour," while she believed the professional nurses were "indifferent to pain." She told her fiancé, who was fighting on the Western Front, "There is something so starved and dry about hospital nurses—as if they had to force all the warmth out of themselves before they could be really good nurses."[11]

The Last sisters were typical of the orderlies recruited to work at Endell Street, and their experiences mirrored those of VADs in military hospitals elsewhere. Like Nina, many Endell Street orderlies had already served as VADs in other hospitals. Regardless of their experience or background, all were meticulously grilled at interviews by Murray and Anderson, who were looking for those particular qualities of intelligence, determination, and good humor that they believed made up the essential ingredients of the Endell Street "spirit." In common with the VAD scheme, Endell Street had its share of moneyed and privileged women who were dropped at the gates each morning in their chauffeured cars before they donned their overalls to scrub floors, empty bedpans, and push trolleys. And while many, like the Last sisters, hailed from the prosperous Home Counties—the shires surrounding London—others came from far-flung corners of the British Isles and beyond.

Women converged from as far afield as Canada, Australia, and South Africa to serve as orderlies at Endell Street. One of them, Frances Lyndall Schreiner, known as Dot, was born in Cape Town, the daughter of a former prime minister of the colony.[12] It was a liberal and enlightened family. Her father had campaigned for the franchise for all Africans regardless of race, while her aunt, Olive Schreiner, was an author and social reformer. Olive Schreiner's book *Women and Labour*, in which she demanded equal working rights for women, was hugely influential in Britain and America. Dot had graduated from Newnham College, Cambridge, in 1910 before returning to South Africa, where she had qualified as a lawyer, but she was prevented from working because women were not admitted to the bar. When the family moved to London for the duration of the war, she worked as a VAD in military hospitals in Britain and

France before joining Endell Street. She would later publish a book of short stories, *Hospital Sketches*, inspired by her experiences.

Whether they had previously served as VADs or not, all the staff wore the pale brown Endell Street uniform rather than the shapeless long blue dresses worn by VADs. And whether they were used to sleeping in silk sheets with a fleet of servants at their command or otherwise, they all now lived together in cold, cramped rooms in the hospital barracks, where they rose at dawn to start their chores.

After putting on her uniform for her first day's work in February 1916, Nina Last reported for duty in the courtyard, where the (male) RAMC sergeant major drilled the orderlies each morning. Rather than working in a clerical role, as she had hoped, she was allocated to three wards in the south block where the most seriously wounded soldiers were nursed. It was nicknamed "the zoo," in another example of dark medical humor, because the groans and screams of the delirious patients, many of them with severely septic wounds, could be heard all over the hospital. Nothing in her twelve months working in the kitchens as a VAD had prepared her for this.

Last began each day at 7:00 a.m., collecting the large bins of soiled dressings from each ward and taking them down one by one in the lift to the incinerator in the yard.[13] Since the wards were stacked one above the other, she began on the top floor and worked her way down. Next she had to empty the bins of ashes from the coal fires on each ward, then return to fill eight coal scuttles from the cellar in the yard and lug these back to the wards. Coughing and spluttering as the ashes blew back in her face, she scraped her knuckles carrying the heavy coal scuttles up the narrow cellar steps. After a hurried breakfast, she was back on the wards to stoke up the fires, empty the ashtrays, and sweep the floors while the moans and yells of the semiconscious patients pounded her ears.

Some of the patients had to be tied to their beds because they were delirious with fever or with morphine, and begged her to release them from their restraints, or from the traction frames above their beds that were used to stabilize their fractures. "I was really very frightened of some of the poor men," Last recalled. With her fear of blood, she found it almost unbearable to witness the men's sufferings when their wounds were dressed each day. Last was not the only one who found the sights, sounds, and smells hard to stomach. At times a fellow "nurse"—as all the orderlies were termed— would faint when she had to hold up a gangrenous leg for the doctor to examine. But the job Last most dreaded was having to wheel patients to the operating theater on the top floor. After delivering a patient to be sedated before surgery, she had to wait in a corner of the theater—careful to stand out of sight of the operation—ready to trundle another unconscious patient, whose operation had just finished, back to his ward. Most worryingly of all, she was told to make sure the man did not start to come round on the return trip and try to swallow his tongue. For the remainder of the day she was "at the beck and call of anyone who wanted any particularly hard or dirty job carried out."

At the end of each day, Last was so exhausted that all she could do was collapse on her bed in the bare dormitory and try to sleep. Yet her nights were frequently disturbed by the sudden clanging of the convoy bell in the courtyard below. Quickly dragging her uniform on over her nightdress and shoving her hair into her cap, she reported in the yard for stretcher-bearing duty. Bleary-eyed and yawning, she lined up with her fellow orderlies to wait for the gray ambulances to roll in. Sometimes, when the convoys were delayed, the orderlies were allowed to lie on the floor and sleep during the wait. In time Last discovered it was easier to volunteer to take the head and shoulders end of the stretcher, even though this was heavier, than to walk backward to the lift holding the end with the feet. Since she was shorter than average, with small hands, and the stretcher handles were designed for men to carry, she struggled to bear the weight of the injured men. On one occasion, carrying a soldier who weighed more than two hundred pounds, she cried out in pain but refused to drop her load. Later she discovered she had badly strained her wrist. After delivering each patient to their allotted ward and waiting for the empty stretcher, which had to be returned to its ambulance, it was often several hours before she could climb back into bed. Even then she would sometimes be woken by the groans of patients in pain. One antidote, she discovered, was reading the novels of Jane Austen. They represented such a "different world" that they possessed a "wonderful power of taking one's mind off unpleasant things."

Most nursing orderlies in military hospitals grew accustomed to the horrors of their patients' suffering surprisingly quickly. Vera Brittain confessed to turning "sick and faint" the first time she helped a sister dress a gangrenous leg wound, which was "slimy and green and scarlet, with the bone laid bare."[14] Two years later, having transferred to a hospital near the front line in France, she was able to drink tea and eat cake amid the foul dressings and human remnants of a fetid operating theater without a second's thought. Many orderlies at Endell Street likewise managed to detach themselves emotionally from their patients' ordeals. Barbara Last—who was put in charge of one of the "zoo" wards on night duty when she was just nineteen—accepted the "grim" reality of nursing at Endell Street. But Nina did not.

At the end of her first fortnight, Last was told to report to the CO. Afraid of being reprimanded—or worse—dismissed, she entered Flora Murray's office. "What had I done or not done?" she wondered. To Last's relief, Murray offered her a transfer to the hospital linens room. For all her strict discipline, Murray was evidently attuned to her orderlies' individual attributes.

One of three orderlies assigned to the linens room, Last was in her element. Although she still had to work long hours doing backbreaking labor, at least she was removed from the wounded patients most of the time. Now she spent her days bagging up vast quantities of soiled sheets, towels, blankets, and military-issue blue pajamas, which all had to be sent out to commercial laundries, since the old workhouse laundry at Endell Street was unusable. She would then apportion the clean supplies for each ward. Since fresh sheets and towels were always in high demand to replace those fouled by blood and mud or infested with lice, Last spent much of her time haranguing the laundries from the telephone in a draughty basement passage chasing up missing items.

According to army regulations, every article of laundry had to be recorded in triplicate as it was sent out and returned. The totals were noted in a huge ledger, which one of the orderlies had to take to army headquarters at Chelsea Barracks to be audited each month. Walking across the huge parade ground at Chelsea, Last felt "very small and shy," but thankful for her uniform. If a mistake was found or an item was missing, the ledger was returned, and the guilty orderly was summoned before Murray. "A few biting words from Dr Murray dashed our spirits for many days to come," she said.

Working six days a week, with only an occasional weekend off, Last found the work so exhausting that sometimes "tears rolled down without my really being aware of them." On the rare occasions when she could escape the hospital, she was often too tired to walk anywhere, so she would board a London bus outside the gates and sit on the open top deck, gazing down numbly on the city streets until it returned to the hospital again. And still she was liable to get called up in the night whenever she was on convoy duty or an air raid warning sounded.

Yet despite the long hours, grueling labor, and tight discipline, Last was having the time of her life. It was fun working and socializing with young people her own age, and she made firm friends among the staff. Her weekly pay of £1 5s seemed "like riches," and whenever she went out in her distinctive uniform, people turned to look—"as I marched past with my nose in the air," she later said self-mockingly.

Pictures of the orderlies at Endell Street published in newspapers and gathered in family albums frequently show exuberant young women linking arms and laughing together as they push trolleys, fold linen, or huddle on the courtyard steps for a well-earned break. It was tough, distressing, and sometimes—in the middle of an air raid—dangerous work, but they were enjoying a degree of liberty and independence they had never before known, along with the financial freedom to enjoy it. Flamboyantly sporting their stylish uniforms, they flashed a daring ankle for the camera and rakishly smoked cigarettes. Freed from the constraints of parents and chaperones, they met up with male friends on leave from the front or flirted with strangers in uniform. On their rare days off, they spent their hard-earned "riches" taking afternoon tea at Harrods and shopping in the stores along the nearby Strand.

In the wartime drive for economy, several London museums and galleries had closed their doors, and motor cars and vans had been replaced by horse-drawn vehicles due to gasoline shortages. Yet the Strand was still "the busiest and most animated street in London," according to *Times* journalist Michael MacDonagh.[15] As he walked the Strand in the summer of 1916, most of the other pedestrians were in khaki—many were soldiers on leave from training camps—and there were women "at work everywhere." Women were driving cars and holding the reins of horse-drawn vehicles, collecting tickets at the Underground stations, and working in hotels. The "lift-boy" had become the "lift-girl," said MacDonagh, while the hall-porter was now "an Amazon in blue or mauve coat, gold-beaded peaked cap and high top-boots." Exemplifying the male chauvinism that was typical of the era, MacDonagh confessed that the latter was "a gorgeous figure that fascinates me," though his favorite novelty was the "conductorette" on trams and buses, who wore a jacket, knee-length skirt, and leather leggings. "I had quite a thrill the first time one said to me as I mounted her moving bus, 'Hold tight, sir, please.'" Shorter skirts—most still hovering around the ankles rather than the knees—had given women the freedom to work in occupations that would otherwise have been impossible, MacDonagh rightly noted. But he could not resist suggesting that while this "skimpiness" did not diminish a woman's attractiveness, "something of her mystery has disappeared."

Something else had disappeared, too. The old codes of decorum that had previously segregated men and women had been replaced by freer relations between the sexes. Working women in their smart uniforms and "skimpy" skirts flirted and joked with soldiers on leave—especially the Australian and New Zealand troops, who were now arriving in London in large numbers after being evacuated from Gallipoli. In their broad-brimmed khaki hats, they were conspicuous on the streets and in the cafés. As MacDonagh observed, "'Flappers' attract them, and they attract 'Flappers.'"

It was not always a good idea, however, to become romantically involved. Many of the male friends that Nina and Barbara Last met on their days off would never return from the front. One such friend was the only son of the vicar in the neighboring parish to their family home. After joining the Royal Flying Corps, he would be killed in action when his plane crashed over France in 1918, aged nineteen.[16] With the death toll of young men climbing all the time, the sisters resolved not to "think of matrimony" until the war was over. Laboring together at Endell Street, they concentrated instead on their war work.

As the weeks progressed, Nina Last grew to respect and even to idolize the hospital's two founding doctors. "My sister and I were truly terrified of them," she would later say, "though we admired them greatly." Murray and Anderson were so devoted to duty that they were willing to give their lives to the cause, she said. "Their sympathy with the men was unfailing," she wrote, "but they had none for any of us who failed to come up to their standards which were extremely high." While any chastisement felt "crushing," a few words of praise made her feel "uplifted for days." And if they had exacting standards for their staff, the two doctors also had enormous faith in their abilities. "Both Drs Murray and G. Anderson firmly believed that the right kind of girl could accomplish anything irrespective of training," said Last.

On one occasion the Lasts were invited to dinner with their COs. This, they thought, was the "greatest compliment" a member of staff could receive. Simultaneously delighted and petrified, the two girls were charmed when Murray and Anderson treated them as "honoured guests" in their private living quarters within the hospital. The treat was short-lived, however. Dinner was interrupted by the sound of a patient crying out in agony, and Murray immediately went to visit him and offer some pain relief. "They were always terribly busy and as they lived in the hospital, they always seemed on duty," wrote Nina. As women, she said, they could not relax "in the way men do when they should be off work."

Although they maintained their private rooms, Murray and Anderson enjoyed very little privacy and barely any time to themselves.

In the few spare hours when they were not busy at Endell Street, they were still running the Harrow Road children's hospital and managing other medical duties. Anderson had attempted to resign from the New Hospital for Women when Endell Street opened in 1915, but—persuaded by the board to stay—she was still nominally assistant surgeon in 1916.[17] She was occasionally spotted at the LSMW too. Octavia Wilberforce—Elizabeth Robins's young medical student friend—was in the dissecting room working on a leg when Anderson walked in one day. She asked Wilberforce whether she had dissected the sole of the foot yet, as she had an operation the next day and wanted to check the anatomy, because she had "forgotten about the foot."[18] Wilberforce had to disappoint her, so Anderson moved on to ask another student. Murray, meanwhile, still made time to visit Harrow Road once a week, bringing "toys and treats" for the children with her.[19]

In the rare moments snatched between convoys and operations, Murray and Anderson would walk their dogs in the Endell Street courtyard and beyond. In the parks and streets around Soho, the terriers frequently attracted ribald comments for their resemblance to the famous dogs on the Black and White whisky label.[20] They had become mascots at Endell Street. The older of the pair, Garrett, who was black, was devoted to Anderson. Although he was banned from the operating theater, he would wait outside the door pining until she finished each session. Garrett was wary of the patients, but he ran to greet anyone wearing the Endell Street uniform, which he instantly recognized. William, the white dog, was friendly to everyone—except the local cats, which he chased from the hospital grounds whenever they ventured in.

Like their pets, Murray and Anderson were as faithful to each other as ever. On occasions when Anderson's nephew visited Endell Street with his younger siblings, he remembered being spoiled by the young orderlies and fussed over by Aunt Louie, "who was fond of us nephews and nieces."[21] But "Dr Flora," as he called her, never spoiled the children. "Cool and reserved in temperament, she made no attempt to indulge in even deputy-aunt behaviour," he said. "Her love was for Aunt Louie and it was fully reciprocated."

NINA AND BARBARA Last would stay on at Endell Street throughout the war, and their letters home provide graphic descriptions of convoys, air raids, and the desperate conditions endured by both patients and staff—much to the anguish of their parents. Even though the sisters kept quiet about some of their worst hardships, their parents grew increasingly indignant about the harsh regime. They were not the only parents to voice their worries. It cut little ice with the chief officers. Although Murray and Anderson were always strict disciplinarians, they also believed their orderlies should be treated as adults. They demanded complete dedication from their staff when on duty, but they were adamant the women should be at liberty to do as they pleased in their leisure hours.[22] Murray never wrote to an orderly's parents without the orderly's knowledge, even when the parents wrote to her first urging secrecy. Indeed, she was often bemused to receive letters not only from parents but also from uncles, younger brothers, brothers-in-law, and family doctors, who all believed it was their right to advise on a young woman's life, even though she was over the age of twenty-one. Murray was saddened when an orderly was sometimes forced to relinquish a job she enjoyed because her mother was bored at home without her, or because her father "likes to have his girls with him in the evenings." Murray's respect for her orderlies' independence was in sharp contrast to the approach sometimes adopted elsewhere. When Katharine Furse took her VAD unit to Boulogne, she forbade her women from smoking and associating with men. On one occasion, she sent a female ambulance driver home when she became engaged to a serviceman she had met.[23]

THE WAR'S INSATIABLE greed for men had created an unprecedented demand for women to replace them. Objections to women contributing to the war effort in the first few months of the conflict had given way eighteen months later to a rush to recruit as many women as possible. The disastrous defeats of 1915 had devastated Britain's military might, and the flood of men volunteering at the start of the war had dwindled to a trickle. Yet France, which had suffered much heavier losses, was demanding that Britain increase its commitment to the Allied cause, with a major joint offensive planned for the Western Front in the summer of 1916. When the Germans attacked French forces at the fortified town of Verdun in February, causing massive losses to both sides for months to come, this further increased the pressure for Britain to demonstrate its support for its chief ally. Despite widespread misgivings, Asquith's coalition government had little choice but to introduce conscription—initially, from March 1916, for single men aged eighteen to forty-one, later extended to married men. As men were called up and more reservists were sent abroad, so more women were needed to replace them in factories, on farms, and in hospitals. From September 1915 the War Office had urged hospitals to replace all male cooks, clerks, cleaners, and dispensers with women wherever possible, although the response was slow and people were resistant. Conscription now made the imperative for women to take on men's work all the more urgent.

A year previously, War Office bureaucrats had thrown every obstacle in the way of the women establishing Endell Street. They had predicted that Murray and Anderson's venture would fail and discouraged other women from following in their footsteps. Now the War Office held up Endell Street as a model of what could be achieved if women were involved even more. Officers from military and naval hospitals up and down the country began descending on Endell Street to see what women could really do.

Already working day and night to keep the hospital running, Murray had to find time to escort parties of skeptical army and naval officers around and show them women bearing stretchers, carrying bags of potatoes, and organizing fire drills.[24] Some of the visitors still shook their heads forlornly and refused to believe that women could replace men in their own institutions, while muttering about the "hopeless difficulty of the situation." One War Office official, who had the job of inspecting hospitals to ensure that every possible man had been replaced by a woman, returned again and again for advice when hospitals he visited insisted they could not use women in certain roles. He had been assured, for example, that women could not work in the X-ray department because men would find this "indelicate"—until Murray pointed out that the images were taken through clothing and in a dark room. The fact that female orderlies, nurses, and doctors were also giving bed baths, dressing wounds in intimate places, and treating men with venereal disease had seemingly not occurred to him. The poor man told Murray that whenever he tried to counter objections from hospital administrators, by citing the evidence at Endell Street, he would see "a nauseated expression come over their faces."

Another visitor keen to learn from the example of Endell Street in the spring of 1916 was an American doctor, Rosalie Slaughter Morton, who stopped in London on her way to help treat wounded Serbians in Salonika. Born into a medical family in Virginia, she had overcome objections from her father and brothers to follow in the family tradition, qualifying in medicine in 1897. After she married and settled in New York, she had become professor of gynecology— the first female professor in any field of medicine in the city—at the New York Polyclinic Hospital. Now that she was widowed, with nothing to lose and "everything to give," she had resolved to work on the front line in Salonika.

During her two-week stay in London, Morton was astonished to find "every fourth house" had been converted into a hospital or convalescent home. She spent her time meeting other women doctors and visiting military hospitals, where she noted the latest advances. As she walked the London streets, she found "England almost manless, being run absolutely efficiently by women, from street cars to politics."[25] But Morton was already thinking beyond her immediate plan of working in Salonika. Anticipating that America would eventually join the war, she was determined ultimately to organize field hospitals overseas where American women doctors would work. Visiting Endell Street, therefore, was "the centre of my greatest interest," she said. She was not disappointed.

Touring the wards and departments, Morton found "the cooperation, equipment, scientific work, administration and housekeeping were admirable." She was particularly impressed by the X-ray facilities at Endell Street and elsewhere, since this had been largely pioneered by women in the face of indifference from male doctors. Leaving London a fortnight later to spend the next six months in a field hospital in Macedonia, Morton would not forget what she had witnessed.

ALTHOUGH LONDON WAS becoming increasingly "manless," for the moment Endell Street kept its detachment of twenty-two RAMC men—although many of the first contingent were replaced by others less fit to fight.[26] Among those now pressed into active service were the three privates Bishop, Price, and Hedges, who had accompanied the women's corps when they first set off for France. Now they were bound for France again—for the trenches. Another RAMC aide, Corporal Musselbrook, had trained as an operating theater orderly under Anderson's guidance but—to universal regret—was now dispatched to join an infantry regiment as a fighting soldier at the front. On the strength of his training at Endell Street, however, he was transferred back to the RAMC and went on to serve as a theater orderly in Salonika and Russia. Progressing through the ranks, he later attributed his rise to his training at Endell Street and the certificate he acquired there, which he carried with him everywhere. In the meantime, he was replaced by another male orderly, Corporal Washington, who became just as popular with the staff as Musselbrook—especially with one of the women orderlies, who would buy ice creams for both of them from the canteen on hot days.

Many of the male staff who remained at Endell Street—or returned there later to report on their travails—were fiercely loyal to their women bosses and became fervent champions of women workers. They in turn became favorites with the women. One of the most devoted—and the highest ranking—was Sergeant Major Harris, who had assumed command of the RAMC detachment at Endell Street in August 1915, despite the forebodings of failure from his colleagues. He would remain there until the end of the war. Harris, who was in his fifties, had served with the medical corps in the Boer Wars but had little experience in hospital administration. Nonetheless, he worked tirelessly at Endell Street and backed the authority of

Murray and Anderson whenever the need arose. It was Harris's job to drill the women orderlies—like Last—and he looked after them with a paternalistic air. Harris formed a close bond with Murray: the pair would frequently hole themselves up in her office to puzzle over the ambiguities of army regulations. Once they had come to a mutual agreement, they would emerge as a united front to put the rules into force. On occasion, Harris returned from visits to his RAMC barracks to regale Murray with tales of disciplinary scandals at military hospitals elsewhere. According to these stories, convalescing patients from other hospitals habitually stayed out all night on unauthorized leave—whether visiting their families or enjoying other pleasures was left unsaid—and as many as sixty patients required disciplinary action each day. Naturally, Harris took pride in the fact that such lapses rarely happened at Endell Street. In Murray's words, he "adopted" the hospital and "took it to his heart."

As more and more able men were "combed out," in military jargon, for active service in 1916, the orderlies supervised by Harris were increasingly women. One male helper spent four months volunteering as a theater orderly before he was replaced by a woman in early 1916. A drama critic in his fifties, he was more used to raising a toast in West End theaters than to lifting patients in an operating theater. After his stint at Endell Street he professed the "most profound admiration" for Murray and Anderson.[27] His work taken over by "strong, enthusiastic girls," he devoted his spare hours to escorting convalescing patients to matinee performances instead.

Endell Street led the way in demonstrating women's abilities. It not only expanded to 573 beds but opened three auxiliary hospitals in the north London suburbs, to provide nearly 150 extra beds for convalescent patients.[28] One of these, Byculla, was a spacious house whose owner offered the property to the War Office in early 1916. Its airy rooms were converted into six wards, and a bathroom was transformed into a small but "beautifully-fitted" operating theater. Before long, Byculla expanded into the adjacent house, owned by a former Liberal MP, Sir Arthur Crosfield. The combined Byculla and Crosfield Hospital provided 82 beds, staffed by a matron and three nurses helped by 55 VADs. The VADs were supervised by Sir

Arthur's wife, Lady Domini Crosfield, who was pictured on the front cover of the *Tatler* looking suitably devotional in her white nurse's apron with its red cross and a white cap. A second auxiliary hospital, known as Holly Park, opened in a house nearby with 36 beds and a well-equipped theater where relatively serious operations were performed.

The third hospital attached to Endell Street opened in February 1916 in Dollis Hill House, a sprawling country residence in northwest London where guests had once included Mark Twain. When he stayed there in 1900, Twain had enthused that Dollis Hill came "nearer to being a paradise than any other home I ever occupied."[29] Local people adopted the hospital as their own. Well-wishers raised funds at garden fetes, and schoolchildren collected £1,250 (equivalent to more than £100,000 today, or nearly US$125,000) toward its upkeep. As they slowly recovered in the lush gardens with their distant view of the capital—a world away from the trenches—the men must indeed have felt they had found paradise. Although most patients in the auxiliary hospitals were less seriously wounded or convalescing, stretcher cases were still admitted when demand was high—as it would be soon enough.

NOW THAT THEY were in command of four hospitals, providing as many as eight hundred beds at the busiest times, Murray and Anderson had plainly proved that women doctors had a place in the army.[30] Even the hardboiled skeptics in the War Office had been won over. With Endell Street having paved the way, in April 1916 Keogh appealed for forty women doctors to join the RAMC—the first time the army had directly recruited medical women—to work overseas. He was overwhelmed by the response. Three months later, eighty female doctors sailed to Malta, replacing men who were dispatched to frontline medical services in France.[31] Before the end of the year Keogh would appeal for a further fifty women doctors for Egypt and elsewhere.

Their experience was far from plain sailing, however. Based on her own experience as an "army surgeon"—as she now regarded herself—Anderson urged the War Office to grant the women doctors the rank of officers and provide them with military uniforms, to ensure they commanded authority with both their patients and fellow medics. Her advice was ignored. The women arrived in civilian clothes and were paid inferior flat rates—in contrast to the doctors at Endell Street, who were graded as captain or lieutenant—on temporary twelve-month contracts, with disastrous consequences. Upon arrival at their army camps, the women found they had no rights to living quarters, rations, or transport and no status. Since they were regarded as junior to the lowliest RAMC stretcher-bearer, they had to appeal to superior officers to enforce their medical orders. When traveling, they had to sit in third-class carriages under the guise of "nurses" or "soldiers' wives." In Malta they were often excluded from officers' messes, and in Egypt they were sometimes turned out of trains altogether. Indeed, as one doctor put it, their experiences were "daily humiliating annoyance."[32] Worst of all, no doubt, was the fact that there was virtually no work to do. They had been sent to the region to boost medical services in expectation of a new Mediterranean theater of war, but the projected campaign never happened.

Despite these demeaning experiences, the supply of medical women at home could not keep pace with demand. Already a large proportion of the one thousand or so women on the medical register were undertaking some form of war work—serving in military hospitals at home and overseas, working as medical officers in munitions factories, and deputizing for male general practitioners—but more still were needed.[33] In one instance, reported with surprise in the press, a woman was appointed to a hospital post over a male candidate. The LSMW had doubled its intake of medical students for the year 1915–1916, and even mainstream medical schools began opening their doors to women. St Mary's Medical School in west London admitted women students from December 1915, chiefly in order to stay open. Charing Cross Medical School, which had turned down sixty applications from women in 1915, agreed to admit female students in 1916, as did the Royal Dental Hospital in Leicester Square.[34]

There were even signs that Asquith might be converted to approving votes for women on the basis of women doctors' contributions to the war effort. Writing to him in May pressing her case for women's suffrage in recognition of their war work, Millicent Fawcett, an astute parliamentary observer as ever, cited the example of the NUWSS-backed Scottish Women's Hospitals, which now had a dozen units in France and farther afield, but made no mention of her niece's work much closer to home.[35] Asquith assured her that he deeply appreciated "the magnificent contribution which the women of the United Kingdom have made to our country's cause," and promised that this would be taken into account when future legislation on the franchise was considered.

The press weighed in with support for women's expanding roles in medicine. When Cambridge University still refused to open its medical examinations to women, the *Daily News and Leader* condemned the decision as "shortsighted," arguing that "it is obvious that the more doctors are now trained, men or women, the better from the national point of view, since the war has made, and will continue to make even after the war, the demand for doctors greater than the supply." Not only were there going to be fewer male doctors returning from war service, but there were clearly going to be more disabled and maimed men needing medical care. Now that mainstream hospitals had opened their doors to women doctors, the *Daily Telegraph* confidently asserted, they would "never be closed to them again."[36] The cause was bolstered by a stream of enthusiastic articles, such as one applauding the "Wonderful Work of Brave Girls in War Hospitals," and photo spreads promoting the work at Endell Street—all carefully pasted into Murray's scrapbook.

A series of photographs depicting daily life at Endell Street, probably commissioned by Murray herself, appeared in various newspapers in early 1916. Among other scenes, they showed two women pharmacists weighing medicines in the dispensary, a female radiographer preparing plates for the X-ray machine, and a "lady dentist" drilling a patient's tooth.[37] For many readers, these pictures provided their first sight of any medical woman. They were featured alongside photographs of cheerful women orderlies pushing a patient in his bed across the courtyard and checking stores in the linens room. One picture showed Mardie Hodgson opening the hospital's black iron gates while a special constable stands to attention beside her. By April, according to the *Daily Chronicle*, the Endell Street uniform was recognized all over London. The hospital's patients wondered, it added, "if there was ever a day when women fought with hatpin and umbrella for recognition of their rights."[38] The only sour note was sounded by the *Yorkshire Post*, whose editor protested at the "many scores of times" he had read about Murray and Anderson's work and said, "General Keogh must be weary of the praises lavished on him for his appreciation of their ability."[39]

BY MAY 1916, the first anniversary of Endell Street opening, almost 1,500 operations had been performed—most of them by Anderson—and the hospital was admitting between 400 and 800 patients a month.[40] Among them was Harry Barter, a private in the Grenadier Guards, who was said to be the tallest man in the British Army.[41] Barter, a farmer's son from Devon, measured 6 feet 8¼ inches when he enlisted in 1911 at the age of eighteen. Five years later, when he was admitted to Endell Street, he had added another inch to his height—at least according to a fellow patient, who wrote to the *Daily Mail* with the news. Barter had been wounded near Ypres, probably in one of the relatively minor battles in February. For his recovery, he had to have an especially large bed made for him. By contrast, Edwin Bostock, another private, was only 5 feet 4 inches tall—just an inch over the army's minimum—when he had enlisted in the early months of the war. A cabinetmaker from London's East End with four children, he had fractured his ankle in France by "falling over a brick" and was admitted to Endell Street in March. Treated by Winifred Buckley, he was sufficiently recovered by June to be allowed ten days' furlough to visit his family. Nine months later his wife gave birth to twins.

As well as treating the sporadic convoys of men who fell sick in the trenches or were wounded in the minor actions on the Western Front in the first half of 1916, the doctors at Endell Street were busy running the casualty department, where an average of five thousand patients a year—soldiers from local barracks and depots—arrived at all hours of the day and night.[42] While most of them had fallen sick or injured themselves while on leave—and sometimes when absent without leave—a large proportion were drunk, and some were inevitably violent. According to Murray, intoxicated men were constantly brought in by the police or in London ambulances—entirely crewed by women from mid-1916—and some became "habitués" of the Johnnie Walker ward. A few had suffered broken bones in jumping from windows or falling into basements while trying to evade capture by police. In one mysterious case of June 1916, a Canadian private who was on leave arrived unconscious at Endell Street after falling from the first-floor window of a nearby hotel. He died of a fractured skull soon after admission. At the subsequent inquest, where Anderson gave evidence, it transpired that he had booked into the room with a fellow soldier after a night's carousing and fallen—or was pushed—from the window in the early hours.[43]

As the days warmed—and the introduction of British summer time brought later daylight hours—convalescing patients were allowed to take the air in a nearby park, where they played on the children's swings in their blue suits.[44] On sunny afternoons the men piled into river steamers to enjoy trips up and down the Thames, courtesy of the Port of London Authority. They smoked, drank tea, and ate sandwiches as they passed famous landmarks. For those deemed likely to regain full health, time was running out. As pressure mounted to increase British forces in France, the men were discharged as soon as they were fit to train for the front again. Their beds would be needed before long.

More doctors were needed, too. In May, the radiographer Eva White left Endell Street; she was replaced by Ethel Magill, another LSMW graduate, aged thirty-five, who took charge of the busy X-ray department.[45] At the same time, three of the assistant surgeons—Gertrude Gazdar, who had been with the corps since Paris, Morna Rawlins, and Gertrude Dearnley—also left. They were replaced by three new arrivals fresh off the boat from Australia.

Like medical women in Britain, Australian women had struggled to obtain a medical education and then faced the same obstacles securing jobs.[46] When war broke out, several of the 129 women on the Australian medical register had volunteered to serve as army medics, but, as in Britain, had been refused. When Keogh had appealed for doctors from the Commonwealth to join the army medical service in 1915, more than one hundred Australian doctors enlisted, but it was made plain women were not required. To dispel any ambiguity, notices were placed in newspapers advising that women doctors were not wanted. But just as in Britain, Australian women doctors found alternative routes to contribute their skills to the war effort.

Eleanor Bourne, Rachel Champion, and Elizabeth Hamilton-Browne arrived in London after perilous voyages through the Suez Canal and the Mediterranean. Bourne would remember cheering as her ship passed Australian troops camped on the banks of the Suez, then threading a zig-zag route through the Mediterranean to dodge German U-boats. Born in South Brisbane, Queensland, in 1878, she had excelled at her girls' grammar school, but had to switch to the local boys' school to study the science subjects she needed to apply for medicine. She won a national scholarship to Sydney University, becoming the first woman from Queensland to study medicine. After graduating in 1903 she had returned to Brisbane, where she specialized—owing to the usual obstacles—in women's and children's health. It was Bourne's younger brother George who planted the idea that she might go to England to work in a military hospital. He had enlisted in 1914, but fell ill with dysentery after five months in Gallipoli, and was then evacuated to a hospital in London. Writing to "Nell," he suggested, "I wonder if you would like to get into a Hospital here?" adding that there was "plenty of work to be had."

Indeed there was. Bourne, who was thirty-seven, was thrilled when she heard she had been accepted at Endell Street and set out in January 1916. Booking into a hotel in Bloomsbury, she reported for work in the gloomy-looking Endell Street hospital. There she met Rachel Champion—known as "Ray"—who was significantly younger, at twenty-five, and had only been qualified for two years. Born in Melbourne in 1890, Champion had studied medicine at Melbourne University, where she was one of only three women among fifty students. Pretty, lively, and self-confident, she made an impression on her tutors—especially on Charles Gordon Shaw, known as Gordon, who was five years her senior. The pair had become close and worked together at the local hospital before war intervened. Gordon enlisted in the Royal Australian Army Medical Corps and left Australia in October 1914, working in hospital ships at Gallipoli and field hospitals in Egypt before being dispatched to France in March 1916. Following hard on his heels, Ray arrived in London two months later and made her way to Endell Street.

Elizabeth Hamilton-Browne, who was thirty-four, was already hard at work, having paid her passage from Australia by working as a ship's surgeon in March.[47] She had graduated from Sydney University's medical school with first-class honors in 1909, one of the first three women ever to do so. She then worked as a pathologist at Sydney Hospital—the first female doctor in residence there—before being sidelined into women's services. All three women would come to regard the next few years as some of the best of their lives.

THAT SUMMER, RACHEL Champion, Eleanor Bourne, and Elizabeth Hamilton-Browne, along with Nina Last and her sister, Barbara, would squeeze together on tiered benches in the hospital courtyard with the rest of the orderlies, nurses, and doctors, and the twenty-two RAMC men, for a remarkable panoramic photograph featuring the entire Endell Street staff.[48] Flanked by these rows of more than 160 women and a handful of men, Murray and Anderson sat side by side in the center, with the matron, Grace Hale, directly behind them, and Mardie Hodgson crosslegged on the ground in front, her dog, Eepie, clasped in her arms.

The arrival of the Australian doctors was timely. In June, hospitals throughout Britain received orders to discharge all convalescent patients. By the end of the month, hospital wards all over the country stood ready, with row upon row of empty waiting beds.[49]

7

Pioneers, O Pioneers!

The Somme Valley, near Albert, July 1, 1916

Dawn broke and a light mist drifted across the battlefield.[1] The sun rose into a cloudless blue sky with the promise of a fine day ahead. As they waited for the whistle, the men of the Lincolnshire Regiment placed their ladders against the trench walls. For the past week, British artillery had shelled the German lines without mercy, and it seemed almost impossible that any enemy troops could have survived. The waiting men had been assured that the bombardment had cut through the thick German barbed wire and devastated the system of enemy trenches, so that crossing the few hundred yards of "no-man's-land" would be easy. The British guns reached a crescendo and fell quiet. In the momentary silence, birds were heard singing. Private William Bilton stood ready with his comrades for the "Big Push" on the first day of the Battle of the Somme. At 7:30 a.m., the first platoons scaled the ladders and launched themselves over the top of the parapet into the full force of German firepower.

Almost twenty thousand men were killed and forty thousand wounded on the first day of the Somme advance—the highest single-day casualty toll of the entire war and in British military history ever. Only half the men who took part on July 1 survived unscathed. The majority were fresh young recruits with no battle experience; all were volunteers. Packed off to France as soon as they were trained, then drilled and rehearsed on French soil, they did precisely as they had been taught. Advancing in waves at intervals of one minute, they walked slowly toward the German lines across a front stretching eighteen miles and were mown down in the thousands. Those who managed to reach the first German trench system—and only about one-third did—quickly discovered that the barbed wire, up to thirty feet thick in places, remained largely intact. The Germans' sophisticated system of deep trenches and bunkers, much of it reinforced with concrete and steel, had barely been touched. The enemy's second line of defense—a further system of trenches—was even more impenetrable. And since German troops had simply taken refuge in their dugouts during the past week's bombardment, hardly any had been killed. Over the next few days the casualties would continue to mount as German guns scythed down the advancing British while rain, which began on July 2, filled shell holes and drowned many who lay there wounded.

As they swept forward on that first day, the Lincolnshires suffered heavy losses, but they succeeded against the odds in breaching the first German lines. Bilton was fortunate—for the moment—since his battalion, the 1st, had been assigned to wait in reserve. But six hours after the first men went over the top, Bilton and his fellows followed in their wake, carrying ammunition supplies. As they crossed the cratered no-man's-land in the beating sun, amid the roar of falling shells and the patter of machine-gun fire, they stumbled past the mutilated bodies of the dead and wounded. Since they were under strict orders not to stop, they ignored the cries for help from those trying to crawl back to safety or sheltering in shell holes. When they reached the German lines, Bilton and his fellows unloaded their ammunition stocks at a prearranged drop point. Then they were ordered to reinforce troops attempting to hold two captured enemy trenches under bombardment from German guns. By the end of the day, more than one hundred men in Bilton's battalion—roughly one in ten—had been wounded, and three had been killed. The shelling continued through the night and into the second day as the men held their ground, although at the cost of fourteen more casualties. Soon after dawn on the third day, orders came to press forward and seize two copses, Birch Wood and Shelter Wood, where German soldiers had taken refuge in heavily reinforced dugouts.

William Bilton had survived the first two days of the Somme assault unharmed. At 9:00 a.m. on July 3, he fixed his bayonet to his rifle as the order came to advance on Shelter Wood. Scuttling over the rough ground, Bilton and his comrades charged into the dense trees in the face of heavy fire. As they drew close to the enemy bunker, German soldiers streamed out to their firing positions, cutting the British down with heavy machine guns and grenades. It was at this point that Bilton, who was five feet six inches tall, came face to face with a German gunner more than a foot taller. Bilton shot him at close range and was turning back to look for his friends when he was hit by a volley of machine-gun fire. Bleeding from his hand and arm, he fell to the ground. By 2:00 p.m., the 1st Battalion had succeeded in taking possession of Shelter and Birch Woods, though not without substantial further casualties. Nine men were killed and more than two hundred wounded in the battle. For Bilton, the next forty-eight hours were a blur. Two days after being shot in Shelter Wood, he found himself in a bed at Endell Street.

PRIVATE BILTON WAS one of three hundred wounded men sent back from the Somme who arrived at Endell Street in those first few days of July. Born in Grimsby, he had enlisted with the Lincolnshires a year earlier at the age of twenty-one. A single man, he had still been living with his mother. On July 6, his story was headlined in the *Daily Sketch*, which called him the "Tommy who took part in four charges in four days"—although in fact, it was an even more impressive three days. A photograph accompanying the story shows Bilton with his left arm in a sling and a dazed expression on his face. He was possibly shell shocked; nearly 30 percent of stretcher cases wounded at the Somme showed signs of that ailment.[2] Invited in by Flora Murray, the *Sketch* journalist had interviewed Bilton and several others who had arrived from the Somme the previous day.

All the patients played down their experiences and joked about their injuries with customary fighting bravado—or at least they did in the heavily censored and embellished columns of the wartime press. An Irish soldier whose hands had been "filled with machine-gun bullets" described his part in the push "with a smile." Hit by a dozen bullets within twenty minutes of going "over the top," he was no doubt relieved to have escaped so quickly. A Birmingham man with an injured arm and bullet wound to his mouth was "merry," despite his wounded lip feeling "as big and heavy as a motor 'bus." But the greatest attention was reserved for Bilton—"perhaps the most remarkable man in the hospital"—whose experiences behind German lines were related in detail. Asked whether he had bayoneted his German opponent, he replied, "Oh, no; I wasn't taking any chances," and added: "I am only a little 'un. . . . So I just shot him." But the men, according to the newspaper, were far more eager to talk about their doctors than to dwell on their ordeals.

As the *Sketch* reminded its readers, Endell Street had been viewed with suspicion when it had first opened just over twelve months earlier. But thanks to the magnificent work of its women doctors, the hospital was now "perhaps the most popular in London." To prove its point, the *Sketch* devoted its entire front page that day to a picture spread of soldiers wounded at the Somme, all being carried on stretchers by women orderlies and assessed by women doctors in the Endell Street courtyard. The headline declared, "Our Wounded Heroes in Woman's Tender Hands." The largest photograph shows Flora Murray crouching beside a stretcher, notebook in hand, as she assesses a new arrival. Still in his khaki uniform, the soldier's head rests on a pillow and his eyes are shut. She appears to be loosening his collar, though she was probably trying to read the label attached to his jacket, which would have identified his injuries and previous treatment.

The Somme offensive brought the war directly into the heart of London. The seven-day bombardment preceding the advance was so intense it had been heard in parts of the capital, more than 150 miles from the front.[3] The first reports in the evening newspapers on July 1 were characteristically optimistic about victory, but when *The Times* described the advance in more somber tones the following day, the mood soon changed. Although most of the press continued to varnish events, it was impossible to conceal the scale of the bloodshed, as unprecedented numbers of casualties began arriving in the capital on July 4. Ambulance trains carried so many wounded from Southampton that there were not enough platforms at Charing Cross to unload them, and trains were diverted to Paddington. Two days later, on July 6, hospital ships had their single busiest day of the war, conveying more than ten thousand wounded across the English Channel.[4] Crowds jammed the streets around railway stations, clamoring for a glimpse of the arrivals. Some were looking for a familiar face among the stretchers, while others simply threw flowers as tears ran down their faces.

As the staggering toll of dead and wounded continued to rise, readers scoured newspaper columns for any mention of a loved one and waited with dread for a knock on the door. Vera Brittain, now a seasoned VAD nurse at a hospital in south London, had been working ceaselessly as stretchers arrived without pause when she heard, on July 5, that her brother Edward had been admitted to an officers' ward in her own hospital.[5] He had been hit while leading his company in the advance near Albert—where William Bilton had been fighting—and dragged himself seventy yards to safety. Edward would survive to fight again, but many, of course, would not. A number of those tending the wounded at Endell Street had family and friends involved in the advance, even if they weren't necessarily soldiers. Gordon Shaw, the fiancé of Australian surgeon Rachel Champion, was in charge of a tented hospital for ANZAC soldiers who reinforced British troops from late July.

The convoys would continue to deluge London hospitals throughout July and August. Before the advance, medical officers in France had anticipated 10,000 wounded a day. The reality was beyond anyone's expectations. Even on the quietest day in July, there were twice that number of casualties, so that frontline medical staff and transport services were utterly overwhelmed. Since beds in the casualty clearing stations filled immediately, stretcher-bearers had to lay men in rows in the surrounding fields.[6] By the end of July, the wounded had exceeded 120,000, and the majority of them had been shipped back to England.[7] A further 52,000 casualties arrived in

August. The strain on medical services, according to official reports, was "without parallel."

As the convoys arrived in the Endell Street courtyard throughout the summer, Louisa Garrett Anderson worked tirelessly in the operating theater, often for twelve hours at a stretch, with only a few minutes' break to eat.[8] Flora Murray frantically cleared beds to make space for new admissions. The continual demand meant that patients had to be transferred to convalescent care as soon as they could be moved, and beds were turned over at a rate of one hundred a week.

All leave was canceled for the nurses and orderlies. It was impossible to take a day off, Barbara Last told her mother, because "we are most awfully busy."[9] All thirty-three beds on her ward were full, and an extra bunk had been set up for a man with shrapnel wounds and scabies. Many of her patients needed constant care. One was extremely ill with fever—malaria or typhoid, thought Barbara—as well as completely deaf. He needed artificial feeding every two hours, and all conversations with him had to be written down.

On one typical day, Barbara was alone, in charge of her ward, when a convoy arrived. She had just finished giving all the men bed baths—usually done on waterproof sheets to protect the bedding—when one of the doctors came to change the men's dressings. To her horror, not a single sterile bowl could be found, so she had to "fly & boil them up & get the dressing trolley ready." In the middle of the panic, Anderson and Murray arrived to examine the new admissions. After dispatching three men for X-rays, Barbara had to send three more to theater—luckily, a second orderly had come on duty—before serving the men tea. But soon after the first patient returned from surgery, she discovered he was hemorrhaging. While she was trying to staunch the blood, the second man returned to the ward, and he, too, was hemorrhaging. Her fellow orderly ran for the doctors while Barbara hurriedly sterilized instruments and bowls. By the time she had finished her shift at 8:30 p.m., exhausted and traumatized, she had missed supper.

Even the hospital library was feeling the pressure. Beatrice Harraden had moved into a club for women in the West End so she could be closer to Endell Street during the "fearful rush," since work was "so heavy."[10] Writing in August to Elizabeth Robins, who had been almost forgiven for swanning off to America earlier in the year, Harraden said the library's workload had "grown & grown" as a result of the frequent convoys. The new arrivals were "reading every kind of book under the sun—technical, literary, scientific"—as well as the inevitable Nat Goulds. As Harraden made her ward rounds, ascertaining the reading tastes of the battered and befuddled men plucked from the Somme battlefields, she felt grateful to be among the living. Despite her exhaustion, she told Robins, "I'm still alive & if I weren't I should only have followed very humbly in the footsteps of thousands who have perished in this awful cataclysm."

Determined to divert the men from the nightmare they had experienced, Murray kept up the entertainments and rounds of visiting dignitaries. Queen Alexandra visited Endell Street twice that summer.[11] In July, she talked to patients lying on their beds in the courtyard, giving her parasol to one man to shield his eyes from the sun, and her monogrammed handkerchief to another, who was dying, to wipe the sweat from his face. On her second visit, in August, her car was held up at the hospital gates because a convoy had just arrived. Once she was allowed through, she spoke to two of the soldiers who had just been unloaded from the ambulances. The Queen Mother was visibly moved as she talked to men who had been severely wounded—some of them permanently disabled—at the Somme. She gave one man, who had been hit in six places, a book bound in scarlet and gold, and asked others what she could send them. The following day gifts of cigarettes, pillows, and walking sticks arrived. The men were clearly touched by the royal presence—and presents—but it was little compensation for the horror they had endured and the disabilities many would have to live with for the rest of their lives.

William Bilton was not untypical. He recovered from his bullet wounds sufficiently to go home to his mother in Grimsby in November, but he would never fight again. He was discharged from the army in February the following year and died ten months later of bronchial pneumonia. Despite the claims of the *Sketch*, his story was not even the most remarkable of the Somme soldiers treated at Endell Street that summer. John Joseph O'Donoghue, a gunner with the Royal Garrison Artillery, had served eleven years in the regular army before the war.[12] Born in Cork, John-Joe, as he was known, was one of the gunners who had helped mount the week-long bombardment that had preceded the Somme advance. Six weeks later, he was hit by a shell during the bombardment before the Battle of Flers-Courcelette. In shock and bleeding from severe wounds, O'Donoghue was so weak he could not speak. Comrades propped him up against a graveyard wall to wait for help. When stretcher-bearers found him, they assumed he was dying and joked that they could save time by throwing him over the cemetery wall. He blinked frantically to convince them he was alive and was sent to a base hospital before arriving at Endell Street on September 24. Although he lost a lung, he recovered sufficiently to settle in London, where he married an Irish woman and lived into his nineties, a much-loved father and grandfather renowned as a "great story teller."

At least the men enjoyed the novelty of their situation. Many of the patients wrote home to describe their surprise at finding themselves in a hospital staffed by women. Lance Corporal James Lyon, who was with the cyclist battalion of the Highland Light Infantry, had been processed through four hospitals in France before he arrived at Endell Street.[13] He had been knocked unconscious and half-buried on September 23 by a shell burst. His hearing was damaged, and his chest badly bruised, and he was also diagnosed with shell shock. After two months at the front, he was delighted when the doctor treating him in France announced that he was going to "Blighty." James told his father: "I could hardly believe it till I was put on a stretcher and carried away," adding, "This hospital I am in is completely managed by women—women doctors and everything."

For those men who went over the top at the Somme, the chances of being killed or wounded—and the degree of injury when they were wounded—were a complete lottery. Like James Lyon, many of them welcomed a "Blighty" wound, an injury serious enough to merit being sent home to England.[14] "Blighty" was a corruption of the Urdu word for a foreign land, *bilayti*, originally used by British

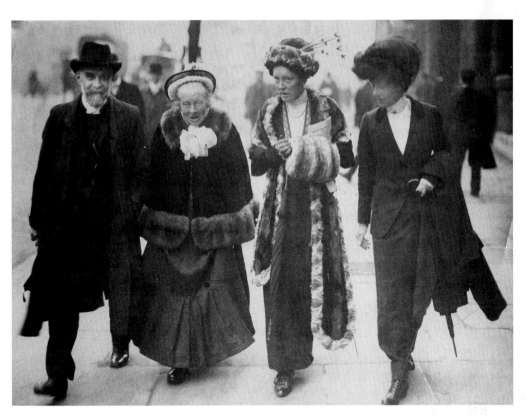

Louisa Garrett Anderson (second from right) on her way to see Prime Minister
Herbert Asquith with her mother Elizabeth and two others in 1910.

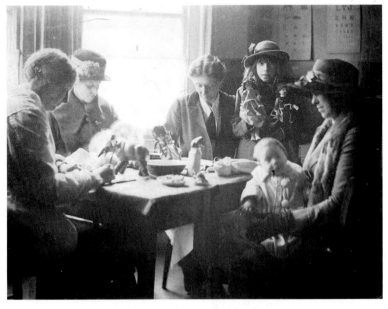

Flora Murray (third from left) in a busy outpatients' clinic at
Harrow Road children's hospital.

Flora Murray
at her desk at
Claridge's, Paris.
(ANDERSON FAMILY)

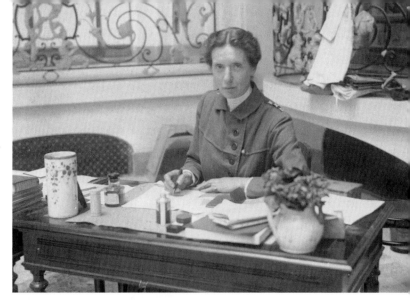

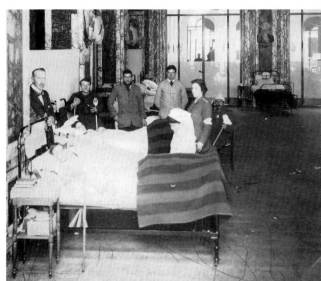

(Left) A ward at Claridge's.
(ANDERSON FAMILY)

(Facing Page) A surprise
encounter at the Château
Mauricien depicted in *Punch*.
(PUNCH, AUGUST 4, 1915)

The Women's Hospital
Corps in Paris. Murray
(seated, far right) and
Anderson (seated, second
from right) with fellow
doctors and orderlies on
the Claridge's courtyard
steps. (ANDERSON FAMILY)

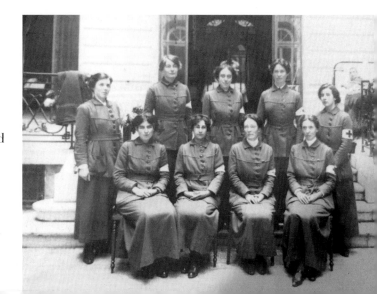

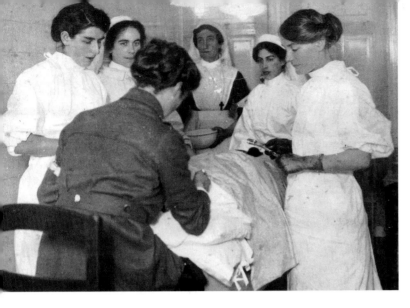

An operation
in the converted
ladies' cloakroom
at Claridge's.
(IMPERIAL WAR
MUSEUM)

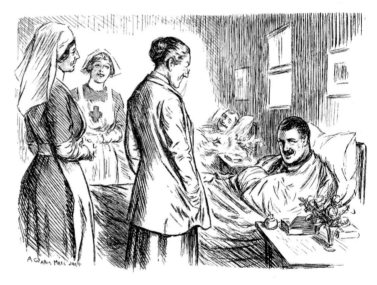

EMMINENT WOMAN
SURGEON, WHO IS
ALSO AN ARDENT
SUFFRAGETTE
(TO WOUNDED
GUARDSMAN): "Do
you know, your
face is singularly
familiar to me.
I've been trying to
remember where
we've met before."

GUARDSMAN: "Well,
Mum, byegones be
byegones. I was a
police constable."

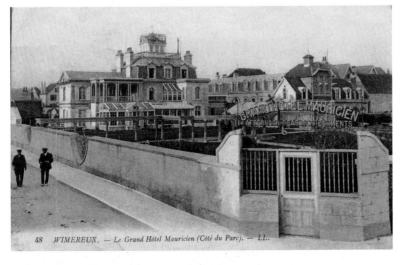

The Château
Mauricien in
more peaceful
times from a
picture postcard.
(COOK-DICKERMAN
COLLECTION)

48   WIMEREUX. — Le Grand Hôtel Mauricien (Côté du Parc). — LL.

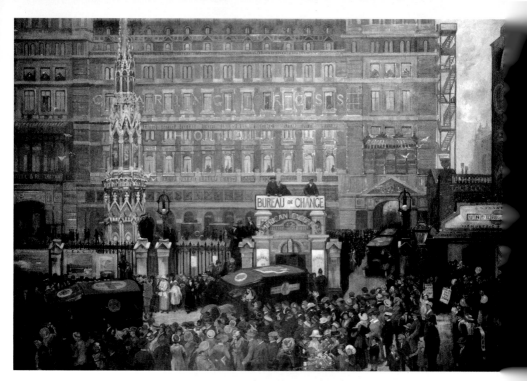

Ambulances collecting
casualties at Charing
Cross station, oil by
J. Hobson Lobley, 1919.

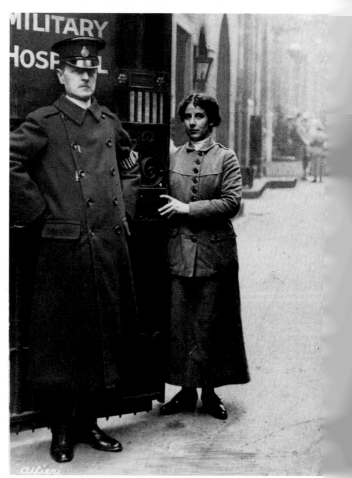

Mardie Hodgson and
special constable at the
gate to Endell Street.

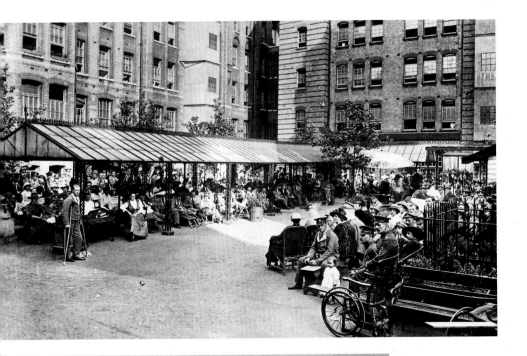

Bank holiday festivities for patients and families.

DAILY SKETCH.

GUARANTEED DAILY NETT SALE MORE THAN 1,000,000 COPIES.

No. 2,286.   LONDON, THURSDAY, JULY 6, 1916.   [Registered as a Newspaper.]   ONE HALFPENNY.

OUR WOUNDED HEROES IN WOMAN'S TENDER HANDS.

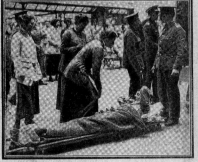

Women doctors busy taking particulars of the nature of their new patients' wounds.
—(Daily Sketch Photograph.)

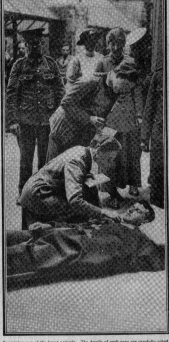

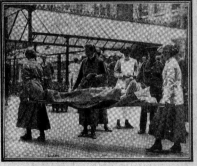

Wounded soldiers who have taken part in the great advance arriving at Endell-street Hospital, which is run entirely by women.—(Daily Sketch Photograph.)

Examining one of the latest arrivals. The details of each case are carefully noted before removal to the wards.—(Daily Sketch Photograph.)

Many of the wounded heroes of the great offensive have been brought straight from the battlefield to the Endell-street Hospital, where they are being doctored as well as nursed by women's tender hands. Staffed entirely by women, the hospital is doing a splendid work in the relief of our soldiers' sufferings. It is one of the most striking examples of the share which the women of Britain are taking in the war.

Casualties from the Somme arriving at Endell Street, pictured on the front page of the *Daily Sketch*, July 6, 1916.

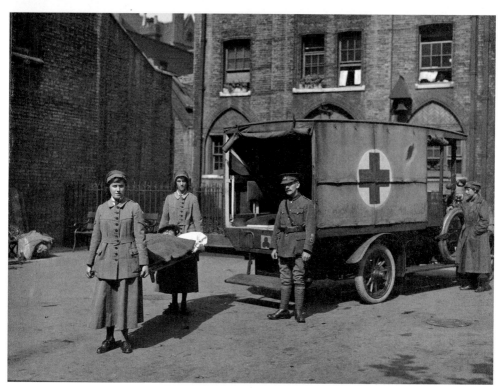

Women stretcher-bearers and Sergeant Major Harris in the Endell Street courtyard.
(COOK-DICKERMAN COLLECTION)

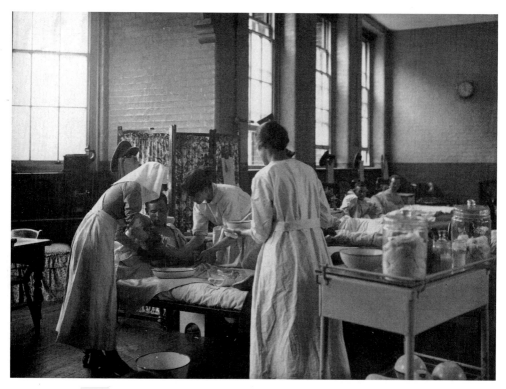

Ward scene. (COOK-DICKERMAN COLLECTION)

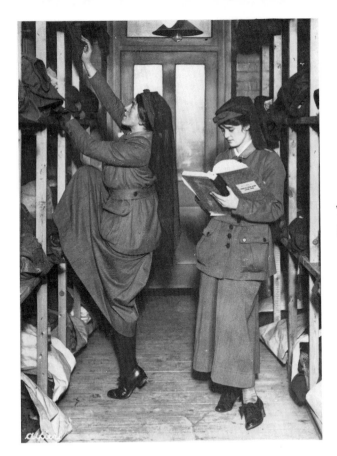

The linens room.
(ANDERSON FAMILY)

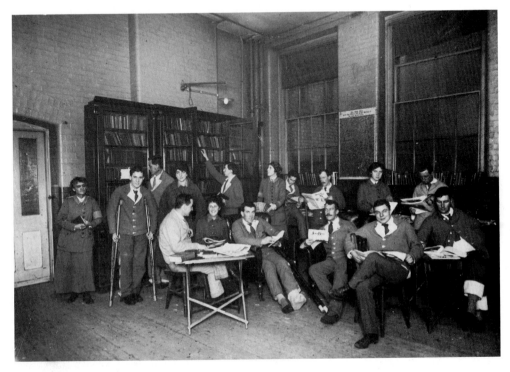

The library. (ANDERSON FAMILY)

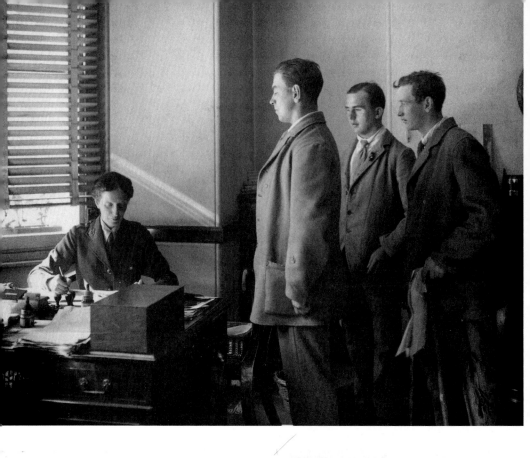

Flora Murray at her desk with men standing to attention beside her.

(COOK-DICKERMAN COLLECTION)

Louisa Garrett Anderson with dogs Garrett and William.

(ANDERSON FAMILY)

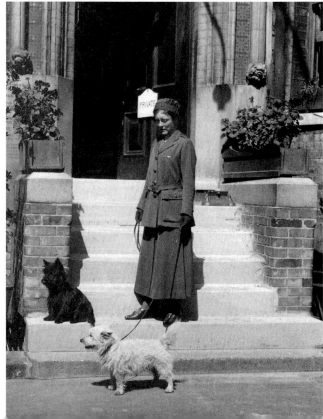

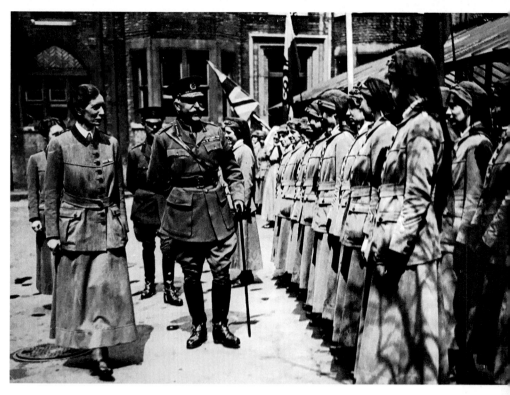

Sir Alfred Keogh with Flora Murray inspecting staff. (BY KIND PERMISSION OF ANDREW WELLS)

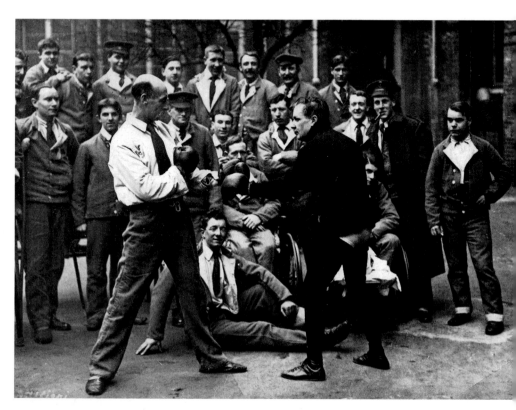

A boxing demonstration in the courtyard. (ANDERSON FAMILY)

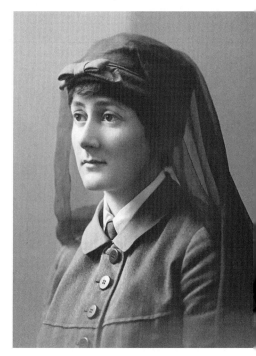

Nina Last.
(BY KIND PERMISSION OF ANNIE FOX)

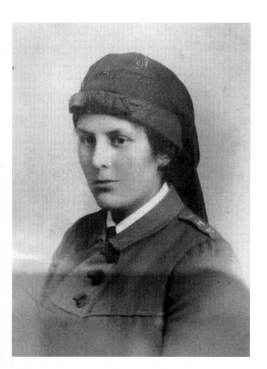

Barbara Last.
(BY KIND PERMISSION OF ANNIE FOX)

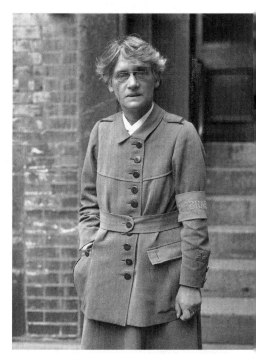

Beatrice Harraden.
(COOK-DICKERMAN COLLECTION)

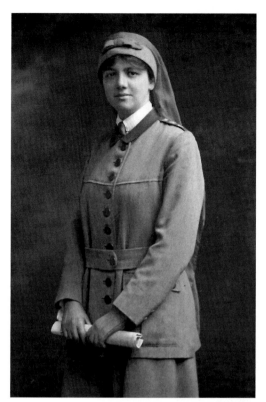

Dr. Frances Evelyn Windsor.
(BY KIND PERMISSION OF DIANA KIM
MCMILLAN)

Dr. Winifred Buckley.
(COOK-DICKERMAN COLLECTION)

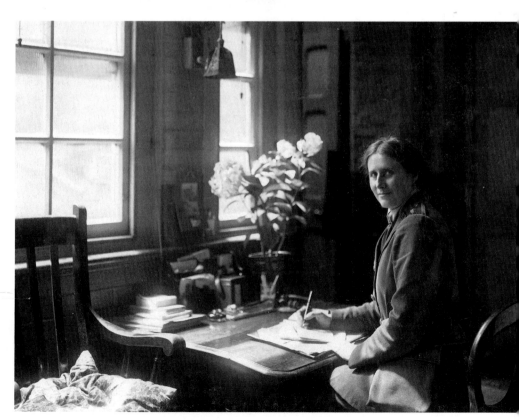

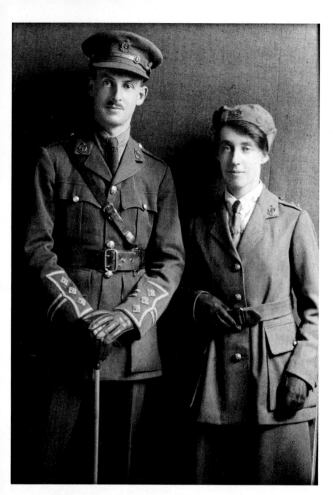

Dr. Vera Scantlebury with her brother Dr. George Clifford Scantlebury.

Nancy Cook (left) with Olga Campbell and patient.

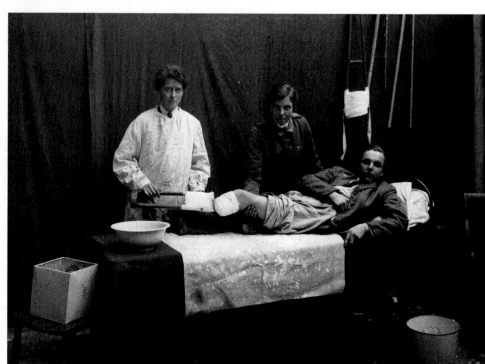

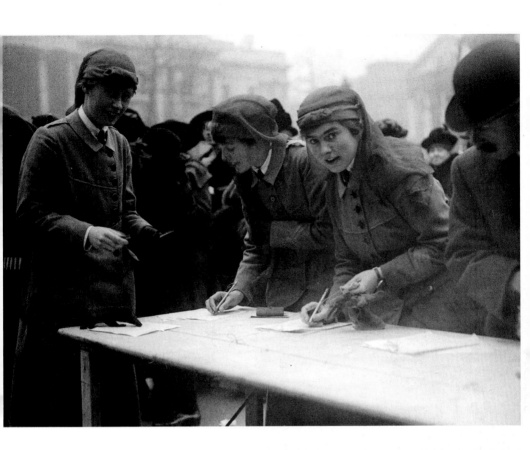

Endell Street orderlies buying war bonds in Trafalgar Square, 1917.

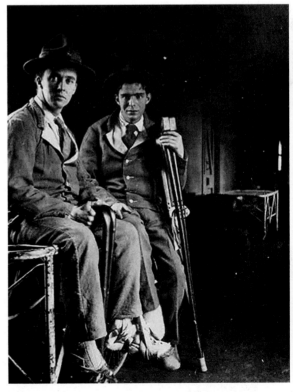

Ernest Beguely (right) with a fellow patient in their "hospital blues."

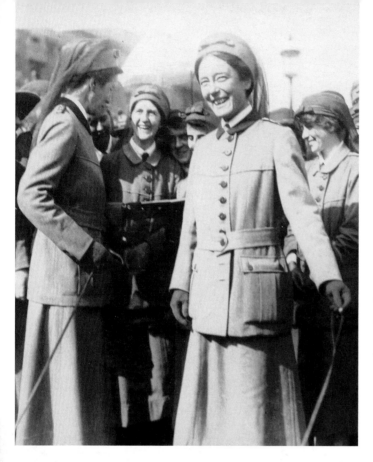

Flora Murray (left) and Louisa Garrett Anderson after receiving their CBEs at Buckingham Palace, 1917.
(ANDERSON FAMILY)

The Endell Street operating theater.
(COOK-DICKERMAN COLLECTION)

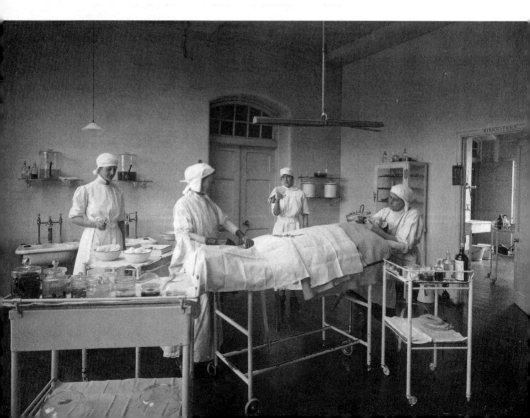

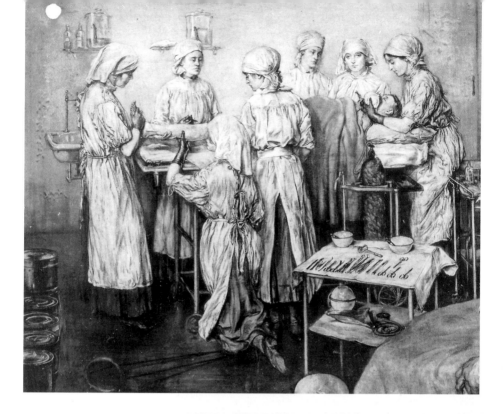

Pastel of the operating
theater, as depicted by
Austin Spare.

(IMPERIAL WAR MUSEUM,
PHOTOGRAPHS 7704-47)

*An Operation at the
Military Hospital,
Endell Street,* oil by
Francis Dodd.

(IMPERIAL WAR MUSEUM,
ART.IWM ART 4084)

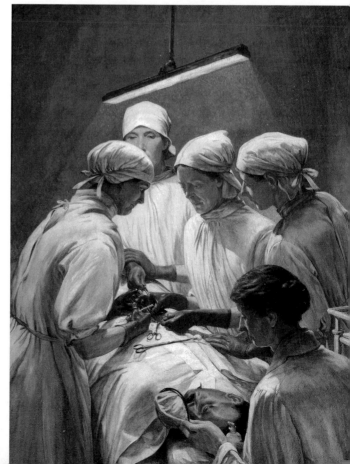

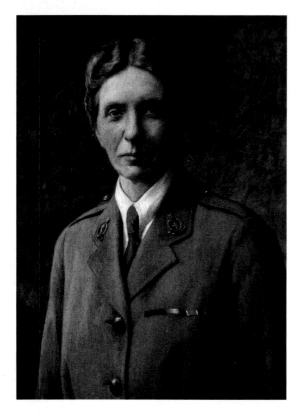

Flora Murray in her Endell
Street uniform, painted by
Francis Dodd, 1921.
(THE ARTIST'S ESTATE)

Louisa Garrett Anderson in
civilian clothes, painted by
Francis Dodd, 1921.
(THE ARTIST'S ESTATE)

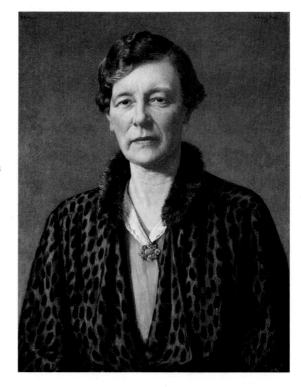

troops stationed in India to refer to home. Some men went so far as to feign illness or to inflict injuries on themselves—shooting themselves in the foot or putting their hands above the parapet were common methods—to escape the trenches, though they risked being executed for cowardice if they were found out. Endell Street received its share of self-inflicted injuries, frauds, and "malingerers," including one man who claimed he had lost an arm, but on inspection, by Anderson, was found to have "the usual number."[15]

Yet many soldiers dreaded receiving the "wrong" kind of wound even more than being killed.[16] The injuries feared most were those that caused a life-changing disability, such as the loss of one or more limbs, facial disfigurement, or damage to sexual functions. More than one million British men would suffer some form of permanent disability or sickness as a result of the war; about 240,000 suffered partial or total loss of one or more limbs, another 9,000 lost one eye, and nearly 800 were completely blinded.[17] Seventy percent of those who lost a limb were under the age of thirty. Many had joined the army at nineteen or even younger, relatively fit and with long working lives ahead of them; some were already married with young families, and others were hopeful of marrying in due course. To find themselves suddenly with a permanent disability or disfigurement was utterly devastating. Not only did such injuries limit their chances of making a living and leading normal lives, but they drastically damaged their self-esteem. Many amputees, in particular, felt emasculated and helpless, diminished by their lack of independence, and convinced they were no longer "real men." One man said that disabled soldiers—"with half our insides and half our limbs gone"—felt they no longer counted as men.[18] The scale of the perceived impact of different disabilities was reflected in the government's pension scheme, which began in 1915. Men suffering the loss of two limbs or more, the total loss of sight, or severe facial disfigurement received a 100 percent disability pension, while smaller pensions were awarded for losing one leg or one arm and other injuries.[19]

As the war progressed, medical services developed better rehabilitation therapies and more sophisticated prosthetic limbs to help men learn new skills and cope with their changed lives. Robert Jones, a surgeon who had previously treated dockers and ship workers with industrial injuries in Liverpool, set up a dedicated orthopedic hospital in west London in 1916. There, he established occupational activities such as embroidery—as at Endell Street—and "curative workshops," where the men learned skills such as carpentry and mechanics.[20] Some patients were even put to work making artificial limbs for future wounded soldiers. At the same time, surgeons such as New Zealand–born Harold Gillies pioneered revolutionary plastic surgery techniques to repair damaged faces.

While the reality of being wounded was gruesome and lonely, injured soldiers were still cast in a heroic light. The press played its role in promoting the wounded as romantic "heroes"—as in the *Sketch*'s front page—while the government exploited disabled soldiers in posters to maintain public commitment to the war and stir others to enlist. One soldier, who lost both legs, recalled how, before the war, the authorities had encouraged him to sign up, yet once the war had ended, the state had no use for him—but images of soldiers as symbols of patriotism proliferated. Some women were even moved to visit military hospitals looking for a wounded soldier to marry as a self-sacrifice born of patriotic duty or grief.

Many of the men who fought in the trenches spoke of the gulf they felt when they returned to their families on leave or were invalided out of the army, since it was strange to find civilian life continuing apparently as normal. Often, they felt more affinity with the enemy soldiers than with the people back home, who had no concept of trench warfare. Worse, although many were unable to repress memories of what they had witnessed, they could not talk about their experiences to loved ones. When the poet Robert Graves returned home after being severely injured at the Somme, he found serious conversation with his parents to be "all but impossible," and could not understand "the war-madness that ran wild everywhere."[21] Civilians "talked a foreign language; and it was newspaper language," he said.

The staff who nursed and treated these men perhaps came closest to bridging that gulf. They saw the men's filthy, lice-infested uniforms and their devastating injuries, they heard the stories of failed nerve and unexpected courage—sometimes they even over- heard the men talking in delirium, or as they came round from an- esthetic, of the horrors they had seen—and they smelled the trench mud. It was no wonder that the men formed strong bonds with the Endell Street staff. Many kept in touch long after they left the hospital and returned to the battlefield. Some would later write to Olga Campbell asking her to send them jerseys, socks, cakes, and even musical instruments to France or Salonika—as if they were sons writing home to their mothers. She always dispatched their parcels. As news of the hospital's work spread among the troops, some who were wounded even asked to be sent there. One man seriously wounded at the Somme specifically asked to be taken to Endell Street, saying, "They told me on the other side I'd be well looked after in here."[22]

MURRAY AND ANDERSON were well aware of the power of "news- paper language" both in maintaining national morale and in fur- thering their own ideals. Murray, in particular, always welcomed reporters and photographers to Endell Street, seeing it as a way of bolstering the cause for women doctors and women in general. Her choice of the *Daily Sketch* to cover the post-Somme rush was sig- nificant—the tabloid's populist appeal and wide circulation, which topped one million in 1916, made it ideal for disseminating her message to a wide audience—though she was open to newspapers of all shades and sizes.[23] The press swooped on Endell Street as a convenient celebratory antidote to the horrors of war, and Murray shrewdly manipulated this interest in order to serve her feminist ambitions.

A typical column in the *Tatler* in July described the "noble ladies who manage the Suffragette hospital in Endell Street" as a perfect example of the "New Woman" who was being born out of the war. Its doctors, nurses, and orderlies, it said, were all representatives of "the sex that has come into its own." Struggling to explain this new world order, the magazine exclaimed: "They are men in the best sense of that word, and yet women in the best sense of that word also." For some observers, this very visible change in women's lives carried a distinct sexual frisson. The *Daily Star* declared that of all the uniformed women in London, the "smartest and most delightfully impudent looking are those young Amazons who act as orderlies at the Endell-street Military Hospital." Often spotted "passing busily to and fro in Oxford-street, with a stop-me-if-you-dare expression," they maintained an air of "rather athletic independence" and looked "quite capable of catching up any unruly patient and carrying him bodily off to prison." Their attitude made clear, the writer said, that "this is no amateur hospital, though it may be run by mere women, and without masculine interference."[24]

Although the existence of a hospital run by "mere women" was still widely reported as a curiosity, gradually the work of women doctors was being taken seriously for the first time. An article in the *Daily Mail* in August described Endell Street as "one of the brightest havens in England." The piece, by a female journalist who had previously visited the corps at Claridge's in Paris, argued that Endell Street had disproved two commonly prevailing myths: it had demonstrated that surgical work was not too strenuous for women's physical endurance, and it had shown that it did not "[harden] their hearts or [make] callous their womanly sympathies." She even maintained, rather fancifully, that Anderson and Murray looked healthier after nearly two years as military doctors. Endell Street, she added, had "proved without doubt" that women doctors could go beyond treating women and children, as they were equal to their male counterparts in every field. The *Daily Telegraph* agreed. Pointing out that women were now performing numerous military jobs previously undertaken by men "short of the firing-line," it said there was "no better illustration of what women can do, and are doing, in war-time" than the work at Endell Street.

THE WAR, FOR all its atrocities, was bringing advances in medicine as well as advances for women. The vast number of casualties generated by the Somme campaign provided doctors with unprecedented opportunities to experiment and improve treatment in every field of medical care.[25] Bigger and better-equipped casualty clearing stations enabled surgeons to perform major operations close to the front line, and they developed new techniques to repair the wounds they encountered. Men with severe abdominal wounds and head injuries, who had previously been left to die, were now operated on, and many survived. Since most casualty clearing stations had gained X-ray machines by 1916, bullets and shrapnel could be located and removed more easily. Most surgeons had now adopted Henry Gray's method of excising all dead and damaged tissue so that gangrene had less chance to spread, although the practice was not yet uniform. Better splints were introduced to stabilize fractures during evacuation and recovery. After Robert Jones, the orthopedic surgeon, was appointed director of military orthopedics in early 1916, he championed the Thomas splint, which had been devised by his uncle, Hugh Owen Thomas, fifty years previously. First used in the summer of 1916, the apparatus would save thousands of lives, and amputation rates fell dramatically that same year. Deaths from compound fractured femurs fell from 80 percent in some units to less than 10 percent by the end of the war. Resuscitation methods to counter shock had also advanced enormously, while blood transfusion, first used in 1914, was slowly being more widely adopted. Since methods to store blood had not yet been developed, transfusions were direct from donor to patient, by tube or syringe. The blood was usually taken from less seriously wounded soldiers in the same medical unit, some rewarded with a pint of stout for each pint of blood.

As clinical expertise gradually improved, so medical care became more specialized. Wounded soldiers were categorized as soon as they arrived at Southampton and other ports in order to be sent to the most appropriate hospital for their injury.[26] Blind soldiers were sent to the 2nd London General Hospital in Chelsea, for example, while most men with shell shock went to the National Hospital in Queen Square or the 4th General Hospital in Denmark Hill, south London, where many were subjected to aversion therapy and electric shock treatment. Patients with head injuries and compound fractures were sent elsewhere. Demand for beds grew so intense during the Somme offensive and other big advances, however, that the wounded and sick were frequently sent to any hospital with spare beds. This meant that patients with shell shock, facial injuries, heart conditions, and myriad other ailments continued to arrive at Endell Street. But Endell Street was not only leading the way in employing women doctors: its doctors were also at the forefront of medical research.

HAVING PATCHED UP wounded troops since the outset of the war, Louisa Garrett Anderson was now at least as skilled in military surgery as the majority of army surgeons. As well as treating shell and gunshot wounds, which were often accompanied by fractured bones, Endell Street continued to admit large numbers of men with compound fractures, since three hundred of its beds were designated for orthopedic cases.[27] Anderson commonly had to join splintered bones with metal pins or plates, in addition to suturing damaged or severed nerves. Since steel helmets had become standard issue by the time of the Somme advance, head injuries had been vastly reduced, but Anderson still occasionally performed operations on the brain. One eminent surgeon, Sir John Bland-Sutton, visited Endell Street around 1916 to watch her perform a difficult cranial operation.[28] Surgery on the brain and skull was a relatively recent innovation, often performed under local anesthetic, because ether and chloroform made the brain swell. A veteran surgeon, Bland-Sutton had worked at a military hospital in south London since the outbreak of the war. Watching Anderson's nimble fingers at work, he complimented her on her dexterity. He was not the only male doctor coming to the realization that women's smaller hands might be better suited to intricate surgery than men's: army surgeon Frederick Treves, who had visited the women's corp at Claridge's, admired how Mary Scharlieb, now a gynecologist at the Royal Free, skillfully performed operations.[29]

In addition to Anderson's surgical prowess, staff at Endell Street had become adept at helping its wounded men recuperate. Arthur Campbell, Olga's father, was busier than ever crafting crutches and artificial limbs for amputees, and another volunteer had become renowned for her skill in making lightweight splints for upper arm fractures from *papier-mâché*. Ethel Magill, who had taken charge of the X-ray department in 1916, was an enthusiastic champion of massage and electrotherapy—essentially early physical therapy—to stimulate wasted muscles. As well as overseeing masseuses at Endell Street, who helped men with paralyzed limbs to regain movement and amputees to adapt to their artificial limbs, she trained women from other military hospitals in electrotherapy.[30]

For all the progress, the influx of patients from the Somme created unprecedented challenges. Staff were overwhelmed by the demands involved in treating septic wounds, which generally needed the dressings to be changed and wounds swabbed with antiseptic as often as every four hours to combat the spread of infection. For doctors, nurses, and patients, this frequent changing of dressings was "exhausting," said Murray. It was also excruciating for the patients. In some cases, the process of prising away the encrusted gauze from large, deep wounds was so painful it could only be done under general anesthesia. Both the length of time involved and the ineffectiveness of the antiseptic agents in use had prompted military doctors to search for alternatives.

In the first few months of the war, army surgeons had relied on the principles of asepsis they had learned in medical school, which entailed meticulously sterilizing instruments and wearing rubber gloves and face masks to prevent bacteria in the operating environment from invading wounds. As it quickly became apparent that most wounds obtained on the Western Front were already grossly infected with bacteria, they had to revert to an older system of wound treatment. This meant leaving the wound open and repeatedly applying antiseptic agents in an effort to destroy the bacteria present. But the antiseptics commonly available were either highly caustic or largely ineffective against such virulent microbes.

At one military hospital in Belgium, a French army surgeon, Alexis Carrel, teamed up with a British chemist, Henry Dakin, to test a new antiseptic agent and new method of application.[31] Their system used a dilute antiseptic containing sodium hypochlorite, known as Dakin's solution, to irrigate deep wounds by means of perforated rubber tubes embedded in the flesh. The wound was loosely covered with bandages before being closed several days later. The system, dubbed the Carrel-Dakin method, was gradually gaining acceptance among French and British army doctors by 1916 and seemed to improve recovery rates. But it was still extremely laborious, since the fluid had to be reapplied every few hours, and the dressings had to be changed daily.

An alternative system was advocated by the British pathologist Sir Almroth Wright, professor of pathology at St Mary's Hospital, Paddington, who had established a research laboratory in Boulogne with his protégé, a young doctor named Alexander Fleming. Wright's method involved continuous irrigation of the wounds using a simple salt solution, but this never caught on widely, owing partly to its disappointing results and partly to Wright's bombastic personality. (He was, among other things, a strident anti-suffragist, arguing that women's minds were "inferior and irrational.")

Anderson and pathologist Helen Chambers had taken a keen interest in treating septic wounds since Endell Street had opened— as their earlier *Lancet* paper testified. Dissatisfied with both the Carrel-Dakin and Wright methods, they were eager to try something different. The patients arriving in droves from the Somme provided the perfect guinea pigs. On July 8, 1916, three days after the first wounded soldiers arrived, Anderson tested a new antiseptic ointment for the first time.[32] The ointment, a bismuth, iodoform, and paraffin paste that became known as BIPP, had been invented by James Rutherford Morison, a surgeon at Northumberland War Hospital, who had tried it on some of his patients at the end of 1915. Impressed by the results, in June he asked Anderson and Chambers to trial BIPP on a larger cohort of patients at Endell Street.

Anderson and Chambers leapt on the request. Morison sent Chambers the formula, and she concocted the paste in her laboratory. Then Anderson chose the first candidate, a young unnamed private who had been wounded on the first day of the Somme and admitted to Endell Street on July 6. The man's foot had been severely mangled, most probably by a shell. Three of the five long bones were smashed, the heel bone was fractured, and the wound had become severely septic. It was so painful that when Anderson first saw him she was convinced there was no alternative but to amputate. Instead she decided to try her best to save his foot.

On July 8, the man was brought to the operating theater. Anderson first cut away all the damaged tissue and removed the bone fragments, then cleaned the wound thoroughly with methylated spirit (denatured alcohol) and iodine. Next she rubbed the raw tissues liberally with BIPP and smeared more paste into the cavity. After this, contrary to contemporary practice, she stitched the wound closed and left the dressings untouched for the next four days. To her surprise, when she then inspected the wound, it looked considerably better. So she continued with the same approach, applying BIPP and leaving the dressings in place for up to eight days at a time. Six weeks later, the soldier's foot had completely healed and he could walk unaided. It was a remarkable result: not only had the man's foot been saved, but he could return, undamaged, to normal life.

Encouraged by their success, Anderson and her surgical team adopted the BIPP method throughout July and August to treat septic wounds in some two hundred men who had been injured on the Somme battlefields. Their injuries ranged from shattered bones in the arms and legs to gaping wounds in the neck, scalp, chest, and torso. In every case, the sepsis subsided significantly or disappeared entirely. Fractured bones knitted together "with astonishing rapidity," and wounds healed with surprising speed. The patients included one soldier with a fractured bone and a deep septic wound in his upper arm. The bone began to mend and the injury to heal within three weeks. Another man had a gunshot wound to his right hand, which had been operated on in France but had become septic. His injury began to heal, and he could move his hand within four weeks. Only one of the two hundred patients suffered any ill-effects from BIPP, developing a fever as a result of the paste's potentially toxic effects, but he recovered as soon as the dose was reduced. Many of the men returned to full or light duties in active military service. Reporting the results on six of her first patients to *The Lancet* in September, Anderson concluded that BIPP saved patients "a great deal of pain and exhaustion." The results were "incomparably better," she said, than any other method she had tried. The article was one of the first scientific research papers ever published by a woman doctor, one of seven such papers published by doctors from Endell Street.

Abandoning other methods, Anderson adopted BIPP universally at Endell Street. Since dressings could be left unchanged for as long as twenty-one days, the new approach reduced time spent changing bandages by as much as 80 percent. It "metamorphosed" the work of the hospital, said Murray. For the first time, work on the wards became manageable. The following March, Anderson and Chambers would publish results in *The Lancet* for more than four hundred patients treated with BIPP, including detailed case studies of sixty-two men in which the majority had healed.

Anderson was convinced that BIPP was superior to the Carrel-Dakin method. The latter used a more powerful antiseptic, yet it had to be frequently reapplied because its effect was transitory. BIPP, she argued, was the way forward for wound treatment. Keen to promote BIPP widely, Anderson would later describe a series of successful case studies—complete with X-ray pictures—to fellow women doctors.[33] In one case she used BIPP to treat a nineteen-year-old boy with an abscess in the frontal lobe of his brain, who made an "excellent" recovery. In another, a man with both legs fractured—who was "pouring out pus and with a high temperature"—healed completely after being treated with BIPP.

Championed by both Anderson and Morison, BIPP soon attracted the attention of army doctors elsewhere. As news of the experiments at Endell Street reached the War Office, Sir Alfred Keogh was even prompted to visit in the autumn of 1916.[34] After meeting staff on parade in the courtyard, Keogh toured the wards. Anderson produced one patient after another whose wounds had healed, and Keogh declared himself convinced that BIPP should be used more widely. It was a proud moment. Keogh would not have time to visit Endell Street again, but at the end of his tour he turned to Anderson and said, "I knew you could do it." He added, "We were watched, but you have silenced all critics."

Throughout the rest of the course of the war, BIPP would be widely adopted by surgeons in army hospitals at home and at the front. According to Morison, more than half the patients arriving at his Northumberland hospital by 1918 had already had their wounds "bipped" and on occasions "rebipped."[35] Opinions remained sharply divided, however, as to whether BIPP was truly superior to the Carrel-Dakin system or other methods. While some surgeons were adamant that the Carrel-Dakin method was the most effective wound treatment, others argued that BIPP was equally successful and considerably less time-consuming. Whatever their relative merits, BIPP continued to be used during the Second World War and later. Even today—a hundred years after its first trial at Endell Street—it remains in daily use by surgeons performing ear, nose, and throat procedures, as well as procedures in neurosurgery and maxillofacial surgery.[36]

THROUGHOUT THE REMAINDER of 1916, the convoys of wounded arrived with grim regularity as the Somme offensive faltered on into November. But if the strains on staff were reduced by the introduction of BIPP, their anxieties were now exacerbated by the renewed threat of Zeppelins. The German airships—which by now had increased in size and power—had briefly reappeared in the skies over the London suburbs in March and again in August. Then, in the early hours of September 3, sixteen Zeppelins were spotted crossing the east coast heading for London. One succeeded in reaching the capital. Barbara Last was asleep in her dormitory after another hectic day on her ward when she woke up to a deafening noise.[37] She leapt out of bed in the pitch black and quickly pulled her uniform on over her nightwear, ready to help carry patients from the top floor down to the basement. She knew most of the 150 men in the upper wards were unable to walk. Petrified by the droning noise, one of the other orderlies began to cry. But even as Barbara was still searching for her stockings, the window was suddenly lit up by a blaze of light. The airship had been hit by a British airplane and was brought down in flames over Hertfordshire.

Barbara was disappointed not to see the Zeppelin plummet to the ground—it was the first German airship to be destroyed by British air defenses—since her window faced the wrong way. But she could hear people in the streets cheering and bells ringing. The night nurses and patients on the north side of the hospital, who had a better view of it, were thrilled by the spectacle. The men were "mad with excitement" as they saw the "Zepp in flames in the sky," Barbara wrote home. She added a sketch showing the course of the airship as it had looped close to the hospital.

Her sister Nina was on duty that night when an enormous convoy of wounded arrived half an hour after the Zeppelin had been downed. "It was a most impressive sight to see all of us out there clad in rather a funny way—all with night dresses on somewhere & caps thrust on to hide pigtails," she wrote. The COs, Murray and Anderson, were in the courtyard as usual—"& cheered us on & worked too." It was 3:30 a.m. before Nina got to bed. Eleanor Bourne, the Australian doctor, had watched the Zeppelin fall flaming to the ground from the roof of the hotel where she lodged near Oxford Street. The next morning, she arrived at Endell Street to find that a piece of shrapnel had come through the roof of one of her wards. Luckily, nobody had been injured.

Three weeks later, during the night of September 23–24, three Zeppelins brought destruction to central London—killing twenty-six people and starting thirty fires—before two of them were shot down. Barbara Last was called up again in the night in case the men needed to be evacuated. "We heard them buzzing about around us but there was not much firing & we could not see them," she said. After the beginning of October, when another airship was destroyed by British aircraft, the Zeppelins were just about vanquished—though worse was to come.

Even if the Zeppelins had been all but banished, the workload was no easier. Barbara was again on duty in October when a convoy of twenty-six wounded arrived on her ward at once. The unpredictability was the worst thing, she told her father. "It is much better for one or two to come in every day than none for ten days & then about a dozen during the next two," she said, adding, "One can easily cope with 8 new cases at once in one's ward but 26 is rather a handful."[38]

The relentless physical demands, coupled with the emotional trauma of tending the Somme wounded, were exhausting for all the staff, but especially for their chief officers. Murray and Anderson worked with scarcely a break throughout the second half of 1916. Up early every morning for clinical conferences, followed by ward rounds and long operating sessions, they were frequently roused in the night by the bell announcing another convoy. Like the matron, the nurses, and most of the orderlies, Murray and Anderson continued to live in the hospital building. The other surgeons, at least, stayed in lodgings elsewhere, but they took turns being on duty as the "orderly officer" for twenty-four hours every eight days. During these shifts, when they slept at the hospital, the duty surgeon visited every ward between 11:00 p.m. and midnight, dealt with emergencies that arose during the night, and took responsibility for admitting the convoys.

Any chance to escape, even for a few hours, was relished. When Barbara Last was given a day's leave to attend a funeral in October, she was delighted at the rare chance to see her family and get away from "poky smutty old Endell St" to the country air. "All the men said I looked 3 years younger when I got back," she told her father, though she admitted that was "hardly appropriate considering I had been to a funeral."[39]

APPROACHING WINTER FINALLY brought the suicidal Somme assaults to an end on November 18. By that point more than 130,000 British soldiers had been killed and another 300,000 wounded, many of them permanently disabled, with scarcely any strategic gain. The offensive, which lasted four and a half months, had been the longest and most destructive battle in British history. Although the Germans had been weakened by having to fight on two fronts, the Somme offensive had largely failed. With the morass of mud now turning to ice, further fighting was impossible, and so the year was about to end as it began: in total stalemate, with victory as far away as ever. Taking stock back home, British civilians had been temporarily cheered by the fact that the skies had been freed of the terror-inspiring Zeppelins. But now they faced a long, dark winter of increasing food shortages, restrictions on movement, and curtailment of pleasure.

At Endell Street, the women were drained and dejected, but at least—although the wounded still arrived—there was a chance to rest, or to become ill themselves. Beatrice Harraden found solace in a trip to Cornwall in November.[40] She took a seaside break—to "collect my senses," she said—although the time off failed to have the desired effect, since soon after returning to Endell Street she fell sick with "flue" and was ill for several weeks. Despite her long hours running the library, Harraden had completed her latest novel, *The Guiding Thread*, which had been published in September. She returned to her post in December, when she told Elizabeth Robins—now back in England—that Flora Murray had been "very cordial" in asking after her.[41]

As the army set about recruiting more men to replace those thousands lost, so Endell Street took on reinforcements, too. A Canadian surgeon, Frances Evelyn Windsor, was already well-traveled by the time she arrived at Endell Street in late 1916.[42] A brilliant scholar who had graduated from high school at age fourteen, she had studied medicine at the Women's Medical College in Toronto. Since she was barred from hospital posts in Canada, being female, she had gained experience as a junior surgeon in Baltimore, Pennsylvania, and Detroit. After touring Europe, she had returned home in 1911 to set up practice with a fellow woman doctor in Calgary. As the only two women doctors in the frontier town, they took her colleague's mother along as a chaperone. When war broke out, Windsor had enlisted in the Canadian Army Medical Corps as a nurse—since women doctors were barred. She therefore became the first female doctor to join the Canadian Army, even if she was limited to nursing. Once she arrived in England and her credentials were discovered, the twenty-nine-year-old Windsor was hastily transferred to Endell Street. She started work toward the end of the year.

Another recruit, who joined Endell Street in November 1916 as an orderly, was equally well-traveled. Born into a wealthy family in Brisbane, Australia, Kath Ussher had studied art in Leipzig, London, and Chicago before sailing with her mother from America to England in 1915, spurred to support the war effort by news of the Australian casualties at Gallipoli. While her mother, a keen suffragette, helped pack parcels for war babies, Ussher worked as a secretary for the Royal Australian Navy. She spent her weekends volunteering in a munitions factory and her evenings as a volunteer ambulance driver.[43] When she heard that volunteers were needed at Endell Street, Ussher, who was twenty-five, lost no time applying. She moved into the hospital soon after.

Like Nina Last when she first started, Ussher lugged huge bins of ashes and soiled dressings to the incinerator each morning and helped carry patients between the wards and the operating theater in the afternoon, as well as emptying bedpans and giving bed baths. In her "humble capacity" as an orderly, she was in awe of the Australian women surgeons and said they did "brilliant work."[44] Her sleep was frequently interrupted as convoys continued to arrive from France. Woken by the bell one night in dark December, Ussher lined up shivering with her fellow orderlies in the courtyard at 2:00 a.m. as they waited for what seemed like hours. The orderly officer on duty eventually took pity on the women with their chattering teeth and numbed fingers, and they were allowed to wait in the dingy outpatients department until the tinkling gate bell signaled the arrival of the ambulances "bearing their shattered human burden."

It was little wonder that Ussher dreamed longingly of Sydney as the British winter ground on. Surrounded by the "soot-blackened buildings" of foggy London, she pictured her home city "set like a jewel in its haven of liquid sapphire." Despite the privations, she never questioned her choice. Interviewed in later life, she said, "Well, you felt you were doing your bit. That is all there was to it." Her Endell Street experience did not put her off hospital work. After six months, Ussher followed a friend abroad to a Scottish Women's Hospitals unit in Salonika, where she worked for another six months. The ranks of women swelled even further in late 1916, when 14 of the RAMC men at Endell Street were replaced by 13 women.[45] Only 8 of the total 176 staff members were now male.

The war was at a standstill, but women were advancing on every front. When Queen Mary opened the new extension at the LSMW in October 1916, the medical school was heralded as one of the largest in London, with a record 380 students enrolled.[46] Since Elizabeth Garrett Anderson, its erstwhile dean, was now too frail to attend, Louisa and her brother, Alan, represented her. A telegram from 30 of the school's former students, now serving as surgeons with the army in Malta, sent congratulations. In November the army appealed for a further 50 women doctors to join the 80 already sent abroad.[47] That same month the Medical Research Committee, founded in 1913 as the forerunner of the Medical Research Council, paid tribute to medical women in its annual report.[48] More than 20 women were undertaking important work in pathology, it noted, while women were making strides in other areas of scientific research as well, including the BIPP trials at Endell Street. Sir Donald MacAlister, president of the General Medical Council, warmly sang the praises of women doctors taking on war work at the GMC's meeting that month and called on all female practitioners to join them.[49]

In December, the jubilee of the New Hospital for Women, founded fifty years previously by Elizabeth Garrett Anderson, turned into a celebration of women doctors' war work. The loudest praise came from Sir Alfred Keogh, who applauded the work of Endell Street as a model of medical women's achievements.[50] He made a rousing call for all medical schools and hospitals to open their doors to women "on exactly the same terms as men," and declared unequivocally that whether as surgeons or physicians, women were "the equal of men." Since her mother was still too ill to attend, Anderson made an emotional speech, appealing to women to strive for the education and experience they needed to achieve their ambitions. Quoting the words of Walt Whitman, her favorite poet, she urged: "We take up the task eternal, and the burden and the lesson, Pioneers, O Pioneers!"

Women could have been forgiven for thinking they were close to winning their battle for equal rights—in medicine at least. Looking back over the struggles of the first women to qualify in medicine, the *Daily Telegraph* asked why a profession eminently suited to women's capabilities had kept its doors "resolutely banged and barred" for so long.[51] Confident that those barriers were now down, it asserted: "When a revolution has succeeded, it is no longer called a revolution, but a reform." The *Manchester Guardian* agreed, declaring the Endell Street experiment a "conspicuous success."[52]

Yet the doors were still "banged and barred" in many places. Although the London Hospital added seven women doctors to its staff in November, most of the capital's medical schools still excluded women. In an angry letter to the *Daily Chronicle*, Elizabeth Robins, back in full-blooded campaigning mode, pointed out that many women doctors active in war work had gained their postgraduate experience in "enemy" hospitals, owing to the boycott of women by hospitals in Britain.[53] Women, as Anderson made clear, did not want special treatment—only "a fair field and no favour."[54] And that December, when Murray gave evidence to a government committee on women's war work, she was at pains to emphasize that Endell Street was doing war work—not "women's war work"—on exactly the same basis as men.[55] Earlier in the day, Colonel Arthur Blenkinsop, deputy director of the RAMC, had told the inquiry that despite the fact that women had replaced men in more than six thousand posts in military hospitals in Britain, women's abilities were strictly limited. Women were unable to work in mental hospitals, he said, or hospitals for "various forms of contagious diseases"—a euphemism for venereal disease, a growing problem in the army—and were incapable of significant heavy lifting. The women doctors who had joined the army in Malta could only perform some two-thirds of the work of men, he maintained. This estimate, he admitted, was based on "hearsay" from an American industrialist he knew. Furthermore, women needed special lavatories and sleeping quarters in army barracks.

Not surprisingly, after hearing Blenkinsop's words of wisdom, Murray was rather curt. Answering questions in her no-nonsense manner, very much in the mode of a typical army major, she said, "The Military hospital at Endell Street is exactly like every other military hospital." Its staff dealt with exactly the same cases as elsewhere, she explained, for "there is no distinction drawn when convoys are sent in." Asked by Sir George Newman, the surgeon chairing the committee, whether she believed there was any case of a sick or wounded soldier who could not be "fitly and appropriately and efficiently" treated at Endell Street, she insisted there was not. When he inquired how many men objected to being treated by female doctors, she could not recollect a single one. Newman was not giving up so easily, however. When he pressed Murray on whether she truly believed a hospital staffed by women doctors was "a sound and safe proposition," she retorted, "Absolutely." Tested further, Murray argued that women were "perfectly suitable" as stretcher-bearers and would be quite capable of working at base hospitals and on ambulance trains in France.

Murray could speak from her own experience. "I did no stretcher bearing myself until I went to France," she said, "but I have done a good deal since then." Indeed, she had recently replaced fourteen men with thirteen women because she knew she would get "better work" from the women. She even argued that women could easily run and staff hospitals for men with venereal disease without any embarrassment to the patients. She was cautious about the future, however. Asked by one committee member whether she hoped she was not just running a hospital but "building for a wider application of that ideal elsewhere," she replied, "I think sufficient unto the day." There was still much to prove.

Murray and Anderson invited the committee to watch a demonstration of women stretcher-bearing at Endell Street. Moreover, they were instrumental in bringing together the two women who would jointly run the army's first dedicated unit for women, the Women's Army Auxiliary Corps (WAAC). Mona Chalmers-Watson, a doctor who was Anderson's cousin, was given the task of setting up the corps in early 1917. But since Chalmers-Watson felt unable to leave her two young sons to work in France, Anderson rang a friend from her suffragette days, Helen Gwynne-Vaughan, who now headed the botany department at London's Birkbeck College, and suggested the pair should share the job. Recently widowed and desperately lonely, Gwynne-Vaughan jumped at the chance. After meeting each other in Murray and Anderson's sitting room at Endell Street, the pair would become joint heads of the WAAC.[56]

AS 1916 ENDED, there was little to celebrate in Britain. Rising food prices and shortages of food and coal, coupled with the Somme disaster, had forced Asquith to resign in early December, to be replaced as prime minister by David Lloyd George. With concerns focused particularly on the scarcity of bread, Anderson's brother, Alan, had already been recruited to oversee a royal commission on wheat supplies. As temperatures plummeted and London was cloaked in fog, people braced themselves for one of the worst winters on record. Cynthia Asquith, the daughter-in-law of the now ex-prime minister, was reduced to wearing her fur coat at breakfast. Few felt inclined to indulge in the usual seasonal festivities.

Nothing, however, could deter the women at Endell Street. Staff, volunteers, and patients combined forces to make Christmas, the second at Endell Street, the best and brightest so far.[57] The recuperating men excelled in the now annual competition to decorate their wards despite the wartime austerity. The patients on St Perpetua ward, who were mostly sailors, transformed their room into a mock warship, complete with guns, flags, and a lifeboat. They dressed in naval uniforms, while Winifred Buckley, the ward's medical officer, donned a commander's cap and jacket over a long sparkly skirt. In spare hours the patients busied themselves making wooden toys as presents for the children at the Harrow Road hospital.[58]

On Christmas morning, the men woke early to the sound of singing as a procession of orderlies, clothed in white sheets and crowned with holly, carried lanterns through the wards to light their way in the blackout as they sang carols. After opening their stockings at the ends of their beds, the men tucked into Christmas dinner at long tables in their wards. In the darkening afternoon, the men braved the cold to test their skills at coconut shies and other fairground games in the glow of fairy lights adorning the courtyard. To cap the revels, Bessie Hatton's loyal troupe of actors reprised their performance of Aladdin, the costumes even more elaborate—and the jokes more outlandish—than before.

There was little time to enjoy the festivities. After the shortest of lulls, the New Year would bring more devastation to the Western Front, more convoys to Endell Street, and more air raids to London.

8

The March of the Women

Melbourne, Australia, February 14, 1917

Vera Scantlebury stepped on board the RMS *Morea* for the ten-thousand-mile voyage to the other side of the world with no clear idea of what lay ahead.[1] She had been born in a mining town in southeastern Australia, where her father was a family doctor and her mother a postmistress; soon after, she and her parents had moved to a quiet suburb of Melbourne, where her father's medical practice prospered and three more children arrived. Scantlebury grew especially close to her brother Cliff, who was fifteen months her junior. A family photograph shows them standing together, the serious big sister and mischievous little brother, aged about two and three.

Bright and popular, Scantlebury had been appointed head girl at her high school before enrolling to study medicine at the University of Melbourne in 1907. There she met Rachel Champion, and the pair became good friends. When she graduated seven years later, Scantlebury was one of only four women among fifty-seven students. In her first job, at Melbourne Hospital, she was the only woman on the medical team, and a year later she became the first female doctor in fourteen years at Melbourne Children's Hospital. Soon promoted to senior medical officer, Scantlebury was proud of her work and looked forward to a career in pediatrics. She was also in love with a fellow doctor named Frank Kingsley Norris, who was not only her junior in age but also in rank; the pair had become secretly engaged. War, however, changed all her plans.

The war, which began four months after Scantlebury finished medical school, saw most of her male colleagues leave for Europe, so that almost all the doctors in the hospital where she worked were now female. Most of her male friends from medical school, as well as Cliff, who had followed her into medicine, had enlisted as doctors in the Australian Army and were serving near the front line. Even Norris, her unofficial fiancé, had served briefly as a hospital orderly in Gallipoli before returning home to finish his studies. Scantlebury, now twenty-seven, no longer wanted to be left behind. Since the Royal Australian Army Medical Corps (RAAMC) did not accept women doctors, she had put her name forward to join her friend Champion at Endell Street. An October 1916 letter from Flora Murray offered her a six-month contract as an assistant surgeon, paid at the same rate as a lieutenant in the RAMC. Scantlebury did not need asking twice; she paid the £129 passage herself. As the *Morea* steamed out of Melbourne on its six-week voyage, she embarked on a journey that would form one of the defining experiences of her life.

After navigating the Suez Canal, the ship threaded through the Mediterranean, dodging German U-boats on its way to Marseille. Feeling homesick, Scantlebury began to wonder whether she had made the right decision. As she traveled through France by train she heard the distant guns of the front line. Arriving in Boulogne, she headed straight for No. 13 Stationary Hospital—the old Sugar Store Hospital, now based in huts beside the sea—to look for Cliff. He had enlisted in early 1915, and the pair had not seen each other for over two years. When she heard he had been posted a week earlier to a casualty clearing station near the front she almost wept. Pressing on, Scantlebury crossed the Channel to arrive in London at the beginning of April. Her first impressions were not good.

Having left sleepy Melbourne, with its salty air and exotic flora, at the height of the Australian summer, Scantlebury found London noisy, dirty, smelly, and—even in April—bitterly cold. She was shocked by the number of buses and taxis hurtling through the streets, and the London fog was so dense she almost choked.[2] The city seemed overrun by women, striding in military-style uniforms and barking orders as they clipped tickets on the buses and directed crowds on the Tube. Everywhere, people seemed burdened by depression. Scantlebury was somewhat cheered when an Australian friend took her on a whirlwind tour of the sights from the top of a London bus, and relieved when she saw her old friend Rachel Champion—"Ray"—waiting on a street corner. After a hasty lunch catching up, Champion took her to Endell Street.

The weather had turned wet and gray. And Scantlebury's first sight of the hospital did not improve her mood. The wards seemed enormous and gloomy after her bright, sunny children's wards in Melbourne, and the soldiers in their beds were "huge and uninteresting" compared to the babies and children she normally tended. All the staff looked weary, and when they stressed the "tremendous amount of work" to be done, she wondered what she had let herself in for. She had already decided that the uniform, which she had to pay for herself, was "hideous," with its "silly little cap" and flimsy veil.

When she was ushered in to meet the two COs, her spirits sank further. They were "two pale-faced thin women" with austere manners and strident views, she told her family in letters home. Scantlebury launched into a nervous diatribe on the folly of women traveling except for wartime purposes and was met with a blank silence followed by a tart riposte from one of them. After the informal Melbourne society in which Scantlebury had grown up, the two women seemed aloof, imperious—and distinctly British. So when they asked whether she could start work immediately, Scantlebury floundered. Dismayed by her tour of the wards and the severity of her bosses, she said she could not possibly start until May 1.

Beating a hasty retreat, Scantlebury spent the next three weeks touring the English countryside and exploring London. Then she moved her belongings into new "diggings," a bedsitting room in a house in Wimpole Street belonging to an aural surgeon named Octavia Lewin, as Murray had recommended. The second-floor room provided only a single bed, a gas fire, and a kettle, but at least it was quiet and the communal meals were decent. She even managed to meet up with Cliff, who had wangled ten days' leave to join her. They spent a glorious day in Oxford rowing on the river and strolling through the colleges, then threw themselves into a giddy round of London theaters, shops, and restaurants.

Reporting for duty on April 30—she had compromised that far—Scantlebury joined Endell Street two weeks before its second anniversary. Her arrival meant that four of the hospital's sixteen doctors were now Australian. As the newest, least-experienced, and second-youngest doctor on the staff, Scantlebury became one of six assistant surgeons helping Anderson with operations and ward rounds. She was not the only new recruit. Physician and founding corps member Louisa Woodcock had died of pneumonia, possibly contracted through her hospital work.[3] The fifty-seven-year-old Woodcock had been replaced by Margaret Thackrah, a physician—and suffragist—who was thirty-seven. There was little time for mourning. For as Scantlebury had been warned, there was, undoubtedly, a "tremendous amount of work" to do.

THE EARLY MONTHS of 1917, when the battlefields of the Western Front were icebound, were relatively quiet. But the Allies had been eager to launch a major spring offensive, which they felt sure would bring about a quick and decisive end to the war.[4] Since the disaster of the Somme, the British Army had trained new troops—including the first conscripts—and developed new shells and fuses that could cut barbed wire. Detailed surveillance of German defenses was now being provided by the army's Royal Flying Corps. But the Germans had not been idle either. In February, German troops had begun a planned withdrawal to a significantly stronger and shorter front several miles farther north known as the Hindenburg Line, leaving a trail of destruction and booby traps in their wake. Following the retreating Germans over old battlegrounds, Allied troops had to rebuild roads, railways, and bridges as well as establishing new depots and medical units.

Hopes for a speedy victory in France were made all the more imperative by fears that the Russian allies, who were fighting the Germans on the Eastern Front, might soon surrender in the unrest seeded by the revolution in March 1917. A Russian armistice would allow the Germans to relocate more forces to France. And although the Americans had finally entered the fray, declaring war on Germany in April and arriving in some thousands on French soil from June, it would be another year before US soldiers were involved in their first major offensive. Meanwhile, mutinous uprisings were spreading among French troops demoralized by the long campaign, so that the onus on British, Canadian, and ANZAC forces was heavier than ever. Beginning in sleet and snow on April 9, the Allies' new offensive on the Western Front would bring thousands more casualties to the gates of Endell Street throughout 1917.

ARRIVING FOR HER first shift on the last day of April, as casualties were flooding back to London from assaults at Vimy Ridge and Scarpe Valley, Vera Scantlebury was thrown in at the deep end. Since she was accustomed mainly to treating babies and children, she had little experience of adult male patients and none of military surgery—just like Murray and Anderson in their early days. Yet on day one she assisted Anderson at more than twenty operations and was put in charge of a surgical ward. The following day she performed three operations herself, two on men who were "very ill." Five days later, on May 4, she experienced her first convoy.

Sleeping at the hospital for her first night duty after a busy day's work, Scantlebury was woken up at 4:30 a.m. by the clanging bell in the courtyard. She fell back asleep while waiting for the second bell, until she heard a voice asking if she wanted tea. Assuming it was one of the sisters, she muttered a refusal. It was Flora Murray, standing by her bed with a cup of tea in her hand. Sheepishly, Scantlebury followed Murray down to the courtyard, where the orderlies and nurses were already lined up waiting in the dark. Four ambulances then rumbled in, bearing sixteen wounded men from France. The men had stood the journey well, she thought; many were smoking cigarettes. As she helped Murray examine the new arrivals, she felt humbled by her first direct brush with the war and hoped "that I can do enough for these soldiers."

The pattern of Scantlebury's life was set.[5] After breakfast at Wimpole Street, she arrived at Endell Street at 9:00 a.m. for the daily conference led by Anderson, when the orderly officer finishing her night duty reported on any worrying cases. The rest of the morning was spent on her ward rounds and supervising wound dressings before a break at noon for lunch. After returning to her lodgings or meeting with friends to share a meal, Scantlebury was back at 2:00 p.m. for the afternoon's operating list. When the workload was heavy, as it frequently was in 1917, she might not finish until after 7:30 p.m. And every eight days, she served as orderly officer for the night shift. Yet despite the routine, she could not settle to the work.

From her first day, Scantlebury worried that she was inadequate to the surgical challenges. She had only been put in charge of one ward, rather than the two she had been promised, and was convinced this was because the COs doubted her competence. Writing to her fiancé, Frank Norris, she confided, "Never in my life have I felt more a failure and ignoramus nor yet so tired and depressed." She feared she was clumsy in the operating theater—her "fingers all thumbs"—and added: "I feel it is almost beyond me. I have not the brains or the knowledge or the capacity and I am beginning to wonder about the physical strength!" It was "rather hard to learn military surgery in three days," she reflected. Indeed it was.[6]

As the weeks passed, Scantlebury continued to be beset by doubts about her abilities and anxious about impressing her formidable bosses. Murray was "very clever—tall pale thin—but I like her," while Anderson was "also pale" and "quite English," she wrote to her parents.[7] "They both work like slaves. Put me to shame." She was in awe of her Australian compatriots, too, especially Rachel Champion and Elizabeth Hamilton-Browne, who had both been promoted to the rank of captain. Hamilton-Browne had "an absolutely brilliant record," Scantlebury wrote, having come third in her final year at medical school, and enjoyed the "confidence of experience." In addition to her work at Endell Street, she was in charge of one of the auxiliary hospitals. Her friend Champion was not only "very good" at her work but also "extremely popular." Scantlebury was impressed by Evelyn Windsor as well. A "sweet Canadian girl" with a bright smile and "slightly casual manner," Windsor was kept busy administering anesthetics. Winifred Buckley, the third captain, who lodged in the same house as Scantlebury, was harder to get to know. She was a "nice steady serious girl wrapped up in her work and very seriously minded," but she looked "tired out" all the time, said Scantlebury. After one shift they walked back to their lodgings together in silence because Buckley—"We all address each other by our surnames"—was so exhausted she could not speak and just hummed a tune. It was not surprising Buckley was tired; while Scantlebury managed one ward, Buckley was in charge of two and a half.

As she struggled with the relentless workload, the difficult surgeries, and the strange customs so far from home, Scantlebury was at times on the verge of giving up. But, slowly and fitfully, she began to gain confidence, and even, eventually, to enjoy life at Endell Street—thanks to the discreet nurturing and subtle encouragement of her two COs. When her patients improved, for example, Anderson congratulated her. Scantlebury enjoyed the praise and proudly reported on it amid a litany of anxieties in long, gossipy letters to her family. "I have the greatest admiration and respect for these two women," she wrote home. "They have struggled against fearful odds and have succeeded beyond all expectations against the greatest prejudice." For all their faults, they would "both go to heaven and have crowns and golden harps."[8]

Impressed as she was by her bosses, though, Scantlebury was initially exasperated by their preoccupation with women's suffrage. Since women in Australia had enjoyed the vote for fifteen years, Scantlebury had little concept of—and even less interest in—the suffrage campaign and its struggles in Britain. She gleefully described herself as working in a "nest" of radicals and told her family their "innocent harmless little daughter" was "in the midst of the very militant suffragettes." After Murray lectured her on the suffrage campaign on one occasion, Scantlebury grumbled, "Somehow or other we always get around to that subject again."[9]

Her attitude shifted slightly, however, when she accompanied Murray on a visit to the auxiliary Dollis Hill Hospital and, as they drove past Holloway Prison, Murray described Anderson's time behind bars. This insight into prison life "from a leading suffragette" plainly brought home to Scantlebury some of the stark realities of the suffrage struggle. But Scantlebury thought her two COs went too far when it came to their views on men.

When male friends, doctors in the Royal Australian Army Medical Corps, called for Scantlebury at Endell Street—as they often did—she thought Anderson was cool toward them. A few days later, when Murray invited Scantlebury and Buckley to dinner in her sitting room, Murray warned them both to "beware of men" and never get married. She had been advised, Scantlebury told her parents, to "live in a state of single blessedness all the days of my life" because work was all-important. Since the women at Endell Street were dedicating their time to saving the lives of men, Scantlebury thought Murray's sentiments seemed unfeeling and even joyless. "Sometimes however I do wish they had a sense of humour! It would help matters so much but I suppose it has all been battered out of them."

For all their apparent lack of humor, Murray and Anderson often teased Scantlebury about her work anxieties and her popularity among men. Scantlebury even had to concede that the two women did possess some sense of humor after she learned, from Buckley, that they had dressed up as "the Hon. Mr Dug-out and his Lady" for a recent party thrown for the orderlies.[10] This vision of the COs masquerading as a staid married couple—Murray as a gruff army colonel and Anderson as a simpering wife—made them "even more marvellous" in Scantlebury's eyes. She was delighted, too, when they presented themselves in the hospital staff room one evening dressed for a formal event and Anderson said, "Just look at us ready for the ball!"[11] They were "so excited" and "so were the dogs and so was I," Scantlebury wrote.

Despite the jokes and the playacting, Murray and Anderson were fully attuned to the needs and welfare of their staff. They were plainly aware that Scantlebury was struggling—giving her one ward to manage instead of two was one way of alleviating the load. And at the end of her first fortnight, Scantlebury was touched when Murray and Anderson invited her to spend a day at their country cottage in Penn with Rachel Champion. It was the "acme of kindness," thought Scantlebury. In the midst of her hectic operating schedule, Anderson even took time to write a note telling the two friends they would be met off the train the following day and arranged a basket of food to take with them.

A WORLD AWAY from the air raids and ambulance convoys of London, the country cottage was a haven of tranquillity.[12] After catching a train from Marylebone, Scantlebury and Champion were met on arrival, as promised, by an elderly man named Buckles, who drove them in a pony trap through the lush spring countryside to the little village of Penn nestling in the Chiltern Hills. The two-story cottage was a "gem," Scantlebury declared. Overlooking woods and fields, it was surrounded by clipped lawns and colorful borders blooming with tulips, wallflowers, and forget-me-nots. Inside, the house contained "two of everything." As well as antique curios and expensive china, there were shelves crammed with books on women's rights. "As Ray and I investigated we could not help thinking what a wonderful pair of women these two are," said Scantlebury, "and we wondered if their plans for their big undertaking had been hatched in this peaceful faraway spot." Perhaps they had.

The two friends enjoyed lunch—lamb cutlets with paper tails—prepared by the housekeeper from the basket of provisions they brought with them. Then they set off for a long walk through the woods, where they "laughed and sang and rested and talked until our tongues ached." Scantlebury was entranced by the English countryside. "It was all so fresh and quiet and restful, far away from the rush of London and the hospital with all its boringness," she said. But she had not completely forgotten her patients. "I wished we could put those men in this country place. Some of them would have adored it for many of them love the flowers." In the evening Scantlebury and Champion sat on either side of an open fire on two "comfortable sofas with downy cushions" and gossiped. Then they retired to their separate rooms, each with lavender-scented pillows and "soft downy mattresses," where they fell asleep in minutes. It was a short stay—they had to be back at work in the morning—but a welcome reprieve from the horrors of war.

Slowly finding her place in the Endell Street team, Scantlebury would return often to the cottage at Penn. In early June, she spent a weekend there while Murray also stayed in the cottage, with what Scantlebury mistakenly described as her black and white "spaniels."[13] They walked together through the woods, although Scantlebury felt constrained because Anderson had warned her not to talk much to Murray because she was "resting." They were joined at the cottage by Octavia Lewin—Scantlebury's landlady—and, on Sunday, by Olga Campbell and Mardie Hodgson. Sitting in the garden under the shade of the beech trees, surrounded by the buzzing of bees and the song of blackbirds, Scantlebury was enthralled as Campbell and Hodgson reminisced about their work in Paris and Wimereux. It was "paradise," she said. She returned to Endell Street laden with bluebells and daisies to decorate the wards, freeing Anderson to travel to Penn for a well-deserved rest.

As she grew accustomed to the Endell Street routine, Scantlebury began to take pride in her work and started to enjoy the hectic social life both within and outside the hospital. She was initially surprised when the housemaid at her lodgings told her the doctors wore their uniforms to dine out in public, because "people are proud to be seen with you!"[14] On Empire Day, May 24, when the men gathered around a piano to sing popular songs, she dismissed the festivities as "the usual rather cheesy performances in the court yard"—though she conceded that "the soldiers love it."[15] But a few days later, on Whit Monday, when the courtyard was again crowded with patients belting out choruses of favorite wartime tunes, and those too ill to join them hung their heads out of windows to listen, she had to agree it was "so gay here." Since it was visiting day, some of the soldiers had families with them, and their children joined in the fun. Scantlebury also enjoyed lunches, lectures, and outings with her colleagues.[16] Beatrice Harraden took a break from her library duties to take Scantlebury for afternoon tea at the Writers' Club, and Jessie Scott-Reid, a new Scottish doctor, took her to lunch at the Ladies' Army and Navy Club. Another day she quaffed champagne with two orderlies—served by a butler—in an apartment in Whitehall where one of them lived. But the highlight of the summer revelries was a fancy dress party that Buckley threw at the end of June in the hospital recreation room.[17] The theme was farm life, so Scantlebury and Champion dressed in frocks like those worn by rural children— Scantlebury in pink and Champion in blue—while Buckley adopted the guise of a farmer. Others came as milkmaids, a scarecrow, a pig, and a cow. The guests had to clamber over a stile to enter the room—generating much amusement as the COs did the same—and everyone joined in country dances around a maypole. As the slaughter continued less than two hundred miles away, and the impact of war was ever-present in the ambulance convoys, air raids, and food queues, Scantlebury was keenly aware of the irony that she had "seldom gadded so much." Like so many others embroiled in the war, partying was, to her, a form of survival and self-protection.

YET EVEN AS she found her feet at Endell Street and threw herself into London life, Scantlebury continued to recoil from military surgery, and she still doubted her professional skills. In mid-June, when the injured flooded back from the Battle of Messines, she thought the wounds "so awful" that she admitted, "I am not at all keen on military surgery. At present I think it is horrible."[18] She dreaded her turn as orderly officer, when she was not only on convoy duty but also responsible for air raids, and found the operating sessions grueling. The day after Buckley's party, when she was about to begin a night shift, she wrote: "If I felt two last night I feel 102 tonight. Oh such sick cases. I operated on four poor beggars today." Although she pored over anatomy books in her spare time, she wished she was more knowledgeable and better skilled, so she could heal every one of the men who came to Endell Street. She empathized with her patients—another reason for her distress—especially when they came from her homeland. She visited one Australian soldier when she heard he was homesick and they had a "long talk."[19] The fact that so many of her friends, as well as her dear brother, were themselves in danger cannot have helped to calm her nerves. After one day of patching men up to return to the battlefield, she said, "Poor beggars—it must be abominable going back to France again."[20]

Despite her anxieties, Scantlebury did her job well and lauded the Endell Street medical achievements. To her fiancé, Frank Norris, she described herself moving from bed to bed with a tape measure in hand, readjusting splints and dressing wounds on men with fractured femurs.[21] The Thomas splint was "the latest craze," she told him, and asked whether he had yet tried BIPP; she had sent him the recipe.

Scantlebury performed many delicate and difficult procedures. In one operation, she extracted a piece of shrapnel close to a man's eyelid; in another, she freed the ulnar nerve from scar tissue in a patient's arm, enabling him to use his hand again.[22] She came close to weeping over one youth with a smashed knee who was doing well in surgery but suddenly developed an aneurysm in an artery; she had to perform an emergency procedure to tie the vessel higher up in his thigh. After a busy day in theater when she helped administer anesthetics as well as performing an operation, she was proud to report that her patients were "progressing quite well and I am to have some more patients tomorrow I believe." It was almost impossible to describe "that beehive of an operating theatre," she added, "with its hot stifling atmosphere and white gowned & hooded women moving ceaselessly about and stretchers pushed hither & thither and the sweet heavy sickly fumes of the chloroform."[23]

Yet when she was still in charge of only one ward after six weeks, Scantlebury felt so downhearted and undervalued that she considered offering her services to Great Ormond Street Hospital for Children instead.[24] At one point she argued with Anderson over the treatment of a patient with appendicitis.[25] When she mentioned their dispute to Murray—who inevitably sided with Anderson—she felt crushed as Murray drily retorted, "Oh Dr Scantlebury, I thought you were too young to have any theories of your own." Eventually she confessed to Murray that she did not feel "very useful at military work" and was thinking of returning to treating children.[26] Gently, Murray urged her to reconsider, and Scantlebury, reassured, decided to give herself another chance: "I shall stay. . . . [I]t certainly does buck one up to feel one is really needed."

DESPITE THE SUPPOSEDLY anti-male warnings from the two COs, there was a surprise in store for the Endell Street staff at the end of June. Evelyn Windsor, the Canadian anesthetist, turned up at the hospital early on Saturday, June 30—her day off—and calmly announced she was getting married at ten o'clock that morning.[27] Nobody, apart from Rachel Champion, knew she was even engaged. Her fiancé was on the staff of the Canadian Army in London and the brother of her medical partner in Calgary. As Windsor's colleagues gathered around to congratulate her, Elizabeth Hamilton-Browne informed Anderson, who rushed over, grasped Windsor's hand, and exclaimed, "Well, well, you poor girl, I am sorry for you." The other doctors shrieked with laughter and Scantlebury ran to the office to ask Murray if they could all attend the wedding. True to form, Murray said she could "hardly approve" and hoped "it would not become infectious"—though of course she agreed.

The Endell Street doctors rushed to the nearby St Giles in the Fields Church and took their seats in the pews. The bride and groom, both in their uniforms, were married by a Canadian army chaplain, a friend of Windsor's father, before leaving in a taxi for a fortnight's leave. "It was all over in ten minutes. It was so sudden, we have hardly recovered from gasping yet," Scantlebury told her family later. By the time the doctors returned to Endell Street, the news had spread through the hospital. After her honeymoon, Windsor went straight back to work, administering anesthetics in the operating theater.

THERE WAS LITTLE else to celebrate that summer. The beginning of the Third Battle of Ypres—also known as the Battle of Passchendaele, for a village close to Ypres—on July 31 ensured that the ambulance trains kept arriving with monotonous regularity at London stations with their cargoes of maimed, shocked, and gassed soldiers. There were more casualties shipped from France to Britain in 1917 than in any other year of the war.[28] Evacuation methods had at least improved, so that the first men wounded when the Battle of Messines began at dawn were unloaded from an ambulance train at Charing Cross station by 2:15 p.m. that same day.[29]

Meanwhile, the sustained campaign by German submarines against merchant shipping was creating severe shortages of fuel and food on the home front. Staple foods such as bread, potatoes, meat, and butter were extremely scarce or extortionately expensive, causing long queues and occasional outbreaks of violence at shops.[30] Leading a campaign to encourage people to grow their own vegetables, King George V had the flower beds outside Buckingham Palace dug up and replanted with potatoes.[31] Concerns about bread shortages were so acute that it was made illegal to feed crumbs to wild birds.

On top of the deprivation, attacks from the air brought fresh destruction to the capital in the form of huge Gotha biplanes that could unleash as many as 13 bombs each. The first London raid occurred on a sunny morning on June 13, when 14 Gothas dropped 72 bombs over a wide area of London, killing 162 people and injuring 426.[32] One of the bombs fell in Holborn, a stone's throw from Endell Street.

Scantlebury, as luck would have it, was the orderly officer that day, and was therefore responsible not only for greeting convoys, but also for air raid duty, which included treating any local civilian casualties. She was dressing the wounds of a severely ill man on her ward when she heard a crash followed by the "patter-patter" of answering machine guns, but she was too busy to look out the window. At one point an airplane zoomed directly overhead, and some of the patients saw smoke rising where bombs had fallen. Fortunately, there were no casualties nearby, although Murray stood ready at the firehose in the courtyard as a precaution. Fire drills had become routine at Endell Street. Affecting nonchalance, Scantlebury advised her family not to be alarmed—"Everyone takes these things very phlegmatically"—before she discovered that it had been "a big air raid" after all.[33]

It seemed the Germans had Scantlebury in their sights. For when the Gothas returned on July 7, another bright morning, she was orderly officer again. She had risen early in Wimpole Street to a fine day, but her approaching shift loomed large as the "cloud on my horizon." The clouds not only gathered but burst. In the middle of her ward round, she heard what sounded like "30–40 German aeroplanes"—it was more likely closer to 20—which "flew like birds above our heads." The noise was "terrific" as bombs fell all around the area, British pilots chasing the enemy craft without success.

Scantlebury was kept busy trying to prevent panic from spreading among the men, since many were bedridden, as well as being traumatized by the deafening reminder of the battlefield. Most remained calm, although some "trembled a little," Scantlebury said, while she continued her work—even when some shrapnel crashed through the window of one of the upper wards. This time there were 53 deaths and 182 people injured, mainly in central London and the East End. Scantlebury treated one local man who had been knocked off his bicycle by a speeding motorist in the mayhem, and Champion was called to help a woman who had fainted in the street. Neither were serious casualties, though Scantlebury confessed, "I do feel in the centre of things." Her colleague Eleanor Bourne felt the same. She thought the raid "rather exciting," even when a direct hit on the Central Telegraph Office a mile away showered pieces of burnt paper down on Endell Street.[34]

The resulting outcry over the lack of warnings for the virtually defenseless capital prompted the government to introduce maroons—distress rockets fired into the sky—to raise the alarm when raids were expected, although only during daylight hours. The Gotha attacks would continue throughout 1917, with especially heavy ones in September and October, although these would all arrive at night—without warning. Scantlebury was having dinner with Murray and Anderson when one such raid began.[35] They left her with the dogs while they supervised the evacuation of patients into the basement. She found Murray and Anderson later sitting on some steps beside Sergeant Major Harris. The men were drowning out the noise of the falling bombs by singing popular songs to the accompaniment of a harmonium.

THERE WAS NO letup in August—the busiest month for casualties arriving in London—as the war entered its fourth year. A convoy of forty-five men arrived at 3:00 a.m. one morning in mid-August. Scantlebury, who was on duty, said, "They seemed so pleased to be here, poor old things!"[36] One of the men told her, "You do not know how nice it is to see you English girls again!" Swallowing her Australian pride, she did not correct him. By the end of the month she was thrilled finally to be granted a second ward—it had previously been managed by Champion, who was recovering from an appendix operation—although Scantlebury still worried that some of her patients were taking too long to improve. Nevertheless, in September she signed up for another six months. She felt she could not desert the hospital "for after all I am in the military and this is war."[37] In truth, Scantlebury was also becoming "quite fond of old London." She loved her morning ride to work on the top deck of a bus, enjoyed traveling first class on the trains as a "bloomin' orficer [officer]," and even had to admit that the hospital was "not so bad" at times.[38]

THOUSANDS OF SOLDIERS wounded in the ongoing slaughter in France would have cause to be thankful for Scantlebury's skills and those of her colleagues during 1917. Among them was Harold Adams Innis, one of many Canadian soldiers treated at Endell Street that year. Innis, who had enlisted straight after graduating from McMaster University, was hit by a shell splinter, which penetrated his right thigh, when he was on patrol near German lines. Transported to a base hospital at Étaples, he underwent an operation to remove the splinter before being shipped to England, where he arrived on July 16. Innis would later remember being almost overcome by emotion as he was lifted from the hospital train in London and showered with flowers and cigarettes. After his admittance to Endell Street with a fever, he wrote home to say he was in a hospital "run entirely by ladies," adding, "it promises to be some affair." Writing from his hospital bed, Innis urged his mother not to worry. "There are some very bad cases in the hospital in comparison with which mine is child's play," he said. "One with arms and legs off and what not."[39] But a week later, his temperature was worryingly high—infection had set in—so he had a second operation to clean out the wound, when it was probably "bipped." A day later, the pain had subsided.

After being wheeled around in a chair for some weeks, Innis graduated to crutches. He managed to limp to a concert in the recreation room that featured some "fine singing, [and] violin playing," but since he was keen to continue his studies in economics and earn a master's degree, he spent most of his time reading. Beatrice Harraden was "especially kind to me," he remembered: no doubt she kept him supplied with economics textbooks. After a month, he was transferred to a convalescent hospital, and he returned to Canada the following spring. Innis would become one of Canada's foremost economic historians. More than three decades later, he would still recall "the kindness of the English people" at Endell Street.

Others were not so lucky. Frank Brissenden was wounded in France in February 1917.[40] He spent a month at Endell Street and recovered sufficiently to return to the Western Front a year later. He was killed in action in August 1918, at the age of twenty-six. Another patient, Thomas Manley, who enlisted in 1915, was nursed at Endell Street after being gassed at Ypres in November 1917.[41] It was probably mustard gas, first used by the Germans in July, which caused burns and blindness. He recovered and returned to France only to be killed a month later: he was twenty-one. There were many others who died in their beds at Endell Street despite the best efforts of its staff.[42] Most of them young, many of them little more than boys, their remains were sent home to grieving parents and wives.

For the first time, too, there, were women on the wards at Endell Street as patients rather than staff.[43] The first women recruited to the army's new all-female corps, the WAAC, were sent to France in

March 1917 to serve throughout the rest of the war as cooks, clerks, telephonists, and drivers as well as in other auxiliary jobs. Although they were kept away from the front line, some were wounded in air raids on base hospitals and other medical units, which the Germans targeted from July 1917. Others fell sick through other causes. Belatedly, the army realized it would need hospital beds for its invalided WAACs—and Endell Street provided them, opening a ward on the top floor of a block in August. The beds, later doubled to two wards, were also occupied by members of the Women's Royal Naval Service (WRNS), established in late 1917, and the Women's Royal Air Force (WRAF), founded the following year. In all, Endell Street would treat some two thousand women patients.

At times, Endell Street surgeons had to operate on their own staff, too. In September, one of the nurses, Sister Ethel May, developed an infection in her hand, probably contracted from a septic wound on her ward.[44] May had originally trained at the London Hospital and enjoyed a long nursing career before joining Endell Street when it first opened. A much-loved member of staff, she had run the St Theresa ward from the start. That spring, when she had joined Anderson and Murray at a dinner to celebrate the hospital's third anniversary, Anderson had told her she had "contributed as much as anyone to the success of the hospital" and "helped a large number of very bruised men back to life." That devotion had now led to a life-threatening infection.

As May became dangerously ill with a fever and intense pain, Anderson was forced to amputate her third finger; what was worse, she had to remove diseased tendons in May's palm, which meant she would no longer be able to use her hand. Anderson wrote to May's father, a doctor, to let him know her progress, but confessed she had not yet told May she would never work again. "I think it is better to wait until she is stronger and to let it dawn on her gradually that the hand will be useless," she said. "Her life has been spared and the hand will not require to be amputated—that is all we have been able to do." Anderson said May, who was forty-seven, had been "splendidly brave" and that her work at Endell Street was "a great achievement." She added, "Her influence has been most uplifting and stimulating and she was a perfect surgical nurse." The past tense said it all.

May was not the only staff casualty. Another nurse, Sister Inskip, was seriously ill at the same time with a septic elbow, and colleagues feared she might lose her arm. Since she was still young, her plight seemed worse, thought Barbara Last, for at least Sister May had "the satisfaction of having been so frightfully good up till now."[45]

WHILE THE BEDS filled with soldiers and staff, the round of revels kept pace—often with the slenderest of excuses. When one of the sisters came back from time off in September, her ward, St Perpetua, threw a jamboree to celebrate her return. It included a feast of sandwiches, cakes, and sausage rolls, a rousing sing-along, and a conjuror.[46] The beds were pushed back and men crowded round in their wheelchairs, joined by others who limped along from other wards, to watch the show. The men sang a lusty rendition of "Land of Hope and Glory," led by a young, red-haired orderly. Scantlebury, who came to watch the merriment after finishing her shift, was transfixed when one of the ward cleaners, a "motherly old woman of 50," sang a plaintive song about bravery at sea. As she was singing, the late summer sun suddenly lit up the ward, and the men applauded so loudly that the "roof resounded with cheers and clapping." The men enjoyed themselves so much that they all declared they had forgotten the war.

There was more significant cause for celebration that month. In August, Murray and Anderson had been created Commanders of the Order of the British Empire in the new honors list established to recognize men and women for their war work.[47] On September 27, they went to Buckingham Palace to receive their awards, dressed in brand-new uniforms they had bought for the occasion. They were accompanied by a posse of orderlies from Endell Street, plus, of course, their dogs. As they emerged through the palace gates after receiving their awards from the king and queen, both grinning broadly—and all but holding hands—they were cheered and clapped by their waiting entourage while the dogs yapped excitedly.

Back at Endell Street, the bell in the courtyard rang out and staff hurriedly lined up—not in expectation of a convoy but to form a guard of honor for the hospital's founders. When Murray and Anderson entered the courtyard, they were greeted by a cacophony of whoops and yells from the gathered doctors, nurses, and orderlies—as well as patients in their blue suits. As they showed their medals to their colleagues, the two women looked radiant. All the anguish of three years of warfare and war wounds seemed to fall away, and their usually pale and serious faces were wreathed in smiles. The honors, bestowed with equanimity on both women and men, were the most significant recognition of their work to date—and of women's wartime work in general.

DESPITE THE ADMIRATION for Murray and Anderson, not everyone heeded their advice. For it seemed that marrying was indeed becoming infectious. Three months after Evelyn Windsor's surprise wedding, Rachel Champion was set to marry her fiancé, Lieutenant Colonel Gordon Shaw.[48] Since her appendix operation in August, Champion had been forced to give up working at Endell Street—much to Murray's sorrow. Although Champion was still recuperating, she and her fiancé arranged a hurried wedding in London on October 2 to fit in with his leave. Scantlebury completed a morning's list in the operating theater before setting off to the church, All Souls in the West End, where a party of Endell Street doctors was already gathered. She declared the ceremony "one of the nicest weddings I have ever been to" and Champion the "sweetest bride I have ever seen." The guests repaired to Wimpole Street for afternoon tea. Since sugar was in short supply, the wedding cake was decorated with white heather. The couple left for a week-long honeymoon before the groom went back to France.

Champion would never return to medicine. After all her years of surgical experience, she would settle back in Melbourne after the war, raising a family of four while her husband built a distinguished career as a hospital surgeon with a busy private practice. But memories of Endell Street were never far away. One of her sons would remember his mother's pained disapproval on one occasion. Recalling the war, his mother began, "When I was a doctor . . . " at which point the five-year-old interrupted to say, "You mean you were a nurse, mum," and patiently explained: "Men are doctors, ladies are nurses." Her response can well be imagined.

MANY OF THE staff found the demands at Endell Street during the grim days of 1917 overwhelming. Yet being away was somehow worse. Working during one of the busiest periods in July, Barbara Last had almost despaired. "It is simply awful," she wrote home. "I really do not know whether I am standing on my head or on my heels." Yet in October, when she was transferred to clerical duties for a brief reprieve, she was "simply dying" to get back to her ward. "The Hospital is very heavy," she wrote. "We have had a convoy in every single night since last Thursday week." There was "something awfully thrilling" about the arrival of the convoys, she added: "I love helping to get them in."[49] The only way to cope with the futility of war was by helping to alleviate its worst horrors.

Scantlebury felt much the same. When she was granted two weeks' leave in October, she set off for the cottage in Penn, courtesy of her COs. But after less than a week extolling the autumnal countryside, she was restless and returned to Endell Street. She was still dithering over whether to leave, this time to join a friend at a hospital in Petrograd—at times she could be exasperatingly indecisive—but after a "very painful" interview with Murray and a "tense" shift working alongside Anderson, she committed herself to staying until spring. On inquiring about a transfer to Petrograd, she had discovered the situation was "extremely doubtful"—this was three weeks before the second Russian Revolution—and after all she was "frightfully fond" of her two bosses, even if she did not agree with "one eighth of their views."[50]

By November, as casualties poured back from the Battle of Cambrai, the turnover was frenetic. Scantlebury was looking after eighty patients in two wards, and many of them were not only seriously ill from wounds but had winter coughs as well. No sooner were her patients on the road to recovery than they were moved on to an auxiliary hospital. After one long shift in which she performed five operations, at least she could boast they were "all still alive" the following day.[51]

Good news from the front was swiftly eclipsed by bad. Bells rang out across London to celebrate victory at Cambrai, when troops breached the Hindenburg Line with the support of tanks, but the celebrations were short-lived, as the Germans regained most of the ground a few weeks later. The dark days were brightened briefly when Lieutenant General Sir Francis Lloyd, the commanding officer in charge of defending London, visited Endell Street in November to open an exhibition of the patients' needlework. Having watched many of her patients painstakingly producing exquisite embroidery, some with only one arm, Scantlebury was humbled by their perseverance.[52] She bought one piece—an Australian badge—while another item was bought by the queen.

As Londoners braced themselves for another severe winter, it was hard to beat the gloom. Even Murray and Anderson seemed to be buckling under the strain. They spent a rare weekend together at Penn in December—leaving Scantlebury and Hamilton-Browne in charge at Endell Street. They had "worked themselves fleshless," thought Scantlebury, and were "the colour of parchment."[53] A few weeks later, Anderson was spending a weekend at Penn alone, but she rushed back early when informed by telegram that Murray had been taken ill, perhaps with a winter bug. Scantlebury raced across town to meet Anderson from the train and assured her that Murray was already on the mend, knowing she would be "worried to death" about her "beloved friend."[54]

It was not Anderson's beloved friend, however, but her mother who succumbed to illness that December. Elizabeth Garrett Anderson died on December 17 at the age of eighty-one after being ill for two years.[55] Although the end had been long expected, Louisa was naturally bereft. A memorial service five days later in the church adjoining Endell Street was packed not only with family—including Aunt Millie—but also with fellow stalwarts of the suffrage campaign, medical colleagues, LSMW students, and Endell Street staff.

The following month, Louisa and her brother (who was by now Sir Alan, since he had been knighted in the honors' list) agreed to rename the New Hospital, which their mother had founded in 1871, the Elizabeth Garrett Anderson Hospital.[56] Although it would later be subsumed within University College Hospital, the name survives today in the Elizabeth Garrett Anderson Wing.

IF THE WAR showed no signs of ending, at least it seemed that women's battle for equality had been all but won. The Representation of the People bill, which promised the vote to women over the age of thirty, was lumbering through Parliament. Politicians who had previously sworn outright opposition to female suffrage, including Herbert Asquith, were now among its most vocal backers. Women's contributions to the war effort in munitions factories, in military hospitals, and now in the military services, too, had made it impossible to deny them full citizenship—for some women, at least. As obituary writers had observed, the obstacles that Elizabeth Garrett Anderson had faced some five decades earlier now seemed unthinkable when women doctors were not only working in hospitals at home and abroad, but running them, too. The government had recently invited women doctors to staff one of the biggest military hospitals in Bombay.[57] Yet the advance would be anything but straightforward.

Giving a welcoming address to the new intake of students at the LSMW in October, Louisa Garrett Anderson had assured her audience that medicine was "not only the finest profession open to women," but the best possible training for public life.[58] In an impassioned speech, she urged the students, the next generation of women doctors, to work for the school, for medicine, for women—and "for England." But she sounded the alarm against those calling for universal co-education for medical women. Medical schools that had flung their doors open to women during the war could just as easily slam them shut again, she said. In London, in particular, there was "every possibility" that medical schools would exclude women as soon as sufficient male students became available again.

Murray was equally apprehensive about the future. In December, Agnes Conway, a keen suffragist who was collecting material to celebrate women's war work for a planned national war museum, called on Murray at Endell Street.[59] Conway, a formidable woman who had studied ancient history and archaeology at Cambridge before traveling in Greece and the Balkans, was gathering photographs, documents, and uniforms for a women's section that would eventually take its place in the Imperial War Museum. She had already asked Murray several times to send one of her orderlies to sit for an official photograph, to no avail, so had decided to visit Murray in person. Although Murray now agreed to the photographs, she was emphatic that Endell Street should not be included in the women's section of the proposed museum alongside hospitals run by female lay volunteers, some of which were staffed by men. Despite Conway's assurances that she fully understood the professional nature of the work at Endell Street, Murray ended the interview abruptly by exclaiming, "Hands off our Hospital in the Women's Section!"

As always, it was equal treatment and fair play that Anderson and Murray sought. Even as they were busy running Endell Street, they were taking up cudgels on behalf of women in numerous other areas. At the request of the Medical Women's Federation, set up in 1917, they were pressing the War Office to grant honorary rank to women doctors serving with the army overseas. At the same time they were lobbying the income tax commissioners to allow women doctors at Endell Street to pay the lower tax rate enjoyed by their male counterparts in the army.[60] But it was not just medical women they campaigned for. They were also demanding equal pay for the clerks at Endell Street, who processed the vital information in the voluminous military records system. Murray was adamant that their twenty-five shillings weekly pay was "not a living wage," and infuriated when male government clerks were awarded a raise of four shillings a week while the female clerks were given half that. She was likewise arguing for a pay increase for the hospital's cooks, who had not had a raise for three years, and now earned less than the kitchen maids. Fighting to improve the lot for her women staff on all fronts, Murray accumulated files "full of letters about inadequate pay or insufficient allowances." Anderson and Murray could seem stern at times, but they were battling tirelessly for the women under their command. In accordance with their suffragette creed, they showed their true feelings through deeds, not words.

DESPITE THE BITTER cold and food shortages, Murray and Anderson were determined to make Christmas 1917 a celebration to remember for both patients and staff. Festivities began on December 22, when the Endell Street choir sang carols in the courtyard by lantern light, watched by men from the open windows above.[61] When the familiar air raid maroon sounded, the orderlies hurriedly extinguished their lanterns but carried on singing even as the men were bustled into the basement and the windows quickly closed. The now traditional contest for the best-decorated ward was more keenly fought than ever. In one ward, the men created an English garden in springtime, while another resembled a scene from China. Yet despite all the men's efforts, Murray awarded first prize to the WAACs' ward, since—as Scantlebury reported—"She says she is very fond of girls."

On Christmas Day, Scantlebury joined the men on both her wards for lunch before enjoying her own dinner of turkey and plum pudding as a guest of the COs. Returning to her wards for more festivities, she watched the men play musical chairs—which must have looked as comical as it was tragic—and the week was rounded off with the traditional pantomime. As 1917 drew to a close, Scantlebury reflected on the year, which had begun for her "in heat & sunshine" in Melbourne and ended with snow and ice on the other side of the world.[62] She wondered whether she would end 1918 in the warmth of an Australian summer.

THERE WAS MORE than a ray of sunshine for Murray and Anderson in January, however, when they celebrated the passing in the House of Lords of the bill giving women the vote. The Representation of the People Act of 1918, which gave the vote to men over twenty-one and most women over thirty, was widely regarded as a reward for women's war work. There was some way to go before the suffragists' demands would be fully met. The age differential was intended to ensure that male votes would outnumber women's by three to two; it would be ten more years before women achieved equal representation. For Murray and Anderson, at least, the reform represented a landmark: it rewarded their years of militant campaigning and was a credit to their war work.

Celebrating the event, Murray ordered bunting to be strung up around the hospital and the flags of England, Scotland, Wales, and Ireland hoisted in the courtyard.[63] A few days later the two COs presided over a fancy dress party with dinner for all the staff. Anderson toasted the queen with lemon syrup, and Murray gave a triumphal speech. Then the pair led their staff in a procession around the hospital as they sang "The March of the Women." Written in 1911, the suffragettes' anthem spoke of the "weary days" of the women's struggle and looked forward to a time when the victors would wear "the wreath the brave have worn." But the weary days of the battle they were now braving were not over yet. Endell Street was about to find itself closer to the war than ever.

9

Darkest Before Dawn

Covent Garden, midnight, January 28–29, 1918

German bombs had rained down on London during the autumn and early winter, but since Christmas, the foggy weather had kept the enemy planes away.[1] When the fog lifted to reveal a cloudless night sky on January 28, Londoners feared the worst. As soon as they heard the maroons fired to warn of approaching bombers, people scurried into cellars and air raid shelters. Some were trampled in the rush. Close to 9:00 p.m., three Gotha planes appeared from the east and let down bombs across the City—London's business quarter—as well as the East End and the northern suburbs before disappearing again. In the quiet that followed, people listened for the "all clear" bugles. Some emerged from their shelters to a "dead hush" and tried to reach their homes. Others, like Vera Scantlebury, simply turned over in bed and went back to sleep. In Covent Garden, around six hundred people who had taken refuge in the basement of Odhams Printing Works, a designated air raid shelter on the corner of Long Acre and Endell Street, decided to stay put. Then the rocket signal fired again to warn of another attack.

Just after midnight, a Giant—one of a new fleet of huge four-engine German planes that had first appeared the previous September—was spotted approaching London from the north. After dropping bombs on the East End, killing one person and injuring eighteen, the Giant crossed the Thames into south London and then turned in a tight loop, crossed the river again, and headed north. In swift succession, the Giant dropped four bombs on the Covent Garden area. One of them landed on Savoy Mansions, an office block near the Strand, and another in the middle of the Flower Market. The next fell on Odhams.

Ripping through the pavement at the rear of the printing works, the massive six-hundred-pound bomb exploded in the basement, severing gas pipes and setting fire to the four-story building. Fueled by bales of newsprint, the inferno tore through the interior. Rescuers were quick to reach the scene. Police rushed from nearby Bow Street, and fire crews arrived to tackle the blaze. But as people stumbled into the street, shocked and injured, the rear wall collapsed, taking down several concrete floors, which crashed on top of those still inside. Some trapped in the rubble are thought to have drowned as water from the fire hoses filled the basement.

The inferno killed thirty-eight people and injured eighty-five. It was the worst human cost extracted by a single bomb in Britain during the war. Most of the dead were women and children. One boy, who had been sheltering with two friends, was pinned to the ground by a piece of machinery. He saw women and children "bleeding and burning," and one woman with her dress ablaze who ran over him. His two friends were never found. Within minutes, the injured were arriving at the gates of Endell Street hospital less than two hundred yards away.

Elizabeth Hamilton-Browne was on duty that night.[2] Together with Anderson, who was almost never off duty, she treated dozens of casualties with severe burns, broken bones, and shock until 4:30 a.m. Many of the injured were hurriedly taken to beds on the wards. Flora Murray was recovering from her recent illness and to her distress was unable to help. Since it was forbidden to use telephones during a raid, it was impossible to call in the rest of the medical team, so a message was dispatched by hand to the doctor who lived closest, a recent recruit named Fede Mackenzie, and she raced to the hospital to help.

When Scantlebury arrived for work the next morning, she was horrified to discover she had slept through the disaster instead of being called in. "They were brought to the hospital burnt and shocked and smashed," she told her family, "and we put up as many as we could, the others being taken to civilian hospitals." Throughout the night, mothers had called at the hospital gates asking after children who were missing. Being confined to bed, Murray was "like a caged lion," said Scantlebury, while Anderson "has had just about as much as anyone could stand during these last few months." The ruined building at the bottom of Endell Street, still smoldering as search crews brought out the bodies, looked "like the pictures you see of Ypres." Worse, Scantlebury realized, another second's delay would have meant the bomb falling on the hospital itself. It was a day "racked by sadness and sorrow."

THE ODHAMS BOMB disaster made a tragic beginning to a desperate year. Aware that significant reinforcements from America were due to land in France in the spring, the Germans launched a massive new offensive on the Western Front in March.[3] Bolstered by troops transferred from the Eastern Front following the conclusion of a peace treaty with Bolshevik Russia, the Germans pushed back depleted British forces along a wide front in the Somme region. They launched a second attack in Flanders in April in a last-ditch attempt to seize the Channel ports, regaining ground that had been painstakingly won by the Allies in 1917. To rally his demoralized and outnumbered men, Field Marshal Douglas Haig, the commander of the British Army, issued a solemn message to the troops: there would be no choice but to "fight on to the end" with their "backs to the wall."

Depressed and exhausted, the British feared that defeat was imminent and a German invasion could happen at any moment. "It seems as if only days and hours are between us and our fate!" wrote one diarist.[4] Even David Lloyd George, the prime minister, believed the war was lost.[5] With German U-boats blocking food supplies, rationing was introduced in London in January for sugar, and the following month for butter, margarine, and meat; the system was later extended nationwide, although food scarcities continued. Fear and hunger fueled suspicion and distrust of foreigners, pacifists, conscientious objectors—and anyone perceived to live differently.

In one extraordinary example, a right-wing MP, Noel Pemberton Billing, published an article in his newspaper, the *Vigilante*, in February suggesting that an American dancer named Maud Allan was involved in a secret British cult of lesbians and homosexuals.[6] Billing claimed the Germans possessed a "Black Book" containing the names of forty-seven thousand British men and women with "moral and sexual weaknesses" who were vulnerable to blackmail. The allegation against Allan was triggered by an advertisement for a private performance she was due to give playing the title role in Oscar Wilde's banned play *Salome*, to be staged in London by the theatrical entrepreneur Jack Grein. Both Grein and his wife, Alix, were longtime supporters of Endell Street; Mrs. Grein had written the hospital's Christmas pantomime three years running. Protesting at the intimation that she was a lesbian, Maud Allan sued Billing for libel, but when she lost her claim, crowds inside and outside of the court building cheered wildly. The Black Book was, of course, a fiction, but the homophobia was real. It was one thing to accept women in jobs where there was dire need; it was quite another to countenance breaches of traditional morality such as lesbianism.

Amid this atmosphere of anxiety and recrimination, many of the women at Endell Street were weary beyond measure and tempers were strained to breaking point. "Things began to go from bad to worse," remembered Nina Last.[7] "Shortages of food and of staff were beginning to tell." Working in the linens room six days a week, often on duty alone, Last was sometimes so tired that she did not even realize she was crying when tears ran down her face. With soap in short supply, she had to ration fresh linens for the wards, and finding enough to eat was a constant worry. "It was necessary to get down to breakfast in good time if one wanted any marg, and a pot of marmalade was treated like gold," she said. Meals often consisted of horse meat or "messes of lentils and dried peas." She spent her rare breaks from work hunting down food staples in local shops, although the restaurants, such as Lyons Corner House, offered only tiny portions, "so we were often really hungry," she recalled. Last kept her complaints to herself, however, aware that no matter how tired she felt, life was invariably worse for the nursing staff, including her sister Barbara, who worked long shifts, often at night, and frequently alone.

Last was not the only one feeling downtrodden. Mardie Hodgson was suffering from a "whopping big cold" and "an equally large dose of the blues" that February.[8] Olga Campbell, still in her post as quartermaster, kept up her sense of humor—at least when writing to her brother, who was enduring a long tour in the trenches. Hodgson and Campbell were cheered briefly when their cousin Elizabeth Murray, Flora's niece, came to stay at Endell Street in March on her way back to France, where she was serving as a volunteer ambulance driver with the Scottish Women's Hospitals (SWH). Elizabeth, who was twenty-four, accompanied Flora to a meeting at the Albert Hall celebrating the women's vote and was pleased to report that Aunt Flo was "looking much better" than a month ago, unless she was "only very hot & excited about the meeting."[9]

As Elizabeth sailed for France, staff at Endell Street readied the hospital for a new influx of casualties from the expected German "Big Push." Scantlebury practiced her dissection skills in the LSMW anatomy room and attended lectures on artificial limbs. But the war gloom and food scarcities meant that "everyone is really depressed," she wrote. "The atmosphere is charged with electricity and overworked people go off pop at the least provocation."[10] She herself erupted in fury at what she regarded as the petty bureaucratic demands made by Anderson—"her ladyship"—and bristled with anger when Murray suggested she had no feeling for British history.[11] When Murray asked if Scantlebury would stay another six months, she agreed, but she was hurt when Anderson quipped that Scantlebury might suddenly head off to "Timbuctoo or some such place." It was not an easy decision: Scantlebury's fiancé was pressing her to return home after a year apart. She was even more piqued when Murray ticked her off for laughing during a visit by Queen

Alexandra, despite earnestly explaining that she was only sharing a joke with Hamilton-Browne at the familiarity with which one of the patients was chatting with the royal party.

The laughter stopped, however, when the first casualties from the German advance began arriving at the end of March. As British and Allied troops were forced to retreat, medical posts were overrun and base hospitals came under attack. Flora's niece, Elizabeth Murray, would later receive the French military medal, the Croix de Guerre, for her part in helping to evacuate patients from the SWH's casualty station at Villers-Cotterêts when it was overrun by German forces in May.[12] Along with the thousands of men wounded in hand-to-hand fighting, the convoys arriving at Endell Street now included dozens of women, new recruits to the military services, who were injured by long-range shelling on base camps. Three nurses were killed in one attack on the base hospital at Étaples in May, and nine WAACs died in an air raid on Abbeville a few days later.

Earlier in the year, rumors had circulated in Britain that the WAACs sent to France were behaving promiscuously and even working as prostitutes.[13] One story claimed that two hundred WAACs had returned to England pregnant; another suggested they were employed in brothels sanctioned by the War Office. The claims had been roundly rejected by an official investigation in March. Although there were, inevitably, some illegitimate pregnancies among the WAACs, the rate was lower than in the general population. The exoneration did nothing to stop the sexual innuendos and ribaldry, however. The *Times* journalist Michael MacDonagh guffawed at being asked whether he would prefer a "whack on the head or a WAAC on the knee."[14]

But when the women casualties began arriving at Endell Street, the public response changed immediately. The WAACs were now acclaimed as brave heroes and stoical patients. "The horrors of war are brought home most convincingly by a sight of these devoted women under treatment at Endell-street," said *The Times*, reporting the arrival of a convoy of eleven WAACs. One woman, who had been severely wounded by shrapnel, insisted she had just been "unfortunate," while another, who was less seriously injured, was "equally cheerful and patient."[15] Others had escaped physical injury but were suffering from shell shock. The *Sunday Pictorial*, reporting the same convoy, said one of the women had been knocked unconscious and buried in debris by an exploding shell—"just like one of the Tommies," as she put it. Another newspaper, featuring pictures of smiling WAACs in their beds, declared the women were "prouder of their hospital blue than they were to don khaki." Visiting the women, Queen Mary arranged for nine of those who were least seriously ill to be transferred to a convalescent home in southwest London. Some would never reach there. The Irish-born Kathleen Carroll, who had enrolled in the WAACs in Manchester, died of her wounds at Endell Street in July, aged twenty-seven.[16]

FACED WITH THIS fresh wave of wounded, Murray and Anderson put the welfare of their staff before their own comforts as ever. When Scantlebury arrived late for work one morning after being up all night admitting fifty new arrivals, she found a note from Anderson instructing her to go home immediately and rest.[17] Spring brought little respite. Snow lay thick on the ground in late April as the casualties still streamed in. "We are trying to keep going strong," wrote Scantlebury, "but the war news the weather and the new wounded all are depressing features above which it is hard to rise."[18] A few weeks later, she was up all night trying to comfort a "very sick boy" who shrieked throughout an air raid, bombs, and shrapnel falling, just before a convoy of forty-three patients arrived.[19] It was the last air raid, though not the last convoy.

When May finally brought warmer weather, Scantlebury was momentarily cheered by a bouquet of spring flowers sent by a grateful patient, who remembered her kindness from a year earlier.[20] Yet she was still anxious about her abilities, telling her fiancé, Frank Norris, about her clumsiness in a letter enclosing case notes on three patients. All three had had their wounds treated with BIPP, which, she told Norris, was "used here with great success."[21] One of her patients had a leg wound, which required the skin to be freed up and reconstructed before being dressed with BIPP. The second had a gunshot or shrapnel wound in his lower spine, but—after she had removed the portions of dead bone—he was "very sick" with a high temperature. The third had a fractured shoulder blade and collar-bone with a gaping wound. After removing the dead bone, she had put the man's arm in traction, she told Norris, helpfully providing a diagram of the apparatus above his bed.

A few days later, on the third anniversary of the hospital's open-ing, Murray and Anderson did their best to boost morale, throwing a party in honor of the more than forty staff members who had served at Endell Street since the start. Flags fluttered in the spring breeze as the entire staff and many of the patients assembled in the courtyard. Murray presented photographs of the hospital to those hardy few who had lasted the course, with ten-shilling notes attached to them. Always keen to recognize the contributions of the unsung workers, Murray stressed the importance of the cooks, cleaners, and laundry staff to the hospital's success. In a moving speech, she told them it was "not the special kind of work" they did that mattered so much as "the spirit in which we did it."[22] That spirit was increasingly hard to keep alive.

AFTER THREE YEARS, the strains were becoming almost intolerable. Although the casualties—both men and women—continued to ar-rive in the Endell Street courtyard, staff numbers were dwindling, as some women left to get married or to join the new women's services, while others were forced to stop work on account of illness, or even, on occasion, died. The Australian surgeon Eleanor Bourne left in early 1918 to become medical controller for the WAACs in northern England. She was followed at the end of April by her compatriot Hamilton-Browne, who set sail for Egypt with the Scottish surgeon Jessie Scott-Reid, to take up jobs as army surgeons at a military hos-pital in Alexandria. Scott-Reid had left Endell Street the previous November, but she and Hamilton-Browne had stayed good friends and were eager for further adventure. "She told me about recruiting for Egypt," Hamilton-Browne later recalled, "and I said I'd like to go to Egypt, so she said 'Why not' and I did."[23]

Regarded as one of the best surgeons at Endell Street, Hamilton-Browne would be sorely missed—not least by Scantlebury. Now the only Australian surgeon left at Endell Street, Scantlebury felt "very flat."[24] A few days later, she became the last remaining representative of the Commonwealth when the Canadian anesthetist Evelyn Windsor also left.

Regardless of her COs' patent disapproval of marriage, Windsor—she kept her own name—had stayed on at Endell Street despite becoming pregnant a few months after her wedding. In the early months of her pregnancy, Windsor's colleagues had given her their quotas of orange juice to ensure the baby received adequate vitamins.[25] As she gained weight, she grew nauseated from the sickly fumes of ether and chloroform, but she forged ahead, sitting on a stool to administer anesthetics during the long operating sessions in the spring of 1918. Maintaining her post even in the late stages of pregnancy, she was startled at one point by an unexpected visit to the operating theater by Queen Alexandra. As Windsor struggled to her feet with the rest of the staff, the Queen Mother insisted she remain seated.

Only when she became unwell, with pleurisy, at the end of April did Windsor finally give up her post. Her son Peter was born six weeks later. Since the army had no procedures in place for pregnant doctors—she was probably the first pregnant doctor ever to serve in the British Army—she was officially released due to "ill health." The departing doctors were swiftly replaced by a new raft of recruits. They included Octavia Lewin, Vera's landlady, who joined as a consulting surgeon for ear, nose, and throat disorders.

Even though the spring sunshine brought some much-needed cheer to Endell Street, the long hours, poor food, and germ-laden atmosphere conspired to demoralize and weaken staff both old and new. Many of the women showed signs of ill health in 1918. Bacterial infections in fingers, noses, throats, and gums were common, and, in a pre-antibiotic age, often lingered for weeks. Any small cut or sore was liable to become infected by the virulent microbes brought back from the trenches. Nina Last suffered repeatedly from a "septic nose," while her sister, Barbara, recovered from an infected arm, but then contracted a "septic tooth."[26] Although Murray had recovered from her earlier illness, she had to have half a finger amputated as a result of infection. Some staff members by now simply lacked the stamina to beat these pernicious germs. One of the orderlies, Eva Graham Prior, contracted Vincent's angina, a nasty bacterial infection of the throat and gums commonly known as "trench mouth," and died within forty-eight hours.[27] A lively character who was widely liked for her "sweet disposition," she was just twenty-one.

In June, Murray went away on a two-week walking tour—a much-needed change of scenery, if not quite a rest—while Anderson held down the fort. It was the longest break Murray had enjoyed since first taking command at Endell Street and the longest separation between Murray and Anderson since they had worked in France. When Murray returned, she found the hospital quite different.

AT THE END of June, patients began arriving from the front with worrying new symptoms. "It is a most peculiar disease, not typhoid, not influenza, not meningitis but symptoms of each," wrote Scantlebury.[28] The hospital's casualty department began filling up with soldiers on leave exhibiting the same signs, and before long the strange malady was affecting staff, too. Although it was labeled influenza, the severity of the illness and the speed with which it developed were unprecedented. Its origins were unknown, but the disease spread rapidly among the troops on both sides of the front line in France before crossing the Channel to Britain.

Both Scantlebury and her brother Cliff, who was visiting London on leave, were early victims. Cliff went downhill so quickly during a trip to the theater that he and Scantlebury had to leave at the interval; the next day he was admitted to the military hospital at Millbank. Both recovered quickly, but others were not so lucky. "Tragedies have been happening here," Scantlebury wrote a week later. "The 'flu' of course has run thro' the hospital and one of the orderlies died from pneumonia and another has just turned the corner." The orderly who died had worked at Endell Street since the start. As she tended the victims on her wards, Scantlebury was worried to see her two COs "looking so ill," while she felt overwhelmed by "post influenzal depression which is quite a real thing." Scantlebury remarked that the "little microscopical rod shaped bacillus" that was wreaking havoc throughout Europe might alter the "fate of nations." She was wrong about the microbe—it is a roughly spherical virus, not a rod-shaped bacterium—but her prediction about its impact was uncannily prescient.

THE SUMMER INFLUENZA epidemic imposed an added burden on Endell Street's already embattled and depleted staff. Just as the government extended conscription to include all men under fifty-one to replace casualties lost at the front in 1918, so Murray and Anderson had to draw on all their contacts to supplement their staff. In 1917 they had sent appeals to girls' schools and women's colleges asking for volunteers to give up a few weeks of their summer vacation so the hospital orderlies could take a break.[29] Dozens of girls from the top boarding schools had flocked to Endell Street—and they did so again in 1918. Medical students from the LSMW gave up their vacation time as well to help in the wards, laboratories, and operating theater.

One of these volunteers was Dulcie Staveley, a nineteen-year-old student in her second year at LSMW who spent two weeks in the X-ray room in 1918.[30] Both of her older brothers were already serving in the army, and Staveley was determined to do her bit for the war effort. Later she would remember the "redoubtable" two women, Murray and Anderson, who ran Endell Street. Facilities in the X-ray room were "pretty primitive," she recalled, in common with all X-ray departments of the time. She was hastily instructed in how to use the instruments by another medical student, and warned to stand on a rubber mat to protect against electric shocks. At one point, when a Canadian soldier, who had dislocated his hip in jumping from a third-floor window in the Strand to avoid arrest—he was presumably absent without leave—was brought in for an X-ray, one of the staff members absentmindedly stepped off the mat and everyone in the room, including the patient, received a jolt. Although her stay was short, it would have a lasting impact on Staveley: she would go on to become the first female radiologist at the Royal Free Hospital.

Another recruit was a young black woman who arrived at Endell Street by royal appointment in the summer of 1918. She had written to Queen Alexandra asking to help with the war effort and had been sent on to Endell Street as a nursing orderly. The Queen Mother made a special visit to meet her in August. "We are a cosmopolitan crowd here," wrote Scantlebury.[31]

Schoolgirls, students, and royal protégées all rendered valuable help at Endell Street—just as the older conscripts plugged some gaps at the front—but it was not enough in either case. Allied troops finally managed to stem the German advance by July, at the cost of huge numbers of casualties, but they were desperate for reinforcements. While the Allies waited anxiously for the Americans' first major offensive in France, Murray, too, turned to the United States.

A FEW MONTHS earlier, in April, Murray had written to a friend, Dora Sedgewick Hazard, a philanthropist and suffragist who lived in Syracuse, New York, asking if she could find ten or twelve young women to work as orderlies at Endell Street.[32] The letter was followed a few days later by a cable urging Hazard to send twenty women as soon as possible, owing to the dire difficulties of finding staff at home. The women should be between the ages of nineteen and thirty-two, physically fit and strong, blessed with cheerful dispositions, and attractive, since, Murray confessed, she had a predilection "for good-looking ones." In an interview, she explained, "We are expecting the American boys any day now . . . and we are longing for American girls, fine vigorous young American blood, because we are tired."

Hazard rose magnificently to the challenge. Within two days of receiving the cable, she had mustered applications from thirty candidates, who were put through a rigorous interview process. All of them were from well-to-do families in upstate New York, and were more used to gliding across polished ballroom floors in dainty pumps than with scrubbing hospital floors on their knees. Announcing the mercy mission, the *Syracuse Herald* said the recruits would be exchanging their "afternoon frocks and evening gowns" for the drab uniforms of hospital orderlies. "It is pure drudgery," the newspaper added, "but somebody must do it."

The twenty young women who were selected, nicknamed the "Hazard Unit," crossed the Atlantic in a convoy of thirteen ships containing American troops bound for the front. They constituted the only wholly female American unit to serve in the war. On arrival in London on July 28, they were taken to Endell Street in a double-decker bus. When they entered the hospital gates, they found the courtyard decked with flowers and flags, including a huge Stars and Stripes, and packed with staff and patients. As they walked in, a piano struck up and the choir launched into the "Star Spangled Banner." "We could all have cried," said one of the women, "and some of us did." The Americans were then treated to tea and cakes and shown to their individual rooms. They were expected to work three hours a day—thus receiving considerably more favorable treatment than their jaded British colleagues. After being measured for their uniforms—"quite the prettiest uniforms I have seen" said one—they were granted a few days' leave to see the sights before starting work.

The Americans were certainly welcome both in England and abroad. The sight of US soldiers arriving in force on the Western Front from May onward cheered the Allies and would change the course of the war. Vera Brittain, now working as a nursing orderly in Étaples, was awed when she saw the American troops with their "fearless swagger." They seemed "so god-like, so magnificent, so splendidly unimpaired in comparison with the tired, nerve-racked men of the British Army."[33] The first major battle in which the

Americans took part, at Cantigny on May 28, was a decisive victory, and more triumphs would follow.

THE AMERICANS WERE welcome at Endell Street, too. One of the new recruits was Marion Dickerman, a twenty-eight-year-old teacher from Westfield, New York, who had volunteered with her best friend Nancy Cook.[34] Having met as students at Syracuse University, they had become not just friends but lifelong companions, as devoted to each other as Murray and Anderson. Dickerman was bright and ambitious, while Cook, who was seven years older, was more artistic, with short, frizzy hair and a "high nervous tension" that manifested in a permanent frown. Both ardent suffragettes and pacifists, they had volunteered in the expectation of helping with some light domestic chores.

When they first arrived at Endell Street, Dickerman and Cook made clear that neither of them knew anything about nursing; Cook had never even entered a hospital before. Yet they were immediately assigned to two wards containing seriously wounded cases. Cook was horrified by the sight of the mutilated men, and after a week spent avoiding all contact with patients she was assigned to making artificial legs. A talented craftswoman, she became renowned for her skill in designing crutches and prosthetic limbs and teaching the men how to walk with them. Dickerman, meanwhile, coped as best she could.

Reporting for work on her first day on St Theresa ward, Dickerman was told to prepare a row of patients for their wounds to be dressed. Having no clue what this entailed, she asked one of the patients, a man who had had both legs amputated, what to do. Coached by her kindly patient, a florist named Brook, she soon picked up the procedure. At first the work seemed horrific and exhausting, but before long Dickerman found she was carrying stretchers, changing bed pans, and even giving injections with scarcely a second's thought. With typical Endell Street pragmatism, she said the work "just had to be done, and you did the very best you could."

Once she had mastered the basic tasks, Dickerman was assigned to night duty. She was terrified, initially, by the arrival of the convoys, especially since many of the men were suffering the effects of gas attacks. "The poor men would cough and cough and there was so little that you could do for them," she recalled. She tried to soothe patients who complained that their toes hurt despite having had their legs amputated—a condition known as phantom limb syndrome—and rubbed men's backs with soapy water to prevent bed sores. On occasion she wrote letters for patients to their families and loved ones; after she chided one man several times for not writing to his wife, he whispered that he was unable to write. Eventually Dickerman was transferred to the record office, where she was put in charge of logging the new arrivals, contacting their next of kin, and reporting the daily tally of empty beds to the War Office. Though it was significantly less grisly than working on the wards, the responsibility of the new job gave her nightmares in which she dreamed she had overestimated the number of vacant beds and the corridors became full of men lying on stretchers.

Dickerman and Cook, nicknamed "Dickie" and "Cookie," in line with hospital custom, not only grew used to the demands of Endell Street but came to love the hospital. They would stay for nineteen months, becoming valued members of the staff and close friends with Olga Campbell and others. The matron, Grace Hale, was "a darling," said Dickerman, but she was terrified of the sister in charge of staff accommodations and discipline, Gladys Le Geyt, who she said was "a hellion." She was not the only one afraid of Le Geyt: Nina Last described her as a "hard cruel woman."[35] The two Americans were impressed by their COs' insistence on the highest standards of care. "They had wonderful courage," said Dickerman. "It was a very human hospital." On their days off and occasional longer breaks, Cook and Dickerman enjoyed trips to the cinema and outings to the countryside, including visits to Penn and to Campbell's home in Scotland.

THERE WAS NO doubt the Americans had arrived in the nick of time. Beginning on August 8, with an advance from Amiens spearheaded by Australians and Canadians, the Allies won a series of victories that forced the Germans to retreat. With the backing of more than one million American troops, the Hundred Days Offensive—in reality, ninety-five days—would decide the outcome of the war. But the dramatic gains would be bought at the cost of many thousands more casualties.

As staff awaited the start of this final major offensive at the beginning of August, an uneasy lull descended on Endell Street. The hospital "is very slack," wrote Scantlebury.[36] Working in stifling heat punctuated by violent storms, she worried over some of her long-term patients who were failing to recover, and she felt saddened at sending others to convalescent homes before they were truly fit, in order to empty the beds. She took advantage of the relative quiet by running a baby clinic at the South London Hospital for Women—a respite from military surgery—and attending a theater matinee to raise funds for the Harrow Road children's hospital. Murray had organized the event in her spare time. Scantlebury was cautiously optimistic as news of the first Allied victories filtered through, and buoyed up with patriotic pride by reports of Australian pluck. People's "spirits are rising," she said. The rains having subsided, she gloried in the rare English heatwave. One moonlit evening as she walked home, the searchlights picked out a British plane that shone like a "silver beetle" against the night sky. She knew, however, that the "last push" would soon bring a scale of casualties to test Endell Street to the limits.

The dry spell ended abruptly in torrential rain just as the convoys began to pour in. The wards were "filling rapidly with very sick men," wrote Scantlebury in mid-August.[37] Collapsing into bed at midnight after admitting a large convoy of wounded, she was just falling asleep when she heard the rumble of ambulances announcing the unexpected arrival of a second convoy of thirty men. "Work has begun," she told her family. "Wish me luck."

Within days, the hospital was filled with severely wounded men, and the surgeons were busy operating for six or seven hours without a break. In one afternoon Scantlebury assisted Anderson at eighteen operations and performed four herself, including several amputations. On her ward she had nine new cases, mostly men with chest wounds, and all of them serious. "Oh, why don't we cease all this strife?" she lamented.[38] But there was no ceasing. By early September, Scantlebury was working "without a break," seeing 123 patients in a single morning and assisting at "operations galore."[39]

One week brought ten convoys from France, all of them with desperately injured men, according to an American orderly, Clara Gross.[40] "I never in my whole life worked or dreamed of working as I did yesterday," she wrote home in September. "When my off duty hours come I simply climb into my cubicle and sleep or take off my clothes and rest." One of her patients was a young Canadian, who was "splendid, though totally uneducated, as most of my patients are." He had had both feet amputated as well as other "terrible wounds." His dressings were extremely painful, yet he remained brave. Another man hailed from Brooklyn and was in "much pain" but showed "such grit." Gross brought him some American newspapers for the baseball news and begged some Camel cigarettes for him from some American sailors she spotted in the street. She urged her family to send her long letters from home, because, "after spending two or three hours among the most terrible wounds and seeing big strong men wince and weep because the dressings hurt so cruelly, a letter from home is just peace."

Emergency cots were put up to provide additional beds as the convoys arrived without a break. One ward that normally contained forty beds had fifty-two patients, and men were discharged every day to make space for new arrivals. "This place is an absolute hell," wrote Nina Last in September.[41] "It is simply crammed with frightful cases & convoys keep on coming in every night." The nursing sisters were tearing out their hair because there were "only Americans & Medical Students" left on the wards. Life was scarcely any easier in the linens room, where Last had to process more than five hundred dirty sheets a day, most of them filthy with mud and infested with lice. "My idea of Hell is always changing," she said. "It is now the Dirty Wash, it is unspeakably awful, besides the smell & dirt nearly all the bundles are full of vermin & there is so much of it that we can't forbear groaning aloud in agony." Her ankles were swollen with bites. Her one comfort was that Barbara was spared the rush; she had been sent home unwell, although she plied her sister with queries about the progress of her favorite patients. Nina duly reported that one of them, Symonds, was "still alive," though "too weak to scream except in a feeble way." It was probably not much reassurance. Everyone was having "a terrible time all round," she said, "but let's hope its 'Darkest before Dawn.'"

One of the patients admitted to Endell Street that September was a young Canadian private named Larry Tarrant.[42] Having enlisted in 1916, aged eighteen, Larry was shot in the head, arm, shoulder, and both legs at the beginning of the assault from Arras, which would become known as "Canada's Hundred Days." After being evacuated to a base hospital, where his wounds were cleaned, he arrived at Endell Street on September 11 with his left arm in a Thomas splint. Dorothy Daintree, a new recruit who had recently qualified, was the surgeon on duty that night. She sent Tarrant for an X-ray, which revealed that his elbow was shattered, with four inches of bone completely destroyed. There was every chance he would lose his arm, yet Daintree refused to give up on him. She performed an operation on September 16 to clean out and stitch his wounds, which were "bipped" with the customary ointment, and Tarrant not only recovered, but his arm was saved. He stayed at Endell Street until the end of December, undergoing massage and physical therapy, before being transferred to a convalescent hospital. Returning to Canada the following year with a permanent crook in his arm, Tarrant found work in a paper mill, married, and had four children. In later life he would tell his children and grandchildren that "a young female doctor in England" had saved his arm.

FINALLY IT SEEMED an end was in sight—on the front, at least. September brought news that the Germans had been forced back as far as the Hindenburg Line, and there were even rumors of peace talks. Hearing reports of the victory, Murray rushed into the operating theater, beaming, to tell Anderson and the rest of the surgical team. Together the pair hurried out to buy buns for a celebration.[43]

Struggling with the workload still, Nina Last hoped "it won't be for much longer."[44] The men were "very excited" about the news, she wrote, though they feared it might be a trap. "Anyhow it is good & you never saw anything like the changes in people's faces," she added. "Everyone's wearing a broad smile." Scantlebury, meanwhile, remained skeptical of any imminent peace, though she allowed herself to dream of a future in which she lived a simple life in a hut in the Australian bush keeping goats and catching fish.[45]

When she returned to Endell Street in mid-October after a two-week break in Ireland, Scantlebury found the hospital "full to the brim."[46] The wards were all "tremendously busy" with extremely sick men, and the operating lists were as heavy as ever. In addition, there were more cases of flu rolling in both from France and at home. Snatching a few hours off to visit the Swedish War Hospital, funded by the Swedish Chamber of Commerce in west London, she was flabbergasted to find the surgeon there had an assistant, two sisters, and three VADs to help him in the theater, while Scantlebury struggled with just two orderlies at her side.[47] Her two COs looked "tired out," thought Scantlebury, yet they battled on with a "pluck and perseverance" that filled her with wonder.[48]

In the midst of the madness of finding beds for the victims of war and flu, Murray and Anderson still found time to keep the entertainments in full swing and push their political agenda forward. The recreation hall was packed to the rafters in October as the recuperating soldiers enjoyed a play about Henry VIII; a concert by a Scottish boys' band, in which four lads performed a Highland fling; and a sing-along accompanied by violins. Hearing the men joining in as ever with the chorus to the troops' favorite, "There's a Long, Long Trail," Scantlebury confessed, "I am sick of that trail—it is much too long for my liking."[49] Yet for all her reservations about her COs' suffragette views, Scantlebury wholeheartedly supported their campaign for equal treatment for women doctors.

Anderson and Murray lobbied tirelessly for the rights of women doctors in the army to be awarded military ranks and income tax exemptions, in line with their male colleagues, throughout 1918. Female army doctors had won the right to wear military uniforms in June—thanks to Alfred Keogh—but despite a vociferous campaign by the Medical Women's Federation, the War Office still refused them formal commissions as officers.[50] Although Murray had been promoted in July to the pay grade equivalent of lieutenant colonel—making her effectively the highest-ranking woman in the army—she was still technically junior to the youngest Tommy in Endell Street. In October, Anderson wrote a fiery letter to *The Times* complaining that the doctors at Endell Street and elsewhere in the army carried out exactly the same duties as their male counterparts yet were denied the badge of rank which their patients would recognize as a mark of authority.[51] Even more galling, she said, the Income Tax Commission had refused their appeal for service tax rates, on the grounds that the duties women doctors performed at Endell Street and elsewhere were "not work of a military character."

Incensed by this staggering claim, Margaret Thackrah's husband, Leonard, wrote in support of Anderson, condemning the "heartbreaking stupidity" of both the government and the income tax commissioners. Despite being fully qualified doctors who were successfully running "a great military hospital," he complained, they were deprived of their rank by a "senseless" official dictate. The women were told their work was not of a military character despite being paid directly by the War Office and the fact that "their only patients are wounded soldiers!" Scantlebury thought it was "grossly unfair" to tax women doctors when male doctors paid nothing, and she was furious when the women at Endell Street were ordered, presumably by the War Office, to remove their "pips"—the decorations denoting army rank—from their shoulder epaulettes.[52]

Despite the demands of the military work they were most definitely performing, Anderson and Murray did not confine their concerns to women doctors, or even women in the army. They were also lobbying in 1918 against the pernicious effect on women generally of the government's attempts to curb venereal disease. While Germany provided official brothels for its troops in France, and the French government not only sanctioned licensed brothels but issued condoms to soldiers on its side of the front line, the British government had relied, initially at least, on advising its troops simply to avoid "wine and women." This advice being widely ignored, British soldiers had formed long queues outside French brothels and made abundant use of prostitutes, both professional and casual, in France and on leave in Britain. Many, understandably enough, did not want to "die virgins," in the poet Robert Graves's words. The net result was that more than four hundred thousand British soldiers had been hospitalized for venereal disease by 1918, and that roughly 5 percent of the British troops were estimated to be infected with a sexually transmitted disease.[53] Placing the blame for this epidemic squarely on women rather than men, the government had introduced regulations in 1916, under the Defence of the Realm Act (DORA), to penalize any woman with venereal disease caught soliciting anyone in uniform. By August 1918, seventy-six women had been convicted, and the government was claiming that the removal of these "centres of infection," as the women were termed, had led to a decrease in venereal disease in some districts.

The Medical Women's Federation voted unanimously at its first annual meeting in 1918 to oppose the DORA legislation—on grounds not only of its blatant discrimination, but more particularly its medical inefficacy—and lobbied the government for its repeal. Murray and Anderson had been campaigning since before the war for compulsory notification and compulsory free treatment for anyone—male or female—with venereal disease. Their demand had not only united the archrivals Emmeline Pankhurst and Millicent Fawcett but also garnered support from the prime minister's wife, Margaret Lloyd George, and many prominent doctors. In October, the government rejected calls to repeal the legislation, but agreed to set up a committee to investigate its measures.[54] Murray was appointed one of the committee's members.

WOMEN'S SECOND-CLASS STATUS was forgotten momentarily as the whispers of peace grew louder in the first days of November. Even though the newspapers were filled with reports of German defeats, of Germany's surrender, and of the abdication of the Kaiser, nobody dared believe the war might actually end. When at last the armistice was declared on November 11, 1918, the news seemed impossible to grasp.

In France, the rumble of the guns slowly died away and silence fell. For the first time in four years, men could stand up in the trenches and look over the parapets toward enemy lines without fear of a sniper's bullet. Soldiers stared at each other in disbelief, not sure whether to laugh or cry. In London, the maroons boomed for the first time in six months, and for a moment people panicked in expectation of an air raid. Then church bells started clanging, car horns blared, and people streamed out into the streets.[55] Children poured out of school, workers emerged from their shops and offices, soldiers and civilians grabbed anything with which they could make a noise—tea trays, whistles, toy trumpets, even a dinner gong—intent on creating as much commotion as they could. Women clerks in the War Office threw bundles of official forms out of the windows. Strangers danced together and kissed each other, cheering and sobbing. Flag sellers suddenly appeared selling miniature Union Jacks.

Vera Scantlebury had not allowed herself to believe in the rumors of an armistice. She had been on duty on the night of November 10, receiving a convoy in the early hours, and had fallen into bed at 3:00 a.m. A few hours later, she was in the operating theater helping Anderson with a difficult operation. They were just finishing, stitching the wounds, and ready for the patient to revive when they heard the maroons boom three times. The surgeons, nurses, and orderlies who were bent over the slumbering patient looked at each other, speechless with disbelief. Then one of the orderlies exclaimed: "By Gosh! It's Peace!" And one after another, each of the women repeated the words: "It's peace—I can't believe it!" From the courtyard below the sound of cheering erupted. Murray was making a speech to the gathered orderlies. The dogs, William and Garrett, were joining in the celebration, barking excitedly.

Marion Dickerman was in the records office, filling in forms as usual, when she glanced out the window and saw one of the male RAMC orderlies, Corporal Hubbardson, running across the courtyard. Then she heard church bells ringing in the streets outside. Dropping what she was doing, she rushed to find the patient she had first looked after, the double amputee named Brook, four months earlier. "Oh, Brook," she asked him, "do you want to go down to Buckingham Palace?" Finding a wheelchair, she pushed him, in his blue suit and red tie, out into the mobbed streets. As they edged through the crowds, dozens of people offered to help, and women rushed up and kissed her patient, showering him with cigarettes and flowers. When they reached the palace gates, a band was playing the national anthems of all the Allies as the king and queen emerged on the balcony to tumultuous cheering.

Still at work in the operating theater, Scantlebury assisted at another operation before she made her way down to the courtyard, which was now festooned with flags. Murray had given permission for all the patients who were fit enough to leave their beds to join in the street parties, so the hospital was emptying rapidly. Scantlebury emerged into the thronged streets an hour and a half after peace had been declared to see people waving from the tops of buses and standing precariously on the roofs of taxis. As she scurried to meet a friend for a prearranged lunch, a youth slapped her on the back and shouted, "Hurrah for nursie!" Another grabbed her arm and asked, "And what are you going to do now the war is over?" Failing to find her friend in the mayhem, she ate lunch alone. Tired from her night duty and overwhelmed by emotion, she felt depressed by the clamor and found refuge in a church, where the congregation was singing hymns.

When she returned to Endell Street with Brook, Dickerman met Olga Campbell, who was rounding up volunteers to visit local shops and beg for food for a tea party for the men remaining on the wards. Running from store to store around Covent Garden, Dickerman and Cook returned loaded with treats. Scantlebury, feeling calmer as she emerged blinking from the darkened church, had the same idea. Passing a Lyons tea shop, she bought six enormous cakes and struggled back to Endell Street with her arms full. Back at the hospital, she visited her two wards and spoke to every one of her eighty patients as they shared cakes, chocolate, and bread spread with honey. Some of the men had already been out, joining in the celebrations in the Strand. Murray and Anderson had even commandeered a lorry, in which they toured the streets with a bevy of orderlies waving at the crowds. Recognized by their distinctive uniforms, they were cheered rowdily by whooping passersby.

Not everybody cheered. Many felt they had nobody left with whom to celebrate. Almost everyone at Endell Street had lost a family member or close friend or knew someone who was bereaved. The joy was muted, too, for those who had survived at the cost of life-changing injuries, such as Dickerman's friend Brook. In all, 745,000 British soldiers had died and 1.7 million had been wounded during the four years of war.[56] Worldwide, the war had taken the lives of more than 9 million soldiers and 7 million civilians as well as leaving 21 million injured.

Others felt dazed by the news, unable to imagine a world without war and filled with uncertainty about the future. The journalist Michael MacDonagh was saddened for the millions who had died and the millions more who were bereaved, but he also mourned personally, realizing that, as he put it, "a great and unique episode in my life was past and gone." That sense of living for the moment that the war had "so vividly heightened" was about to expire, so that "tomorrow we return to the monotonous and the humdrum," he wrote. For Elizabeth Courtauld, a surgeon at the Scottish Women's Hospital at Royaumont, the war's end meant that the work of these "gorgeous times," in which women doctors had stood as equals to men, would soon be over.[57] Scantlebury, too, felt detached, with an "almost numbing" feeling at the thought there would be no more fighting. Remembering the air raids of just months earlier, she did not know what felt more dreamlike, "that hideous nightmare or the dream of peace."[58] As she contemplated returning to the country she had left almost two years earlier, she was unsure what she would find there—marriage, a career, or her fantasy of a simple life in the bush. For Nina Last, the sound of clocks striking in the night after years of silence and the sight of brightly lit streets and shop windows after the long blackout were "very cheering."[59]

Yet she found it hard to believe that the misery and turmoil of war were really over.

It was not over yet, not for Endell Street, at least. In the days immediately following the armistice, the hospital remained frantically busy as convoys continued to arrive from the front. "I can scarcely believe it," wrote Scantlebury, "but the hospital goes on as usual and never have we been more busy." There were twenty operations on November 13, eighteen the following day. Last was working "harder than ever," doing twelve-hour shifts in the linens room throughout the armistice week. When she heard at the end of that week that Endell Street would remain open for another year, the news "depressed us awfully."

Determined to celebrate, Murray and Anderson threw a fancy dress party that outdid all their previous efforts.[60] As they reprised their roles as Colonel and Mrs. Dug-out, Murray wore a kilt, which she had borrowed from Alan Anderson, and false red whiskers. After toasting the king's health, she gave a tub-thumping speech in the manner of a battle-hardened veteran that was met with rowdy applause. Anderson, in a lace cap and mittens, played a simpering wife who meekly insisted that women were incapable of public service, to uproarious laughter. But Sir Alan, the evening's guest, earned the loudest guffaws when he objected to Murray denoting him the "stranger within the gates," since "my sister is at one end of the table and my kilt at the other." Then they "danced and danced" and feasted on cold tongue, potato salad, and jellies.

Asked to remain open for another year while other military hospitals had orders to close, the women at Endell Street prepared for their last struggle.

IO

Full of Ghosts

Endell Street, London, November 1918

The church bells that had rung so riotously to celebrate the Armistice were tolling now for funerals. Men returning from the front line, in a state of frenzied joy mingled with bewildered grief, were suddenly taking to their beds. Robert Graves, the poet who had survived battles which had sent many of his comrades to their deaths, went home to Hove, collapsed into bed, and was told by a visiting doctor that there was no hope for him.[1] In Endell Street, patients and staff were developing fevers, aches, and coughs at a rate that had never been seen before. The flu had returned. Having disappeared at the end of the summer, the virus had mutated into a deadlier, devastating new form.

Robert Graves was one of the lucky ones. Having been left for dead during the Battle of the Somme, he "refused to die of influenza" and was better within a week. Many more were less fortunate. The "Spanish flu," as it was inaccurately dubbed, would kill an estimated fifty million to one hundred million people—more than the entire death toll of the war and possibly the next one too—in a pandemic stretching from Cape Town to Alaska and from Delhi to Rio.[2] Its origins were mysterious—and remain a puzzle to this day. It is possible that the virus had first erupted in an army camp in Kansas in March 1918 and was brought to Europe by American troops, meaning

253

that the same men who had helped end the war had seeded an even deadlier enemy. Or it may have emerged earlier, at the British army camp in Étaples in December 1916, aided by the damaging effects of mustard gas, or, conceivably, in China in the winter of 1917, or possibly somewhere else entirely. All that can be said with certainty is that it did not start in Spain, where the first cases only appeared in May 1918. It had acquired its name simply because newspapers in neutral Spain, free from wartime censorship, had openly reported that country's shocking death toll.

After the first wave of relatively mild influenza had petered out, in August the flu had reappeared simultaneously in three places— Boston, Massachusetts; Freetown, Sierra Leone; and Brest, France— then swept across the globe with appalling speed and force. Almost nowhere was left untouched; only Antarctica and the island of Saint Helena were entirely spared. And whereas influenza normally wreaked its worst effects on the very young and very elderly, this virulent new strain mainly attacked young adults—men and women in their twenties and thirties. Indeed, many thousands of soldiers survived the long misery of the trenches only to die within days of returning home from a microscopic virus.

The timing was no coincidence. The mass movement of troops in overcrowded ships and trains during the last months of the war and the ensuing demobilization, coupled with the euphoric Armistice celebrations—when complete strangers hugged and kissed with abandon—provided perfect conditions for the unparalleled spread of the disease. With its rapid onset and swift conclusion, the flu was likened to the Black Death. A third wave, in early 1919, which was more virulent than the first but less deadly than the second, would scythe down millions more. In total the Spanish flu would kill an estimated 3 to 6 percent of the world's population in 1918–1919, though this proportion ranged wildly by country, from about 0.5 percent in Great Britain—where three times as many died in the war—to 25 percent in Western Samoa.

The lethal second wave of flu had first hit Britain in October and peaked at the height of the Armistice celebrations in early November, when nearly thirty thousand people died in a single week. This pattern was mirrored in London, where some sixteen thousand people died between September and December, the majority in October and November.[3] Just as thousands were dancing in the streets to celebrate the end of the war, funeral corteges were slowly winding their way to municipal cemeteries.[4] While the front pages of newspapers were emblazoned with pictures of cheering men and women, the obituary columns were filled with notices of people slain by the flu. The disease was so widespread and so destructive that entire families were struck down at once. Buses and trams were canceled for lack of staff; emergency services were dangerously stretched as police, fire, and ambulance workers fell ill; and hospitals struggled to cope as nurses and doctors collapsed alongside their patients. At Endell Street, there were no more convoys of wounded and disfigured soldiers reeking of mud, gas, and gangrene arriving in the night. Now the beds were filled with choking, feverish men and women dying of the flu.

The first signs that the flu had returned to Endell Street had been almost overlooked in the last push toward victory. Men and women arriving in convoys from France showed influenza symptoms in mid-October, when Vera Scantlebury had returned from a break to find "'Spanish flu' flying round the wards."[5] By the end of that month, with peace just within grasp, cases of the flu were "rolling in," she noted, and the disease had spread to staff. Eleven orderlies had been struck down and admitted to "H" ward, where the WAACs were normally nursed, "not caring one atom who wins the war," as Scantlebury put it. Now that the war's outcome had been decided, the hospital was inundated with flu. Local civilians crowded the casualty room, coughing and sneezing, or arrived by ambulance in a worse state as they fell victim to the disease.[6] By mid-November, "dozens of local sick" had been admitted. Between fifty and sixty patients at a time were seriously ill with pneumonia—often the final stage of the flu. Extra beds were made up on the wards and immediately filled, more nurses had to be recruited to replace those who fell ill, and the doctors worked without breaks.

Just when the staff should have been able to rest and recover at the end of the long, dreary war, they were working harder than ever and—worse, much worse—with the least success. Throughout the war, the Endell Street women had saved thousands of soldiers from death and disability through a combination of surgical expertise, pioneering infection control, skilled nursing, dedicated physical therapy, and their particular brand of motivational spirit. But they were no match for the flu. With no antiviral medicines to combat the disease or antibiotics to treat the ensuing pneumonia, which often caused death, they were powerless to help their patients. All they could offer was aspirin, morphine, and quinine to suppress the symptoms; fluids and nourishment to keep up their patients' strength; and bedrest in the hope that the victims would beat the bug themselves. Many of them didn't.

The death rates shocked nurses and doctors alike. Throughout the war years, in the face of appalling wounds and rampant infections, no more than eight soldiers died for every one thousand patients treated at Endell Street—some two hundred deaths in all.[7] Yet in November and December 1918, twenty-four men and women died of flu; at times, there were as many as three deaths a day. The hospital was thronged with desperate relatives, who paced the courtyard, stood in the corridors, and sat hunched beside the beds as they waited to find out if their loved ones would live or die. Elderly parents traveled from as far afield as Scotland and Ireland to maintain bedside vigils; some of the men "clung to their mothers," said Murray.

The speed with which patients succumbed to the flu, and the symptoms they displayed during its course, were completely alien to the Endell Street staff. "Men died like flies, in the street one moment, then three days later, dead," said Nina Last. "It was more like a plague than influenza." Experienced doctors agreed. Victims first complained of sore throats, headaches, and generalized aches but were very quickly forced to take to their beds. Unable to rise, many developed the tell-tale signs of blue-tinged lips and fingers or plum-colored blotches on their faces as their lungs became congested with blood and struggled to produce oxygen. Some patients' teeth and nails fell out; other patients became delirious and even violent or suicidal. Those who failed to rally succumbed either to the virus itself or, more often, as their lowered immune systems allowed bacteria to invade the lungs, to pneumonia, frequently within three days of showing symptoms. As their lungs filled with bloody fluid, they effectively drowned, commonly coughing up blood and bleeding from the nose or ears. Most doctors assumed the disease was caused by a bacterium; the recently discovered Pfeiffer's bacillus (*Haemophilus influenzae*), which was sometimes present in pathology specimens, was the prime suspect. Not until 1933 would scientists realize that a virus, too small for early twentieth-century microscopes to detect, was the real cause.

Those who had fallen ill in the first wave of flu in the summer—including Scantlebury and her brother Cliff—were immune to its later visitations. Scantlebury therefore sailed through her remaining days at Endell Street, eagerly planning her return home, unaffected by the lethal virus. Other staff members had no such protection. Nina Last fell ill with the fearful signs toward the end of the year and was admitted to "H" ward.[8] Nursed by her colleagues, she was extremely ill for a week, but she recovered. Her sister Barbara fell victim too, and although she revived, she never returned to work, her delicate health broken by the disease and her years of toil.

Marion Dickerman was another flu victim who was nursed on "H" ward.[9] As the fever took hold, she became delirious—a common side effect—and began raving about food and drink. When she saw her friend Olga Campbell at her bedside, she burst into tears and complained that she could not eat anything with the tarnished black spoon she had been given. Campbell rushed out and bought a silver spoon engraved with a bird from a local pawn shop. A few days later, Dickerman woke to see the screens surrounding her bed, placed there to provide isolation: she later wrote that "instead of being depressed it struck me as funny." She would keep her "Dickie bird" spoon all her life, a souvenir of her brush with death.

Battling to keep the hospital running as patients and staff sickened with the flu, Murray insisted that the women must be meticulous about hygiene.[10] A disinfecting hut was set up in the courtyard, and staff were sent there to breathe in steamy vapor twice a day. More usefully, perhaps, she ensured that those with the flu were segregated on special wards, with screens placed around their beds, as for Dickerman, and that doctors and nurses wore face masks at all times. These measures, first tested at Endell Street and a few other military hospitals, would later be made standard practice by the War Office.

Despite the staff shortages and additional strains caused by the flu, in early December Murray managed to escape Endell Street for a few days, traveling to Scotland to support her brother William in his third attempt to win a parliamentary seat.[11] The snap general election, called by David Lloyd George immediately after the Armistice for December 14, was the first time that women were allowed to vote. They had to be over thirty—unlike soldiers, who only had to be nineteen, and other men, who had to be twenty-one—and they had to meet minimum property requirements, but it was nevertheless a momentous occasion for the women who had devoted so much of their lives to securing the franchise. Determined to play her part in this climactic event, Murray spoke at a meeting for women voters to rally support for William. Major Murray, as he was now known, was subsequently elected Conservative MP for Dumfriesshire in the landslide victory for Lloyd George's coalition government.

Although Murray and Anderson, along with many of the other women doctors, were entitled to vote, most of the staff at Endell Street—the nurses, orderlies, and other workers—remained disenfranchised by virtue of their age or the property restrictions.[12] And for all her support of William, Murray had little time either for the Conservative Party or the Houses of Parliament. She would later back Christabel Pankhurst, who stood as a candidate for the Women's Party (the reformed WSPU), at which point Murray proclaimed that the House of Commons had a "peculiar smell." It was dust. "If you look down on those leather benches you will see that half of them are empty and others occupied by gentlemen sound asleep."[13]

There was barely time to celebrate the culmination of more than fifty years of campaigning, and little interest in doing so, as the flu continued its rampage. Having cast her own vote, Murray was soon back at her post. Yet despite the pressures, she went out of her way, as always, to look after the welfare of her staff. Generously, Murray offered to release Scantlebury early from her contract so she could return home to Australia; she even wangled a passage for her, since most of the ships were reserved for returning troops, through Alan Anderson. Scantlebury did not think twice.

AFTER THE TWO years of separation from her family and her work with children, Scantlebury was desperate to leave, though saddened, too. In the midst of the flu crisis in mid-December, the medical staff threw a sumptuous farewell dinner party for her at the Savoy Hotel in the Strand.[14] The fifteen women doctors, all wearing their Endell Street uniforms, gathered around a table in a hotel dining room overlooking the Thames. The menu cards were decorated with images of kangaroos in honor of Scantlebury's homeland. Taking their lead from their two COs, and ignoring the scrutiny of an elderly army colonel, who surveyed them through his monocle, the women pulled crackers and donned party hats to give Scantlebury a rousing send-off. As she counted down the days to her last shift, Scantlebury admitted, "I shall miss it in many ways."

Two days later, Murray and Anderson welcomed Scantlebury to a final dinner in their sitting room, and Murray presented her with an antique gold chain as their farewell gift. Moved almost to tears, Scantlebury would treasure her souvenir. At that moment, the strains of Christmas carols floated up from the courtyard below. It was the hospital choir, practicing in the run-up to Christmas, along with some of the male patients. As the sweet singing of the women orderlies mingled with the deep voices of the men, accompanied by the plaintive notes of a violin, Anderson flung open the windows so the cozy room would be filled with music.

IT WAS A SUBDUED Christmas. Knowing it would be the last one at Endell Street, as well as the first after four long years of war, both staff and volunteers were determined it should be remembered as the best yet.[15] When they toured the wards for the annual judging on Christmas Day, the COs awarded prizes to all—in the new spirit of extended democracy—then toasted the men's health in each ward before they toddled, unsteadily thought Scantlebury, to the next. On Boxing Day the staff decorated a magnificent Christmas tree—a rarity that year, on account of its German connotations—with tinsel and fairy lights. Dorothy Daintree donned a white beard and red suit to play the part of Santa Claus and handed out presents to the children of the hospital's cleaning women, who were invited to a special tea.

But the hospital was overflowing with patients in the grip of flu, as well as those recuperating from their war wounds, and even though the wards were decorated as inventively as ever and there were just as many entertainments, the celebrations were muted. The staff seemed to be going through the motions, wearied by work and grief.

Although the second, most lethal, wave of the Spanish flu had almost run its course by Christmas, the third was quick to follow. No sooner had the decorations been taken down from the wards than there was a new influx of flu cases. As Scantlebury worked her last shift on December 30, on night duty for the final time, sick patients—military and civilians—"rolled in one after the other."[16] While Murray was desperately trying to discharge patients to convalescent beds elsewhere, Scantlebury was admitting dozens more to replace them. "It has its funny side," wrote Scantlebury. "As she sat in her office emptying the hospital as quickly as she knew how she looked up to see processions of men being taken in by me!!" It was easy for Scantlebury to see the comedy in the situation. With her demobilization papers in hand, she sailed for Australia on January 11, 1919, ecstatic at the prospect of seeing her beloved family and homeland again.

JANUARY BEGAN DULL, wet, and windy. It deteriorated further as temperatures dropped below freezing and snow fell. Even the novelty of peace could not dispel the gloom as the flu death rate rose for the third time. At the end of the month, *The Times* warned that the country had been seized by a new bout of flu of "considerable virulence."[17] In London, the deaths climbed to a peak in February of more than 650 a week. In all a total of 6,000 people would die in the capital before the third wave eventually receded in May. Struggling to cope with the new flood of admissions, staff at Endell Street watched the death rate rise through January and hit a record high of 30 deaths in February—the hospital's biggest monthly death toll ever. But the brunt of those deaths was borne by the staff.

Back in the linens room after winning her own battle with flu, Nina Last watched as one after another of her colleagues sickened and, in some cases, died. "Pretty young girls, quite well one day, were dead in three days time from streptococcal germs, or influenza," she recalled.[18] One was Mary Graham, a nursing orderly, who had been working on "H" ward, tending flu victims, when she fell ill and soon after died.[19] Her death was followed by that of another nurse orderly who had been working on the same ward. And then Helen Wilks, a young woman who had worked as an assistant in the pathology laboratory for eighteen months, became seriously ill.

Helen was the adopted daughter of Dr. Elizabeth Wilks, a suffragette friend of Anderson's. She had hoped to become a doctor like her mother and was thrilled when Murray took her on, at just sixteen, in 1917. She died on January 15, following an appendix operation, although the flu may have been a contributory factor. Murray was distraught. "She was only eighteen and full of promise," she wrote.[20] Dr. Wilks wrote a poignant letter to reassure the COs that her daughter had been "completely happy" in her work and that she and her husband had never regretted allowing her to join the hospital. "Endell Street was the great time of her life," she said. But it was little consolation for her early death.

As February brought freezing temperatures and further snow, more staff fell sick. One of them, Joan Palmes—"Palmy"—was a much-loved nursing orderly who had worked at Endell Street since it opened. Weakened by influenza, she developed pneumonia; she was only twenty-seven, and her death cast a deep gloom over the entire hospital. "Last week was the saddest this Hospital has ever seen," Nina Last wrote home. "Somehow we all felt poor old Palmy's death more than the others, partly, I think because she was so much a part of the Hospital & also the C.O's were so shattered

& broken down by her death."[21] Last was shocked when Murray, who had kept so relentlessly cheerful throughout the war, now broke down. When Murray was told that another orderly, whose temperature had hit 105°F, was now on the mend, she wept. The sight of their staunch CO in tears, after so many years of unfailing perseverance, was almost more than staff could bear.

With each of these deaths, the women followed their colleague's coffin into the small church adjoining the hospital, where the staff choir sang the *Nunc Dimitis* prayer bidding her to depart in peace. Then the coffin was carried into the courtyard, where the women gathered around to say a final farewell. "Some of our bitterest moments were seeing those coffins pass out of the courtyard," Last later recalled. The church was packed for Palmes's funeral on February 26, when Murray read from the Bible "beautifully." It was a "wonderful service," wrote Last, and everyone admired Palmes's mother, who was "brave & so good to the C.O.'s."

The deaths of these young women, after their years of devotion to the hospital, hit the COs hard. Inevitably, they felt responsible. Murray would later console herself with the fact that only 22 of the 184 staff members were laid low by flu in 1918–1919. Of those who fell ill, 5—including Helen Wilks—died during the pandemic. It was little short of a miracle, given the daily exposure to the virus and the strenuous working conditions, that there were not more. Murray would later admit that during the flu pandemic the "habitual gaiety of the place was hidden under the cloud." In reality morale had sunk to its lowest level ever, and the two COs seemed to have lost heart in trying to revive it. During the darkest periods of the war, when staff worked night after night, and as the convoys rolled in and bombs fell, that idiosyncratic mixture of patriotic zeal and Endell Street spirit had kept the women going. Now that they found themselves fighting an invisible enemy, to no apparent purpose, they had reached the breaking point.

Palmes's death was the last straw. Having lost the will to continue, Murray asked the War Office to close Endell Street as soon as possible. "Dr Murray whose spirit has never been known to fail before completely broke," Last told her mother, "& she has been doing everything in her power to get this Hospital closed ever since."[22] But whatever the War Office responded, there was evidently no hope of an early end to the trials.

Most of the patients who died in that third wave of the pandemic were young. Though many died far from their homes, relatives and friends often made pilgrimages to their bedsides. One young Australian, Corporal Frederick Waring, was admitted with flu and double pneumonia in April. After an operation to remove congestion in one lung, he improved for a while before taking a turn for the worse. A family friend, who was an Australian Red Cross visitor, was at his bedside when he died. He had been comforted by the hospital chaplain, she wrote in a letter to his mother, and received the best possible attention from the nurses, "who spared themselves no effort on his behalf."[23]

Many more recovered thanks to the care of the staff and more than a little luck. Among them was Vic Jones, a private in the Australian Army, who had been wounded in 1917 but returned to France, where he was still working as a driver at the beginning of 1919.[24] In April he was admitted to a hospital in Boulogne with classic signs of the flu, but then he was transferred to Endell Street, where he arrived on April 16. He spent more than three weeks at Endell Street, but was plainly on the road to recovery after his first week. The remainder of his stay revolved around a dizzying succession of visits and excursions. On admission, he recorded in a diary he kept at the time, he received the "best of attention" from the "Lady Doctors and Dentists." A week later he was fit enough for a whirlwind day that began with a motor drive to watch an ANZAC victory march through London; this was followed by a visit to the cinema, and then dinner at the home of a wealthy benefactor in north London. Four days later there was another outing, this time to Windsor Castle, where Jones chatted with George V about the king's racehorses. There was another chance to talk to the royals a few days later, when Jones was invited to Buckingham Palace for a grand dinner. His hospital stay concluded with a spin in a car belonging to an actor—"a beauty" costing £4,500—before dinner, a concert, and a visit to a club. It was all wildly exciting for a farmer's son from halfway across the globe. Ellen Pickard, who had been newly recruited to the medical team at the age of thirty-six, to help with the flu crisis after Scantlebury's departure, had been his primary doctor.[25] When he left in May and sailed home two months later, Jones brought back his diary along with a calendar for 1920. It showed photographs of Endell Street and its staff, and he would keep it until his death in 1945.

WHILE THE WAR Office hurriedly closed down military hospitals at home and abroad, releasing doctors and other staff members to return to their civilian jobs, Endell Street stayed open. Despite her appeal, Murray was asked in April to keep the hospital open for another six months. The hospital's proximity to major railway stations was no doubt a salient factor, though its popularity and reputation for efficiency must have weighed in its favor too. Another factor may well have been that male doctors were eager to return to their practices, while women doctors seemed somehow expendable. Conscientious as ever, Murray agreed to stay open.

As Endell Street was one of the few military hospitals still open in London, its beds were occupied in turn by patients transferred from other hospitals in the capital as they closed, as well as by sick or convalescing troops arriving from almost every corner of the world. Men who had been stationed in India, Africa, Russia, Salonika, Turkey, Egypt, Palestine, and Mesopotamia were brought back by hospital ship and taken to Endell Street.[26] While some were still recovering from war wounds, others were suffering tropical diseases and miscellaneous illnesses such as appendicitis. Other patients were British prisoners of war released from Germany, who related stories of savage mistreatment in their prison camps. Some of them shrieked with terror when they were told the doctor was coming to see them, said Last, then were astonished to find the doctor was "a slip of a woman with gentle fingers."[27] There was less call for surgery now, but the work was scarcely less demanding. The casualty room, meanwhile, was packed with men on demobilization leave who had fallen ill or needed medical examinations and assessments of their disabilities before they could be released. There was a subtle but disturbing change of atmosphere, too.

As spring turned to summer, the men were eager to pick up their old lives and forget the horrors of warfare. While they convalesced and awaited demobilization, they were impatient to return to their homes, their families, and their jobs—at least for those sufficiently able-bodied and with jobs to go to. Now that they had been granted full rights as citizens, the men had had enough of the army discipline and wartime camaraderie that had kept them meek and obedient in the past. For the first time, said Murray, discipline proved difficult. Some of the men, who had been used to lax rules in hospitals elsewhere, were rude and belligerent, while others were "filled with half-understood desires and a dissatisfaction which they could not explain." Many clearly understood these desires very well. They were simply not willing to be bossed about by middle-aged, middle-class women—or men for that matter—with cut-glass accents, or to bow to army regulations any longer. On some occasions, said Murray, as many as 80 to 100 men would arrive in a single party with their sights set on "giving trouble." It is only surprising the difficulties were not worse. Riots and strikes were breaking out in army camps and other places in Britain and abroad over the slow pace of demobilization and unemployment fears during 1919. In Cardiff, Australians waiting to head home joined a week of violence targeting black workers that left three men dead.[28]

Summer brought 150 Americans who were billeted at Endell Street on their way home from north Russia, where they had been involved in the Allied campaign to support the anti-Bolshevik movement. Since they were not sick, the men were allowed out on leave for a few hours on their second day to let off steam. They straggled back many hours later "drunk and sorry" after painting the town red.[29] As the days dragged on with no orders for their departure, the men grew "restless and rebellious," said Murray. Some attempted to leave the hospital without permission but were restrained by "the persuasive feminine tongue."

Characteristically, Murray played down the problems. In fact, several of the Americans were under military arrest—one had fired at an officer, while another had shot off his own toes—while others were mentally disturbed after their ordeals. At one point, one of the British soldiers charged with guarding the men had the bright idea of asking Marion Dickerman to visit a young lad from Chicago who was depressed, thinking it might help him to hear a kindly American voice.[30] After chatting amiably for some time, the youth suddenly attacked her, knocking Dickerman unconscious. She recovered quickly enough, but Murray was furious that she had been allowed into the man's room—and with good reason. When orders finally came for the Americans' departure, several men had already absconded, and two were in police custody for firing revolvers in the street.

There were even stranger visitors that summer. One ambulance convoy brought a party of French soldiers, also on their way back from Russia via a rather convoluted route, who had acquired a large dog that had been trained to hunt bears—a popular sport with the Russian nobility.[31] Although the hound was gentle toward people, he attacked a bulldog in Tottenham Court Road with such ferocity that he was only just restrained by two men with a strong rope. It was lucky for the dog that he had not gone for William or Garrett. Men returning from postings in the Far East and India brought back even more exotic wildlife. It was not unusual, said Murray, "to meet a monkey or a parrot or a strange reptile harbouring in the wards for a few days."

There were changes among the staff, too. Just as the men were returning to their old lives, so many of the orderlies were now demobilized. Reluctantly, Murray let most of her young women staff members go. These were sad days, as some of them had worked at Endell Street since the beginning. Many of them were exhausted, and some—such as Barbara Last—were worn out by their war work and their bouts with influenza. Yet most had no desire to leave. Returning to their comfortable homes, to the tedium of deciding which frock to wear for the usual calendar of society events, they knew their lives would never be as thrilling again. They had learned skills and gained experiences they could never have dreamed of. One young woman had joined as a messenger at the age of sixteen and left four years later as head financial clerk.[32] They were replaced by male RAMC orderlies, who were now available in abundance, in a return to the hospital's early days. Unused to the Endell Street ways, devoid of the Endell Street spirit, the men made a "poor substitute," said Murray. It was the "first step towards disintegration."[33]

Among the first to leave were the American women. Thirteen of the original "Hazard Unit" sailed back to Syracuse at the beginning of March, while five of those remaining went to France to volunteer for postwar duties.[34] Marion Dickerman and Nancy Cook, who had been effectively adopted as honorary members of the corps, stayed on until August. Meanwhile, Grace Hale, who had been matron at Endell Street since the start, took advantage of the comparative lull to visit the battlefields of Belgium and northern France in May as part of a party of twenty women, who were guests of the mayor of Lille.[35] As they traveled to Lille by train through blackened countryside, unrelieved by a single tree or sign of life, Hale stared out the windows in amazement at the rolls of barbed wire, dugouts, shell holes, and abandoned tanks, and at the many cemeteries filled with small wooden crosses. Over the next eight days she visited the sites of battles whose names she knew so well from conversations with her former patients. Reeling off a litany of places—Armentières, Bethune, Lens, Arras, Vimy Ridge, Ypres—which she now saw for the first time with her own eyes, she wondered how any of the men had emerged alive. "How often have we not heard our men at Endell Street giving the account of the day they were wounded at such and such a place," she wrote. Now those places, "vaguely outlined in one's imagination and heard about with all sympathy," were "real pictures." A second party to Lille a few weeks later included Murray and Anderson, traveling together through the same blasted landscape to view the battlefields familiar only from the lips of men they had treated.[36]

Murray was attempting a partial return to normality. She accepted a post in May as assistant medical officer of health for Bethnal Green in London's East End in charge of maternity and child welfare—a job far below her capabilities—but was forced to resign a few weeks later owing to a "breakdown of her health."[37] Despite her ailing health, however, she continued the melancholy task of winding down Endell Street—and her tireless crusade for equality.

PEACE BROUGHT NO reprieve from the old battles. Having buried their grievances at the outbreak of war to prove themselves equal in any area of work to men, women now wanted some reward beyond the sop of the vote for those over thirty. Anderson and Murray continued their crusade on behalf of women army doctors, demanding equal income tax rates and military rank. The new government made promises about a bill for equal rights, but although the Sex Disqualification (Removal) Act, which would eventually become law in November, entitled women to become lawyers, jurors, and magistrates, it changed little else. Canvassing the House of Commons, with the backing of the British Medical Association and the support of Sir Alfred Keogh, women doctors discovered that MPs who had offered them gushing support during the war years now proved evasive.[38] They won their demand for equal income tax rates, backdated to 1915, but lost the claim for equal rank. Winston Churchill, now secretary of state for war, outlined the government's objections in no uncertain terms.

Churchill had evidently not forgotten the indignities he had suffered at the hands of the suffragettes. In a stinging response to the Medical Women's Federation, he insisted—despite all the evidence to the contrary—that women doctors did not deserve equal rank because they were simply not capable of undertaking the same tasks as men in war. They could not work in the trenches, or treat men with venereal disease, or command a medical unit with sufficient discipline; nor had they proved equal to men in war zones in Malta and Egypt, he said. In addition, he claimed that soldiers would object to medical examinations by women, despite the abundant evidence that they had not done so at Endell Street or elsewhere. He thought that such a breach of convention would provoke a public outcry, although public reactions had proved nothing but positive toward Endell Street. Bluntly, Churchill maintained that it was "beyond refutation that Medical Women cannot perform all tasks which are at present undertaken by Medical officers." Furthermore, he asserted, demobilization meant that medical women were no longer needed in the army: "nor will their services be required beyond the present emergency." The message was clear. Women doctors had served their purpose; their talents were no longer wanted.

Despite short shrift from Churchill, Murray and Anderson devoted themselves to improving conditions for women. Murray lent her voice to an appeal by the Social Institutes' Union for Women and Girls, a charity that funded clubs where working-class women could obtain affordable meals and have access to activities and education, to raise funds for a hostel in London for working women between the ages of sixteen and twenty.[39] The war had provided thousands of young women with a wage to enable them to eat decently for the first time, she said. Now those women needed a hostel providing "liberty with discipline" and a "strong esprit de corps"—a re-creation of Endell Street, in other words—in the heart of London.

Men were not forgotten either. Anderson joined her old friends Sir Alfred Keogh and Sir Arthur Sloggett in calling for a fitness drive for young men and women in a bid to improve the nation's health. One of their goals was to offer healthy diversions from the temptations of alcohol and other evils during the "transitional stage between the old world and the new."[40] They urged the newly created Ministry of Health to set up a system to promote sports, especially in industrial areas. Anderson even joined a range of prominent public figures in signing a petition to David Lloyd George demanding the release of conscientious objectors from prison, now that hostilities were over.[41] While Murray and Anderson had been willing to support the government of the day unswervingly during the war, it was plain they were flexing their muscles again now.

When the Peace Day celebrations took place in July, at least one newspaper questioned why staff at Endell Street had been excluded from the "feminine contingent" in the procession.[42] Whether they had been excluded by government authorities or had removed themselves—no longer willing to dance to the government's tune— was unclear. Yet there was no doubt, as Churchill had made plain, that the women of Endell Street had outlived their usefulness.

ORDERS TO CLOSE Endell Street, by the end of October, finally came through from the War Office in September 1919.[43] Although the command had long been expected, still it came as a "shock to us all," said Anderson. It was greeted with "very mixed feelings of relief and sorrow." The last lingering patients were discharged to their homes or to hospitals farther afield. As the wards fell vacant, the remaining nurses and orderlies were gradually demobilized. By mid-October, only the two COs and a small core of a dozen staff remained.

As she walked the echoing corridors and visited the empty wards, once thronged with patients and staff, noisy with concerts and shows, bright with flowers and colored quilts, Murray felt desperately sad. The wards were "dreary," she said, and "miserable in their loneliness." The few women left behind spent the last weeks itemizing kitchenware, furniture, bedding, medical equipment, and even the assorted pianos for their return to army supplies. Every loss and breakage had to be accounted for. In the linens room, Nina Last counted and sorted thousands of sheets and pillows. Having been promoted to sergeant, with three staff working for her, in early 1919, now she was alone again. "It is very dismal with no men," she wrote home. "It is an awful place to live in when nearly empty & full of ghosts of the past."[44] While she worried over how to turn "1,000 sheets into 3,000," and sorted the pillows into feather, flock, or hair, she could not help remembering the thousands of men who had passed through Endell Street and those few hundred who had died, the hundreds of staff members who had worked there, and those who had given their lives in that service. By the end of October, the hospital was "ghastly" and the few remaining staff members were "in a morbid state of fright."[45] She told her mother: "No one will go into a Ward alone & in fact we are nervous of being alone anywhere."

Only Beatrice Harraden, who was busy packing up books in the library to sell them on, seemed unaffected. She was "awfully busy," she told her old friend Elizabeth Robins, but at least the task was "a cheery and pleasant one."[46] After four and a half years working loyally at her job, she was exhausted and "not frightfully well," but she looked forward to returning to her old writing life. The sale of books raised £60 for the Harrow Road children's hospital.

In November, the workmen arrived to clear out the final remains. As the men smoked and spat, played football in the courtyard, and barged into offices without asking permission, Murray—who had been so used to being in command and treated with deference by the previous male incumbents—could barely cope. Hiding away in her old sanctuary of the office, she cringed whenever she heard the foreman ringing the bell in the courtyard, the former harbinger of nightly convoys, to summon his men from their breaks. It was "almost more than flesh and blood could bear," she wrote. At the end of November, the last few remaining members of the staff said their goodbyes. Nina Last went home to her parents in Buckinghamshire. Olga Campbell and Mardie Hodgson returned to their families in Scotland. Grace Hale went back to her old post as matron of the Elizabeth Garrett Anderson Hospital.[47] The doctors gathered for a final farewell dinner, followed by a somber trip to a nearby theater. And on January 8, 1920, Flora Murray and Louisa Garrett Anderson handed the keys of the old St Giles's and St George's Workhouse back over to the Office of Works.

IN THE FOUR and a half years since it had opened in May 1915, Endell Street Military Hospital had treated more than twenty-six thousand patients, most of them men. While the majority were British, they included more than two thousand Canadians, two thousand Australians and New Zealanders, and two hundred Americans, sent from every battle zone of the First World War.[48] A further twenty thousand men and women had attended its casualty room as outpatients. Its surgeons had performed more than seven thousand surgeries in the operating theater, the majority undertaken by Anderson herself, as well as many more minor procedures carried out on the wards. And despite the gloomy forebodings of War Office staff, the hospital had not only survived but won accolades from the public, the profession, and the press.

The only army hospital run entirely by women during the First World War, Endell Street had proved that women doctors were every bit as capable of undertaking military surgery as men. Endell Street had been acclaimed in press reports not only as "perhaps the most popular" hospital in London but also the "most efficient hospital in existence."[49] Renowned for its cheerful atmosphere and lively spirit, the "Suffragettes' Hospital" had likewise been acknowledged for its professional and disciplined approach. Its reputation had spread far and wide. Women had sailed from Australia, Canada, Africa, and America to join its ranks; men wounded at the front had appealed to be sent there for treatment; army doctors and military officials had flocked there to watch and learn from its staff. Its doctors and nurses had saved thousands of men—and women—from death and disability and helped thousands more to adapt to a future with life-changing infirmities.

It had all started with a daring gamble. When Keogh had first announced his plan to let women run an army hospital in London, he had come under intense pressure to change his mind. On his retirement in January 1918, he wrote a poignant letter thanking Anderson and Murray for their work, not only for the country, but for him personally. "I have often talked of you and heard your work discussed, and it has always been to me a great pride to know how successful you have been," he said. "I should have been an object of scorn and ridicule if you had failed but I never for a moment contemplated failure and I think we can now congratulate ourselves on having established a record of a new kind." The success of Endell Street, said Keogh, had probably done more for the cause of women "than anything else I know of."[50]

Keogh was right. Endell Street provided the clearest possible illustration of the significance of the motto "Deeds not Words." The hospital, as Anderson told Winifred Buckley, had been "a landmark" for professional women, "and we may all feel proud as well as happy for the share we have taken in it." As Murray and Anderson walked away from Covent Garden empty-handed, Murray reflected that Endell Street Military Hospital was now nothing more than "a wonderful and cherished memory."

II

The Soft Long Sleep

60 Bedford Gardens, London, March 3, 1920

Flora Murray was furious. The work of the Women's Hospital Corps was due to be commemorated in June at the opening of the Imperial War Museum in Crystal Palace, along with the contributions of thousands more men and women who had helped win the war. Yet the picture intended as the centerpiece to celebrate the women of Endell Street was, in Murray's view, a travesty. Not only did she want it banned from display, she was determined it must be destroyed.

The picture, a large pastel by an artist named Austin Osman Spare, depicted seven women, all clothed in white gowns and with their heads covered by white scarves, performing an operation on an unconscious soldier in the Endell Street operating theater.[1] Spare, a staff sergeant employed as an artist in the medical section of the planned museum, had already created several portraits of Endell Street staff members from the photographs Murray had grudgingly allowed to be taken in 1917.[2] One of them shows a stern-looking Murray writing at her desk as a man in "hospital blues" stands to attention beside her. Unlike these small portraits, however, Spare had drawn his operating theater scene from life.

Spare's group portrait, probably produced at some point in 1918, bears no clear resemblance to any of the staff. Indeed, the seven

273

women pictured look remarkably homogeneous—all young and slim with pretty, feminine features and wistful, dreamy expressions.[3] There is no sign of blood, no glimpse of a wound, no semblance of urgency. Although the medical equipment and paraphernalia are competently drawn, the figures look more like schoolgirls playacting a hospital drama than professional women performing major surgery. Yet it was not Spare's romantic vision that had upset Murray. Her objections centered on far more serious, and potentially damaging, concerns.

In February, soon after she and Anderson had moved back into their Kensington house, Murray had already written to Colonel Frederick Brereton, head of the Imperial War Museum medical section, demanding the picture's destruction because it "caricatured" women's work. Since Brereton had disclaimed responsibility for the picture's fate, she was now writing to Lady Priscilla Norman, who chaired the women's work subcommittee. Spare's picture contained "gross errors," she complained, which made it "an object of ridicule" to anyone with professional knowledge. "It is very painful to all of us who worked at Endell Street to see such a picture hung," she wrote. "We would rather have no record of our work than a false record." Having little regard for Spare's creative talents, she conceded to allowing his other sketches of Endell Street staff to be displayed, since "bad portraits" did not affect the value of women's work. But in the operating scene, she insisted, "the credit of women surgeons is at stake."[4]

Murray and Anderson's concerns were genuine. Although Spare insisted he had portrayed the scene exactly as he had seen it, the two women were mortified that he had featured a number of items that would not normally be found in a well-run operating room. They included a hastily discarded splint, a couch pushed into one corner, and some haphazardly stacked sterilizing drums. Under the rushed, messy circumstances of wartime surgery, there's every likelihood that the Endell Street operating theater contained all these things, and quite probably other stray items that did not properly belong in a sterile surgical environment. But in the cool aftermath of war, Murray and Anderson knew that any violation of perfect medical standards might not only tarnish their own reputations but threaten the future livelihoods of all women doctors.

Despite Spare's protestations, Murray and Anderson prevailed. Since Spare refused to alter his picture, in May the women's work subcommittee commissioned a new work from the official war artist Francis Dodd.[5] A genial man and talented artist, Dodd had produced more than one hundred portraits of British generals and admirals during his visits to the Western Front and naval bases. His careful pictures of serious, thoughtful men had marked him as a skilled and sensitive portraitist, and his large painting of British officers questioning a German prisoner of war, *Interrogation*, had become one of the nation's favorite images of the war.

There were just two major hitches. No matter how fast Dodd worked, he would not be able to produce a picture in time for the Crystal Palace opening. The Imperial War Museum's first public collection was duly opened by George V on June 9. Over the next twelve months it would attract some 2.5 million visitors, who wandered among the potted palms marveling at more than 100,000 items, including a full-scale model of a dugout complete with tins of bully beef and condensed milk. The section devoted to women's work, which had been squeezed into a "very unattractive corner," contained a model depicting the surgeon Elsie Inglis in a field hospital in Serbia, along with pictures of women munitions workers, WAACs, and VADs.[6] But there was no trace of the Endell Street operating theater or any other aspect of the hospital. More problematically, since Endell Street hospital no longer existed, it was plainly impossible for Dodd to depict an operation in progress there from life.

Dodd was nothing if not resourceful. Starting work in September, he gained access to the empty workhouse building, braving whatever ghosts might still be haunting its corridors, and sketched the derelict operating theater. He then visited the Elizabeth Garrett Anderson Hospital and sketched an operation there on a woman patient, by its senior surgeon, Louisa Aldrich-Blake, and her assistants. In his studio he used these figures as models for Anderson, Murray, and Winifred Buckley, as well as two assistants, and changed the sex of the patient from female to male. The resulting oil painting, entitled *An Operation at the Military Hospital, Endell Street,* was finished by April 1921.[7]

Dodd's picture of an operation that never took place would become the most striking tribute to the women of Endell Street as well as one of the most remarkable images of the entire war. His carefully composed study in pale green and white shows the five female figures tightly grouped around an operating table. Illuminated by the ethereal glow of an overhead light, Murray holds a chloroform mask to the face of a mustached soldier who slumbers peacefully as Anderson performs an abdominal operation, assisted by Buckley and two nurses. Excluding almost all the normal paraphernalia of an operating theater, the picture presents a far more idealized and romanticized scene than Spare's. Yet by emphasizing the five women's faces, all concentrating intensely on the operation in progress, and their gloved hands working in harmony, Dodd conveys the combined professionalism and humanity of the surgical team far better than Spare's static attempt. Without ever visiting the hospital in action or witnessing an operation taking place there, Dodd had captured the quintessential spirit of Endell Street.

The picture certainly found favor with Murray and Anderson. Anderson enthused that Dodd had taken "infinite trouble" over the composition of the group and technical details of the operation.[8] In fact, they were so impressed that they commissioned Dodd to paint their own portraits in oils. The twin portraits, showing Murray in her neat Endell Street uniform and Anderson in a more feminine purple gown, would later hang side by side in the Royal Free Hospital medical school.

Murray and Anderson clearly had been prepared to go to extraordinary lengths to eliminate a picture they believed showed women doctors in a poor light. Now that Endell Street was only a "cherished memory," they were determined to protect its legacy. But their fears were not misplaced. When they insisted that the credit of women surgeons was at stake in the years immediately after the war, they were absolutely right. Spare's picture may have been consigned to a dustbin, but it was the scene depicted in Dodd's painting—women surgeons operating on a male patient—that was set to vanish. Just as women's war work had been shuffled into an "unattractive corner" of the Crystal Palace by 1920, so women everywhere were being herded back into their prewar roles.

THE WAR HAD changed everything, and nothing. Women in Britain had proved they could do the work of men—on the land, in factories, on the buses, and in hospitals—with at least as much skill, stamina, and dedication. Roughly two million women had taken on jobs previously done by men—albeit at substantially lower pay—to release men for the battlefield.[9] Thousands of women had donned khaki to join the WAAC, the WRNS, and the WRAF, and many more had served as military nurses and VADs in France and at home. More than one hundred thousand had enrolled in the Women's Land Army to flex their muscles on farms and in forestry; aided by a fine summer in 1917, women had brought in a record wheat harvest. And as many as one million women had worked in munitions factories, producing the shells and ammunition that helped win the war. In addition, women had filled vacancies as coal heavers and dockers, lamplighters and gardeners, funeral directors and ambulance drivers; they had kept banks, offices, government departments, and emergency services running throughout the war. In short, women had undertaken every conceivable role, with the sole exception of frontline combat, that had previously been done by men. Some had given their lives to that fight, including four hundred women who had died in accidents and from poisoning in munitions work.

Life for women would never be the same again. Wartime earnings had enabled many women to enjoy new leisure activities, such as the cinema and dancing, and the relaxation of social norms had changed entrenched attitudes toward clothing and behavior. Women had adopted shorter skirts and shorter hair, they were openly smoking and wearing makeup, and some had even taken to wearing trousers. According to Millicent Fawcett, who had finally relinquished her role as president of the NUWSS in 1919, at the age of seventy-two, the war had "revolutionized" the industrial position of women. "It found them serfs," she said, "and left them free."[10]

Medical women had led the way in embracing that freedom. Seizing on the war as an opportunity to demonstrate their abilities as well as to do their patriotic duty, they had run hospitals, joined the army, and served in every war zone. Women doctors at Endell Street and elsewhere had broken the taboo on treating male patients. They had proved they could perform military surgery, handle trauma and emergency work, and command military establishments with just as much competence as their male colleagues. On the home front, women had run hospital departments, taken over general practices, and carried out clinical research with the same diligence as men. Women doctors had been accepted by male patients, even for intimate complaints, despite all the previous objections. Some men had even found they preferred being treated by women and specifically asked to be sent to Endell Street or other women-run units, choosing them over mainstream military hospitals. No longer was it possible for the male-dominated profession to argue that medical women were incapable of the same tasks as men. War had proved the worth of women doctors; but peace had seemingly brought their value to an end. They had won their argument but gained nothing.

As men slowly returned from the front, they demanded their jobs back in the factories, on the farms, on the buses—and in the hospitals. The legions of women who had fed Britain, armed its troops, and kept the country moving were expected meekly to return to their own kitchens. The women's military branches—the WAAC, WRNS, and WRAF—were all disbanded by 1921, and would not be reestablished until the next world war. Most of the women who had taken on men's jobs in industry and other spheres were forced to give them up—even though some employers were eager to retain them, since their skills were more up-to-date and their wages often lower. In rare cases where women were kept on or secured new jobs, they were often vilified for depriving men—especially veterans disabled by the war—of their livelihoods. One journalist complained that "girls were clinging to their jobs" to earn "pocket-money" to buy frocks, even though many were war widows struggling to feed their families.[11] By the end of the war, more than half of all civil service employees were female, but over the next few years the vast majority were dismissed in favor of men.[12]

Many women were happy to return to their homes and families, but some—especially young single women relishing their newfound economic freedom—were not. One pioneering female engineer said after the war that it was widely accepted that men should enjoy shorter hours, higher wages, and more leisure time, yet women were "merely told to go back to what they were doing before," regardless of their desire for economic independence and better living standards.[13] Another woman complained that she had spent more than thirty years in clerical work before the postwar world decided that women workers had been "an experiment."[14]

More significantly, perhaps, the mood toward women had changed. The sudden ending of four years of unprecedented brutality over a strip of foreign land, at huge human cost for seemingly no gain, had unleashed a surge of anger and violence in men returning home.[15] Early signs of this unrest had materialized at Endell Street in 1919, when Murray noted that the normally docile patients had become hostile and difficult. Much of this male rage was targeted at women, particularly women workers, in a rash of bitter jibes, physical attacks, and even sexual assaults. Not only were women castigated for stealing men's jobs, but even their wartime contributions were undermined and trivialized. In the impulse to wipe out the worst memories of the war, men wanted women to return to their prewar domestic roles and submissive behavior.

It was not possible to turn back the clock entirely. Although some 750,000 women lost or left their jobs within a year of the war's end, the overall total of working women was still higher than before the war, and this number would continue to climb through the 1930s.[16] Yet almost invariably, these women would suffer worse pay and conditions than their male counterparts for decades to come. When George V opened the Imperial War Museum at the Crystal Palace in 1920, he voiced the hope that its contents would remind visitors that the horror of war belonged to a "dead past."[17] Like the tins of bully beef and condensed milk, women workers were seen as part of that dead past.

WOMEN DOCTORS FACED the same obstacles as women in other jobs.[18] Male doctors returning from war service expected as of right to resume their former posts in general hospitals, medical schools, and private practice. Women doctors were expected to return un-complainingly to treating only women and children in women-run hospitals, just like before the war. Their war service counted for nothing. With medical posts in short supply, competition was fierce, and men invariably won priority. The president of the General Medical Council, Sir Donald MacAlister, who had urged women doctors to join the war effort in 1916, now announced that their services were "less in demand" and warned them to expect "disappointments."[19] Hospitals that had depended on female doctors to stay open during the war now turfed them out and refused to appoint any more. Even when a new hospital opened to treat women for venereal disease, the two medical posts went to men. Since hospital appointments were made by boards composed entirely or almost entirely of men, women candidates were simply ignored. That did not stop some women doctors from trying.

One woman doctor was offered a junior post at the London Hospital in 1922 but never started work, because the hospital's male doctors threatened to resign if she did.[20] Another was accepted for a research fellowship at the St Mary's Hospital pathology institute only on two conditions: that she would keep silent in the anatomy department, and that she would never stray into the building's "male territories."

Faced with exactly the same hostility and prejudice they had encountered before the war, women doctors were sidelined again into low-status, low-paid jobs in maternity and child care, factories and schools, asylums and workhouse infirmaries. Often, they were paid lower salaries than men in equivalent posts, and employers commonly refused to employ married women. Like many local authorities, the London County Council operated a bar on employing married women that it only abolished in the 1930s. One woman who had spent four years as a surgeon with the Scottish Women's Hospitals during the war, operating under extreme conditions in France and Salonika, was turned down for jobs in mainstream hospitals purely because she was married.[21] She would have fared better, she noted wryly, if she had chosen "to live in sin." Very few women who worked as military surgeons during the war remained in surgery afterward; those who did operated mainly on women and children. It is no surprise that many medical women looked back on their wartime service as the happiest time of their lives. The odds stacked against them, some simply retired or went abroad. The future for young women wanting to enter medicine was even bleaker.

One after another, the London medical schools, which had welcomed female students during the war, now again barred them. St George's Hospital, which had only accepted female students on the understanding that it was a temporary measure, was the first to close its doors in 1919. The school was not big enough to "harbor" women, explained one St George's man, when it could now recruit enough men.[22] The London Hospital, which had opened its doors to women in 1918, slammed them shut again in 1922. Defending the decision, Lord Knutsford, who chaired the hospital's board, said he had been converted to accepting female students in the war after visiting Endell Street, which, in his view, was not only equal to the best military hospital in London but "the most popular of all."[23] Nonetheless, the school had decided to exclude women because male students preferred to be taught in all-male classrooms. Two years later, St Mary's Hospital, which had only avoided closure during the war by recruiting women students, put up the barricades after male students signed a petition declaring they did not want to be taught alongside women—partly because this jeopardized the school's record at rugby. Charing Cross, Westminster, and King's College Hospital all followed.

Rejecting protests from medical women, leading male doctors argued that educating female students was a waste of resources because roughly half were likely to marry after they graduated. Medical women made "admirable wives," explained one doctor, so they were "snapped up" by discerning men.[24] In fact, less than one-third of women doctors were married, and many of those were prevented from working by marriage bars. One prominent male medic argued that mixed education was undesirable due to the "inevitable distractions that cannot but arise" when attractive young men and women freely associated. The experiment of co-education had been tried, he said, and "proved unsatisfactory."

Although medical schools elsewhere in Britain continued to accept women, albeit often in limited numbers, by 1928 only the LSMW, attached to the Royal Free, and a dozen places at University College Hospital were open to female students in London. Mainstream hospitals likewise gave men priority for postgraduate training posts, so that young women doctors were again forced to seek clinical experience in women-run hospitals. After a petition from LSMW graduates in 1919, the Royal Free agreed to give preference to the school's graduates for its junior posts where two candidates had equal merits—although it still insisted that two of the six jobs should normally go to men, regardless of their merits.[25] Although medicine had started to be seen as a promising career for bright young women during the war, it had now become a risky prospect.

IN THIS NEW climate, the women who had worked long, hard hours at Endell Street now faced dismal futures. Despite the acclaimed achievements of their wartime work, only a handful of doctors who served with the Women's Hospital Corps in France and London went on to any significant professional success.[26] Most notably, Helen Chambers, the pathologist who had helped pioneer BIPP, enjoyed a distinguished postwar career.[27] Returning to her prewar research into cancer at London's Middlesex Hospital, she became a widely esteemed oncologist, pioneering radiotherapy for women's cancer, and helped found the Marie Curie Hospital in north London. Staffed by women, it became the main center for women's cancer in Britain. Devoting her life to cancer research, especially the treatment of cervical cancer, which was the leading cause of death among women at the time, she achieved the best survival results in the world. Sadly, her own life was cut short by breast cancer in 1935, when she was just fifty-six, possibly as a result of exposure to the radium with which she had worked. New pathology laboratories that opened at the Marie Curie Hospital two years later were named in her honor.

A few other doctors achieved a measure of success. Hazel Cuthbert, the young recruit who had worked at Claridge's and the Château Mauricien, became the first female senior physician at the Royal Free and later headed its children's department.[28] Majorie Blandy, who had joined the corps in Paris and worked at the Sugar Store Hospital in Boulogne, as well as in Wimereux, had initially followed Cuthbert to the Royal Free before joining Great Ormond Street Hospital for Children in 1917.[29] She was dismissed from that job when the hospital resumed its prewar policy of barring women doctors—to the regret of the senior physician who wrote her reference—but she became the first female registrar at the National Hospital in Queen Square, London.

More conventionally, Gertrude Dearnley, who had joined Endell Street in 1915, enjoyed a long and distinguished career in obstetrics and gynecology.[30] Working as a consultant gynecological surgeon at the Royal Free, in 1937 she established London's first fertility clinic. Octavia Lewin, who had joined Endell Street in 1918 as an aural specialist, became a physician at the Central London Throat, Nose and Ear Hospital.[31] Pursuing a rather less traditional route, Morna Rawlins—who worked at Endell Street from 1915 to 1916—became a specialist in venereal diseases in women at the Elizabeth Garrett Anderson Hospital and, unusually, at Guy's Hospital in London.

The majority of the thirty-nine women doctors who had worked for the corps in France and at Endell Street, however, returned to low-status jobs treating women and children, moved abroad, or gave up medicine entirely. None continued in mainstream surgery or treated men. Winifred Buckley was fairly typical. Having worked as assistant surgeon at Endell Street from the day it opened until the day it closed, helping Anderson perform thousands of complex operations, she gave up surgery entirely.[32] After trying to establish herself in general practice in Brighton, she returned to London, but had to supplement her income from private work with posts in schools and infant welfare clinics. Her chance came again in the Second World War, when she moved to Berkshire as an assistant in general practice, no doubt replacing a male doctor who had joined up. She died, unmarried like most of the former Endell Street doctors, in 1959.

Those women doctors who had crossed oceans to serve at Endell Street met exactly the same prejudices when they returned home. Arriving back in Australia in 1919, Vera Scantlebury was refused her old job at Melbourne Children's Hospital because priority went to male doctors returning from war service.[33] Confessing herself "quite depressed," she took on an assortment of part-time posts in children's and women's care before being appointed, in 1926, as the first director of a new infant welfare department for the State of Victoria. The post was designated part-time in order to comply with the marriage bar on full-time women staff, because she got married two weeks later to a lecturer in electrical engineering, Edward Byam Brown. In reality, the job was far from part-time. Over the next twenty years, Vera Scantlebury Brown, as she became, developed a model network of baby clinics and kindergartens that transformed children's health throughout the state. Down to earth and gregarious as always, she won intense loyalty and deep affection for her tireless work. Vera and Edward had two children, Edward and Catherine, but Vera died of cancer in 1946, at the age of fifty-six.

Elizabeth Hamilton-Browne took rather longer to return to Australia. Having left Endell Street in 1918 to seek adventure in Egypt, she came back briefly to England at the end of the war before taking passage for India.[34] She intended to spend a year there but stayed for more than twenty because she "fell in love with the place." Traveling widely, she worked for the Indian women's medical service—which was originally set up under Queen Victoria to provide female doctors for Indian women—and taught surgery at the women's medical college in Delhi. She was eventually promoted to assistant inspector general of hospitals in the Punjab—albeit with responsibility for women's care. Retiring in 1944, she finally returned to Australia, where she died, forty-one years later, at the age of 103.

Almost as intrepid, Evelyn Windsor returned to Canada with her husband and baby son in 1918 and struggled to pick up her career in Calgary, where she had two more children, a girl and a boy.[35] After separating from her husband, who assumed guardianship of their two older children, in 1928, she became medical superintendent to the Blackfoot (Siksika First Nation) tribe at their reservation fifty miles from Calgary, where she remained for twenty years. Although poorly paid and poorly regarded, the post provided a regular income and accommodations. Living there with her youngest son, Windsor frequently drove through winter blizzards and summer dust storms to reach isolated parts of the territory in medical emergencies. While respecting Siksika customs, she established baby clinics and raised funds for a tuberculosis wing at the reservation hospital. As a mark of esteem for her dedication, Windsor was made an honorary member of the tribe. She retired in 1948 and died eighteen years later, at the age of seventy-eight.

PROSPECTS FOR THE orderlies and other women who had devoted up to five years of their lives to wartime service at Endell Street and in France were no brighter. The vast majority had no choice but to return to their humdrum, cosseted middle-class lives and idle away their days until they married, or to dedicate themselves to voluntary work. A few did their best to subvert expectations.

Olga Campbell, who was awarded the MBE (Member of the Order of the British Empire) for her five years of stalwart service as the Endell Street quartermaster, returned to the family estate in Scotland to look after her now ailing father, Arthur, and resume her place on the county social scene. Writing to her friend Marion Dickerman in America, she confessed that although she had always enjoyed a "good time" when mixed with work, "as a sole occupation it bores me stiff." Sir Alan Anderson, Louisa's brother, came up with the solution. When he complained to Campbell about the lengthy turnaround time for his ships in port, she retorted that he needed a woman in the job. Campbell was promptly appointed "chief housemaid"—in charge of crew welfare—to the Orient Line. Rising to the challenge just as she had done in her army role, Campbell told Dickerman, "It is such a change for me to be thrown entirely among men after five years of Endell St but I think I shall like it & get on well with them." Living in London with her cousin Mardie Hodgson and another female friend, she commuted daily to her office, which was "fitted like a ship's cabin," at Tilbury docks in Essex. The sole woman employed there, she was quickly accepted. On one occasion, in an attempt to persuade the company's directors to replace the men's uncomfortable bunks, she insisted they all try the beds for size; the bunks were soon changed.[36]

Despite her strike for independence, Campbell yearned for married life. Before the war she had fallen for Horace Byatt, a diplomat in the colonial service who was sixteen years her senior; they had met on the ship when Campbell was returning from Ceylon in 1913. Her father had seemingly opposed them getting married, so Byatt had spent the war in Malta, then Africa, earning a knighthood for his service. When they met again in 1919, Campbell was devastated that Byatt did not propose. Learning that he was about to sail for a new four-year posting in Africa, she told Dickerman she felt "numb & aching." Five years later, when Byatt was appointed governor of Trinidad and Tobago, he summoned up courage at last; the pair were married in 1924.

After her husband died, in 1933, Olga moved with her three young sons to Elgin in Scotland, where her brother taught at the new and progressive Gordonstoun School. She became billeting officer for evacuated schoolchildren in World War II, but did not live to see the end of the war. She died in 1943, at the age of fifty-two.

Mardie Hodgson inherited the family estate in Scotland, where she managed a pedigree dairy herd.[37] Having lost a boyfriend in a submarine disaster during the war, in 1924 she married a former army chaplain, the Reverend Reginald Kemble Wells, and they ran a succession of schools for boys. After giving birth to the first of three children, her hair fell out—it would never regrow—yet she never lost her ebullience. At the age of eighty-five, Hodgson still swam naked in the pool at the family home.

Although they returned to America in 1919, Marion Dickerman and Nancy Cook never forgot their Endell Street experience or the friends they made there. On arrival in New York, Dickerman discovered that she had been put forward as a Democratic candidate for the New York State Assembly—becoming the first woman to run for the New York legislature.[38] She lost the election, but, with Cook as her campaign manager, she made a strident case for women's rights and welfare reforms. Devoting their lives to political activism, Dickerman and Cook became friendly with Franklin D. Roosevelt, and especially his wife, Eleanor. When the Roosevelts separated, the three women shared a house on the Roosevelts' estate at Hyde Park, New York State, where they ran a furniture-making business. After FDR's election in 1932, Cook and Dickerman were frequent guests at the White House, until a rift with Eleanor ended their friendship. Settling in Connecticut, the two remained lifelong partners until Cook's death in 1962. At the age of eighty, Dickerman still reminisced about her days at Endell Street. She died in 1985, aged ninety-three.

Nina Last returned to her parents' house in Buckinghamshire at the end of 1919 feeling "dazed and unsettled."[39] Her last few months in London, when her duties at Endell Street were light and her army pay generous, had passed in a whirl of cinema trips, theater outings, and dances. "Our smart and attractive uniform made me feel somebody," she said. Back at home, aimless and bored, she felt "a poor little nobody." During the war she had steeled herself against romantic involvement; now, aged twenty-four, one of many "surplus" single women, she thought she would never marry. But in 1920, on a countryside trip with friends, she met a young man named Ronald Courage who had just been demobilized. They married—on the anniversary of Armistice Day—that November. Despite producing two daughters, the marriage was desperately unhappy— he was abusive and kept a mistress—and after several attempts she obtained a divorce in the 1940s. Spending the rest of her life with two female friends—her childhood nanny, Netta, and housekeeper, Ella—Last became a magistrate, for which she earned the nickname "the Battleaxe." Nina died in 1972, aged seventy-eight, and was buried beside Netta. Her Endell Street uniform was consigned to a dressing-up box for her grandchildren to play with.

Quieter and less impulsive, Nina's sister Barbara never fully recovered her health after leaving Endell Street.[40] In 1924 she married an army chaplain, the Reverend Charles Wright, who had been badly scarred in a gas attack in the war, and they had a daughter. After taking charge of a parish near Carlisle, he was killed in 1933 in a road accident that also left Barbara in a coma for six weeks. When she recovered, Barbara and her daughter went to live with her younger brother Charles, who was also a vicar, to help look after his parish. Although she rarely mentioned Endell Street, she kept a 1916 photograph of the entire hospital staff hanging on the wall of her bathroom for the rest of her life.

FOR LOUISA GARRETT Anderson and Flora Murray, life after the war could never hope to match the thrills and dramas of Endell Street. Having left for Paris in 1914 with no experience in military surgery, they had not only set up and run two military hospitals in France but founded and managed Endell Street, along with three auxiliary hospitals in London, with nearly two hundred staff at their command. They had saved countless lives, repaired broken men, and— even more remarkable—won the approval of the army, the medical profession, and the public. During the war years they had been inundated with plaudits, but in peacetime their experience and talents were no longer deemed to be of consequence. Just like most other women after the war, they were considered surplus to requirements. Endell Street had become merely a historical curiosity, another remnant of the "dead past."

Worn out and worn down by the strains and stresses of their war work, Murray, who turned fifty in 1919, and Anderson, forty-six, had tried to pick up their old threads. Having moved back to Kensington, at first they carried on as before the war, working mornings at their consulting rooms in Mayfair while continuing to run their Harrow Road children's hospital, now renamed the Roll of Honour Hospital for Children, in the afternoons. At the same time, Anderson resumed her post on the consultant staff of the Elizabeth Garrett Anderson Hospital. A female journalist who called at their Mayfair practice in 1920 to interview Murray confessed to a "childish awe" at seeing the twin brass plates beside the door inscribed with the names of two women—"Dr. Flora Murray, C.B.E." and "Dr. Garrett Anderson"—who had "risen to the top of their profession."[41] Asked about the future for women doctors at a time when medical schools were fast bolting their doors, Murray declared the prospects were "excellent"—although these prospects, she admitted, were chiefly in public health or overseas. In reality, as Murray well knew, prospects were far from excellent even for women at the "top of their profession." Few private patients beat a path to their Mayfair door, and their children's hospital was struggling for survival.

Despite having expanded to twelve beds, the small hospital was hopelessly overwhelmed by demand from poor families in the neighborhood, with an average of one thousand new patients cramming its outpatient clinic each month, and a staggering eighty thousand total attendances in 1919.[42] The lack of space meant that staff frequently had to turn away sick babies and children with tuberculosis, heart complaints, and other serious conditions, many of them wasted by malnutrition.

Launching an appeal in 1920 to build a bigger hospital, Anderson and Murray wrote to former staff and patients of Endell Street seeking donations. Contributions flooded back from as far afield as Australia, New Zealand, South Africa, and America. Some ex-patients sent pitifully small sums in threepenny and sixpenny pieces, with scrawled notes of thanks for their treatment, while others enclosed money collected from friends and colleagues. One man sent fifty shillings from a collection at his workplace; another raised five pounds by organizing a village dance. One former patient wrote to say he had been wounded twice since leaving the hospital, but insisted, "I wasn't cared for anywhere else so kindly as I was at Endell Street."

Money arrived from bereaved relatives, too. One widow sent one pound—a significant sum to a woman left alone—in memory of her husband, who had recovered from his wounds at Endell Street only to die of Spanish flu just three weeks after being demobilized. He often talked about the staff, she wrote, and insisted that "there was no hospital as good as Endell St. to him . . . & he never forgot them." Despite the generosity—and the support of Sir Alfred Keogh, who joined the hospital committee in 1920—the children's hospital was forced to close for lack of funds in 1921. More than half a million children had been treated there.

In the meantime, Murray wrote a book, *Women as Army Surgeons*, detailing the story of the Women's Hospital Corps and its work in France and at Endell Street—or at least that version of the story that she was keen to promote. Determined to maintain a tight grip on Endell Street's legacy, Murray painted a rosy picture of heroic women battling to serve their country in the face of the hostility and stupidity of men at the War Office. Although she charted the many trials and obstacles the women had negotiated in order to succeed, she made no mention of the tensions among the staff and paid little attention to the contributions of the professional nurses or women doctors from overseas. Elizabeth Hamilton-Browne, for one, was peeved at the failure to name any Australian doctors.[43] She would have her revenge—later burning a stack of letters from Anderson and a "lovely picture" of Murray. Beatrice Harraden was still nursing a grudge, too. Although she wrote a glowing preface to the book extolling the corps' pioneering work, she told Elizabeth Robins it was "not an easy task."[44]

There is no doubt that Murray's sentiments were sincere. In an inscription addressed to former staff, she noted that although she said "little in praise, yet if you will read between the lines you will find there a very genuine affection for each one of you, and admiration and pride for your courage and endurance."[45] Paying tribute to the women who had died in the cause of the corps' work, she quoted lines from the poet Algernon Charles Swinburne: "Time takes them home that we loved, fair names and famous, / To the soft long sleep, to the broad sweet bosom of death." Murray dedicated her book to Anderson with the words: "Bold, cautious, true and my loving comrade." Taken from a poem by Walt Whitman describing a message left by a soldier for his fallen friend, the quotation was a clear reference to Murray and Anderson's own battles both in their suffragette cause and in the Great War. It was also a brave declaration of their enduring love for each other.

Murray's book won praise in *The Lancet* as an important record of "indubitably valuable work," while *The Scotsman* declared that the book would be "highly prized by everyone who comes up against the lingering prejudice that war service is the exclusive business of men."[46] Yet now that women's war work was being roundly disparaged, her jaunty tone seemed jarring to many; her story had become inconvenient. Hailed as heroines in the war, now Murray and Anderson were out of step.

Dusting off their suffragette banners, Murray and Anderson made a tentative return to feminist politics. But whereas before the war the women's movement had been staunchly united in its demand for the vote—if divided over tactics—now women activists were split into factions dedicated to different aims.[47] While some women concentrated their energies on extending the vote to all women and furthering equal rights, others were more concerned with pacifism or social reforms. Now that most women over thirty could vote, and women over twenty-one could stand for Parliament—the first female MP to take her seat was elected in 1919—party allegiances created further fractures.

At first, Murray and Anderson pinned their hopes on persuading Emmeline Pankhurst to make a triumphant resurgence and lead the women's march toward progress once again. Murray rallied former WSPU members in 1919 to create a fund to support Emmeline Pankhurst in her mature years.[48] The appeal raised £3,000, sufficient to buy a cottage in Devon, though much less than anticipated. But Pankhurst, now in her sixties, rarely visited, preferring to remain in Canada and leave campaigning to younger activists. Standing firm with their old suffragette comrades, Murray and Anderson steered clear of Aunt Millie's former NUWSS, now renamed the National Union of Societies for Equal Citizenship (NUSEC), which focused its demands on special rights for women, especially for mothers. Instead they became founding members of the Six Point Group, launched in 1921 by former WSPU stalwarts as a rallying point for those campaigning for equal rights.[49] More radical than the NUSEC, the Six Point Group demanded changes in the laws to secure equal rights, equal pay, and equal opportunities for women. Murray and Anderson dutifully signed their names to letters in the press and graced society luncheons to support the group, but their energies were at a low ebb. Wearied by their war work, their hearts were no longer in campaigning.

After closing the children's hospital, Murray and Anderson sold their London house and retired to their cottage at Penn. By then, it was 1922. For the first time since the outbreak of the war—for the first time ever, perhaps—they were free to tend their garden, walk their dogs, and enjoy each other's company at leisure. Apart from occasional trips to London for political and social events, they could escape the bitter tensions of the postwar world and relax with family and friends. Briefly, Murray considered standing for Parliament, after her brother William suggested it in September 1922. He thought she might put herself forward in his place for the General Election that November, as he was resigning his seat through ill health. She would "gladly" accept if asked, she told him, even though she was unsure how to label herself—perhaps "moderate progressive" allied with the Conservative-led coalition, she thought.[50] But ten days later she confessed herself relieved that the idea was abandoned. Freed from obligation, she set off with Anderson on a trip to Paris—by plane—for a chance to revisit the romantic streets where they had strolled under the searchlights eight years earlier.

The peaceful idyll would not last. By early 1923 William was gravely ill with cancer, and in a last-ditch attempt to recover his health he traveled to the south of France, where he died on March 5.[51] When she heard the news, Murray set out to bring back his body. By then, Murray was seriously ill herself. Diagnosed with rectal cancer, she underwent an operation at a nursing home in north London, where she died six days later, on July 28, 1923.[52] The date was Anderson's birthday. Murray was just fifty-four.

She was buried four days later, on a sunny, blustery day, in a quiet corner of the churchyard at Penn. The church was packed for the funeral service with old suffragette comrades, former medical friends, and colleagues from Endell Street. An Endell Street nurse stood throughout the service at the foot of Murray's coffin, which was draped with a Union Jack, and a eulogy was read by a former Endell Street chaplain. In a mark of esteem for her wartime work—and recognition of her honorary rank as lieutenant colonel—the War Office was represented by Sir William Leishman, successor to Keogh as director general of army medical services. As her coffin was lowered into the ground, a bugler played the "Last Post." Then Anderson stepped forward and threw a sprig of rosemary—the emblem for remembrance—into the grave.

Murray's will was short. She left everything to Anderson, her lifelong friend, comrade, and partner, to dispose of "as she thinks best." Friends and acquaintances alike were stunned by her early death. For all their differences, Beatrice Harraden declared the "utmost grief" when she heard the news. Many were convinced Murray had sacrificed her life to her war work. Nina Last would later say that Murray "literally gave her life for the wounded."[53]

News of her death filled columns in newspapers and journals in Britain and abroad, from her home town in Dumfriesshire to New Zealand. Obituaries charted her extraordinary journey from being a reviled enemy of the state as the suffragettes' chief doctor to the highest-ranking woman in the British Army. In running Endell Street, Murray had broken "entirely new ground," said the *Manchester Guardian*. Writing in the suffragist journal, *The Vote*, Harraden said Murray's name would stand out "illustriously" for her contributions to the women's movement. As well as being a "fighter and a reformer," Murray was a tender physician with a "boyish" sense of humor, Harraden remembered. In *The Observer*, Elizabeth Robins recalled her days in the Endell Street library and declared that Murray had run the hospital in the teeth of difficulties "which would have broken a spirit less valiant." But it was Louisa Garrett Anderson, the friend and partner who knew Flora Murray best, who provided the most complete and poignant portrait. Both graceful and gracious, Murray was an "ideal physician," she said, who loved the science of medicine but "never forgot the human being."[54]

LIVING ON AT Penn, Anderson faced the future alone. Characteristically, she refused to descend into melancholy. Instead, she threw herself into public service and county politics—serving as a magistrate and raising funds for the local Conservative Party—while continuing to support women in medicine and other causes close to her heart.[55] She chaired an inquiry on child assault for the Six Point Group that made farsighted recommendations in 1925, including anonymity for children in court and inspections of residential children's homes.[56] Faithful to her mother's pioneering work, she continued to support the LSMW and Elizabeth Garrett Anderson Hospital, often attending events with her brother, Alan. When she learned that a cousin was planning to write a biography of her mother, Anderson wrote her own version and then burned her parents' love letters.[57] She even traveled again, visiting Palestine in early 1928 with her aunts, Millie and Agnes, who were now in their eighties. During an intrepid expedition into the mountains, their car ran off the road into a snowdrift.[58] As they waited to be rescued, with darkness approaching, Anderson feared the worst, although the aunts were unperturbed. Later that year she ventured as far as Australia, arriving in Melbourne in November for a joyous reunion with Vera Scantlebury and Rachel Champion.

Greeting her old CO after a gap of ten years, Scantlebury was overwhelmed.[59] As Anderson stepped off the boat, she was treated almost as an international celebrity and surrounded by journalists. Throughout her stay, as Scantlebury and Champion shepherded her around the sights, she was inundated with invitations from "the whole women mob of Melbourne." Traveling on to Sydney, Anderson was feted as guest of honor at a lunch held partly in gratitude for her treatment of thousands of Australian and New Zealand men at Endell Street.[60] In an impassioned speech, she said the suffrage movement had trained women for their war work. That experience had "made men understand that women could lead women, and that women should trust other women," she said. "When war came, and our weapons became Red Cross bandages . . . we found the training we had undergone of very great help to us." Returning via Ceylon, she met up with Aunts Millie and Agnes—Millicent's final adventure before she died the following year—before sailing home.[61]

When war came again, Anderson was ready to serve once more. Moving back to London in August 1939, as the Second World War loomed, she volunteered to help treat air raid casualties at the Elizabeth Garrett Anderson Hospital.[62] Now sixty-six, she performed surgery during the London Blitz just as she had done at Endell Street in the midst of the Zeppelin raids more than two decades earlier. Her duties were light, however, so she whiled away the empty hours by attending lectures at the National Gallery and meeting Alan for weekly lunches.[63] She had left her dog, no longer Garrett or William, but an Aberdeen terrier named Roddy, with her nephew Colin in the countryside, so he would not be frightened during air raids.[64] She gave her meat ration cards for Roddy and greeted him on their reunions by rolling around on her nephew's doormat clutching him in her arms.

Tending casualties at the hospital named in her mother's honor as bombs fell on London again, Anderson's thoughts turned back to one of her oldest friends, Evelyn Sharp, the journalist and fellow suffragette she had barely seen since the start of the last war. Sharp had finally married Henry Nevinson, the love of her life, but eight years later, in 1941, Nevinson died. The women had scarcely had a chance to rekindle their friendship when Anderson, too, became ill in early 1943. After suffering with back pain for several months, she was diagnosed with a rare form of cancer, retroperitoneal sarcoma, and treated at the Elizabeth Garrett Anderson Hospital—placing her faith in women doctors to the last—but an operation was unsuccessful.[65]

After she was admitted to a nursing home in Brighton, Anderson wrote in October to tell Sharp she was dying. She felt profoundly grateful, she said, to be spared a "solitary old age," and she looked back on her life with "real happiness."[66] Drowsy with morphine, she watched the sea from her bed and remembered the "very happy memories" they had shared in their youth. She would not have missed the WSPU or her prison sentence or their vacations together in Scotland "for anything," she said. She was not receiving any more visitors.

On November 15, Anderson died, just hours before Alan arrived after dashing back from America to see her one last time. She was seventy. Her body was cremated and the ashes scattered on the South Downs. A few days later, her friends, family, and colleagues, including dozens of women doctors and "a forest of nurses" from the Royal Free, Elizabeth Garrett Anderson, and Endell Street hospitals, gathered in St Pancras Church, London, for a memorial service.[67] The parson recalled Anderson's work during the First World War yet made no reference to her suffragette actions. Newspaper obituaries chiefly remembered Anderson as the daughter of Britain's first woman doctor. Amid the all-consuming war, her own pioneering work in an earlier one had faded into obscurity.

There was no mention, either, of Anderson's beloved partner and companion. In her will, dividing her cottage, artworks, and jewelry among family and friends, she left diamond rings to her "nieces in love"—Flora Murray's three nieces, Elizabeth, Vivian, and Eleanor. Anderson's name was added beneath Murray's on her tombstone at Penn with the words: "We have been gloriously happy."

TOGETHER LOUISA GARRETT Anderson and Flora Murray had battled through two great wars: the war for women's rights, and a world war. They had stood shoulder to shoulder in the suffragettes' fight for women's enfranchisement, and when Britain went to war in 1914, they had put down their placards to serve their country as doctors saving soldiers' lives. Confounding their critics, they had run a hospital at Endell Street that was acclaimed as the most efficient, most popular, and even the most successful in the British Army. As commanding officers, they could be difficult, intimidating, even uncompromising, but they never wavered in their faith in women. Now they had both succumbed to the soft long sleep as another war raged across the world, their contributions largely forgotten. And yet their legacy lives on.

Ever since Elizabeth Garrett Anderson became the first woman to qualify as a doctor in Britain in 1865, women in the United Kingdom and beyond have persisted in the battle to enter medicine and work as doctors on an equal footing to men.[68] Even though hundreds of women doctors proved they could perform just as well as men during the First World War, the peacetime backlash meant they lost almost all the ground they had gained. At the outset of the Second World War, the War Office guaranteed equal pay and conditions to women doctors who joined the army, but they were still denied commissions as officers. By 1944, a year after Louisa Garrett Anderson's death, women still constituted only 20 percent of the medical profession, a number that went virtually unchanged into the 1960s.

After the Second World War, in 1947, all British medical schools were forced to open their doors to women in order to qualify for state funding, although many insisted on a 20 percent limit for decades to come. Only with the passing of the Sex Discrimination Act in 1975 were British medical schools and hospitals finally forced to accept women on an equal basis. The proportion of female medical students rose to 50 percent soon after and continued to climb to a record level of 62 percent at the dawn of the twenty-first century, before stabilizing at around 55 percent today. Lagging slightly behind, the number of qualified women doctors rose to 48 percent in the United Kingdom in 2018, and as that rise continues, female doctors are predicted to outnumber men by 2022. Yet despite these gains, women are still underrepresented at the most senior levels in medicine as well as in specialties such as surgery. Worldwide, the picture varies widely, with women forming more than 70 percent of doctors in some Eastern European countries, but still only 39 percent in Australia, 34 percent in the United States, and 20 percent in Japan.

Nothing now remains of Endell Street Military Hospital but a few artifacts, memories, and ghosts. The old workhouse building was demolished and replaced in the 1980s by public authority housing. Only the courtyard, the little square where the bell once tolled to announce the arrival of ambulance convoys, where blue-suited patients once sat in summer sunshine under striped umbrellas, and where the hospital choir sang Christmas carols, still survives today. A plaque with the motto "Deeds not Words" is the only reminder that the hospital existed. Yet the story of Endell Street continues to provide inspiration for women in medicine—and for all women— today. The women who founded Endell Street, and all the pioneering women who worked there, are still proof of what women can do in deeds and words.

Acknowledgments

Writing about the women who worked at Endell Street Military Hospital and the men and women who were treated there has been an honor and a delight. I feel blessed to have had the chance to learn about their lives and tell their story. For that privilege I am indebted to many organizations that have provided assistance as well as to countless individuals who have helped with information, advice, and material. First and foremost I owe an enormous debt of gratitude to Dr. Jennian Geddes, who has been my guide, my adviser, and my friend throughout this journey. Having researched and written about the Endell Street women for many years, Jennian has been unstintingly generous in sharing her knowledge, her material, and her time. This book could not have been written without her.

I am grateful to Lady Antonia Fraser, DBE, and honored to have received the first Antonia Fraser Grant through the auspices of the Society of Authors, which has helped to fund my research.

Various people have advised me on aspects of the First World War and other issues. I would especially like to thank Mick Crumplin, Pete Starling, and John Ellis, who each read the draft and advised me on military matters. Likewise, I am thankful to Heather Sheard, who provided information on the Australian women who worked at Endell Street, and to Lucy Byatt, who advised me on Olga Campbell's life. I would also like to thank Sara Haslam for her timely advice, engrossing conversations, and warm friendship as we jointly navigated the intricacies of Elizabeth Robins's and Beatrice Harraden's scrawls. I'm grateful also to Alison Ramsay of Digital Drama for her kind help.

Many individuals and families have generously shared their memories and material in helping me to research the lives of the staff and patients of Endell Street. I am extremely grateful to Anthony and Caroline Murray and their family for their kindness and hospitality in inviting me to their home at Murraythwaite and allowing me to trawl through family papers for information on Flora Murray. I'm grateful also to Sue Byrne for her insights on Murray. For permission to access the Garrett Anderson family papers, I wish to thank Robin and Rose Carver, Catriona Williams, and Jenny Loehnis. I owe a huge thank you to Andrew Wells for sharing family papers belonging to Mardie Hodgson and for his hospitality. Likewise I wish to thank Robin and Jilly Byatt, Fiona Byatt, Lucy Byatt, and Diarmid Campbell for sharing the papers of Olga Campbell as well as for their interest in the project and their hospitality. Warmest thanks to Annie Fox for sharing her papers and memories of Nina Last and to Nancy and Anne Prentis for sharing those of Barbara Last.

Many more people provided information on ancestors who worked at Endell Street, including Christopher Haviland (on Evelyn Clemow); Dr Michael Grant (Ernestine de Longueuil); Michael Fellows and other members of the Fellows family (Evelyn Windsor); Elizabeth Simpson (Elizabeth Exell); and Kate Staveley Down (Dulcie Staveley). Additionally, I am indebted to many descendants of patients who were treated at Endell Street for sharing their knowledge. They include Kate Kendall (on John Joseph O'Donoghue); Barb Angus (Larry Tarrant); and Miles King and Mrs. Reece King (Vic Jones).

My thanks are also due to many people who have offered expertise and advice in a wide range of areas. They include Louise Bell, Rose Brown, Ian Castle, Sarah Chaney, Elizabeth Crawford, Alan Cumming, Ross Davies, Patricia Fara, Charlie Forman, Dr. Julio Grau, Peter Higginbotham, Mark Honigsbaum, Paul Jiggens, Angela John, John Langton, Ruth Richardson, and Anne Thomson. In

France I was thrilled to be invited to visit the Château Mauricien at Wimereux by its current owners, Jérôme and Sandrine Lanoy, who kindly shared their knowledge and research. I am grateful to the staff at Claridge's Hotel, Paris, for taking time to show me around the hotel. And thanks to Kit Bevan for showing me Dudley Court courtyard—all that survives from the Endell Street hospital.

As with all my books, this story owes its existence to the dedication and hard work of numerous staff members of libraries, museums, and archives in the United Kingdom and abroad. My thanks are especially due to staff at the Women's Library at the London School of Economics (especially Gillian Murphy), the Imperial War Museum, the Wellcome Library, The National Archives, the British Library, London Metropolitan Archives, the Museum of London, the Bodleian Library Oxford, the British Red Cross Society, the Royal College of Nursing, Newnham College Cambridge, and the National Army Museum. I wish also to thank staff at the British Medical Association; Royal College of Physicians; General Medical Council; Florence Nightingale Museum; Royal College of Obstetrics and Gynaecology; Royal Free Hospital School of Medicine; Royal London Hospital Archives and Museum; Museum of Military Medicine; Suffolk Record Office, Ipswich branch; Churchill Archive Centre, Cambridge; Leeds University, Brotherton Library; Queen Mary University of London; University of Birmingham, Cadbury Research Library; National Library of Scotland; Queen's University, Belfast, McClay Library; St Leonard's School; Cheltenham Ladies' College; Bedales School; Dorking Museum and Heritage Centre; Devil's Porridge Museum, Dumfries and Galloway; Surrey History Centre; and Staffordshire Archives and Heritage. In America I am extremely grateful to archive staff at the National Park Service, Hyde Park (especially Tara McGill); the Fales Library, New York University (especially Nicholas Martin); and the Harry Ransom Center, University of Texas. In Australia I am thankful to archive staff at the University of Sydney; the University of Melbourne; the State Library of Queensland; and the Geoffrey Kaye Museum, Melbourne.

I have been extraordinarily lucky in enjoying the best possible support and guidance of experts in the publishing world. For their tireless enthusiasm, shrewd advice, and careful editing I am indebted to Karen Duffy and Clare Drysdale at Atlantic Books in the United Kingdom and to Claire Potter at Basic Books in the United States. My thanks also to Tamsin Shelton (UK) and to Kathy Streckfus (US) for their patient and meticulous editing. Most of all, I am supremely grateful to my agent, Patrick Walsh, for his unfailing zeal for this book and for my writing. Finally, I want to thank all my friends and family members for keeping me going throughout the journey, especially Peter, Sam, and Susie for being there always.

Selected Bibliography

Manuscript Sources

Bodleian Library, Oxford—Papers of H. W. Nevinson; Papers of Evelyn Sharp

British Red Cross Society—VAD records; Joint War Committee Summaries of Work

Churchill Archive Centre, Cambridge—Lord Esher's War Journals

Imperial War Museum, London—Private Papers of Sir Henry and Lady Norman; Papers of Women's Work Sub-Committee; Women's Work Collection; Department of Art Collection

Leeds University, Brotherton Library—Liddle Collection, interview with Kath Ussher

London Metropolitan Archives—Women's Hospital for Children (Harrow Road), annual reports, in King Edward's Fund Collection, annual reports from London hospitals and charities; Elizabeth Garrett Anderson Hospital (New Hospital for Women), annual reports and other records; Royal Free London NHS Foundation Trust collection; London School of Medicine for Women and related collections; South London Hospital for Women and Children and related hospital records

Museum of London Library—Suffragette Fellowship Collection, Frances Bartlett Papers

The National Archives, London—Armed forces service records; British Army medal index cards, 1914–1920; British Army war diaries, 1914–1922

National Army Museum, London—Papers of Helen Gwynne-Vaughan

National Park Service, Hyde Park, New York—Marion Dickerman Papers

Newnham College Cambridge—College archives

New York University, Fales Library—Diary of Elizabeth Robins; Letters of Elizabeth Robins

Royal College of Nursing archives, Edinburgh—Papers of Evelyn Clemow

Royal London Hospital Archives and Museum—Papers of Ethel May

State Library of Queensland—Eleanor Elizabeth Bourne Papers; George Herbert Bourne Papers

Suffolk Record Office, Ipswich—Papers of Elizabeth Garrett Anderson; Papers of Louisa Garrett Anderson

University of Birmingham, Cadbury Research Library—Edith Barling album; Papers of Cynthia Mosley

University of Melbourne archives—Papers of Vera Scantlebury Brown

University of Sydney archives—Papers of Dr. Elizabeth Hamilton-Browne

University of Texas, Harry Ransom Center—Elizabeth Robins Collection

Wellcome Library—Medical Women's Federation archives; Iconographic collection

Women's Library—Papers of Elizabeth Garrett Anderson; Papers of Louisa Garrett Anderson; Papers of Millicent Garrett Fawcett; Records of Women's Tax Resistance League; Papers of Nina Courage (née Last); Papers of Katie Gliddon; Papers of Kitty Marion; Papers of Gertrude Lind Setchfield; Papers of Ellen Isabel Jones

Private Collections

Letters of Mardie Hodgson, by kind permission of Andrew Wells

Letters of Olga, Keir, and Arthur Campbell, by kind permission of Diarmid Campbell

Memoir of Sir Colin Skelton Anderson, courtesy of Robin and Rose Carver

Murray family papers, Murraythwaite, by kind permission of Anthony and Caroline Murray

Published Sources

Abel-Smith, Brian. *A History of the Nursing Profession.* London, 1960.

Alberti, Johanna. *Beyond Suffrage: Feminists in War and Peace, 1914–1928.* Basingstoke, 1989.

Anderson, Louisa Garrett. *Elizabeth Garrett Anderson, 1836–1917.* London, 1939.

Atkinson, Diane. *Elsie & Mairi Go to War: Two Extraordinary Women on the Western Front.* London, 2010.

———. *Rise Up Women! The Remarkable Lives of the Suffragettes.* London, 2018.

Balfour, Frances. *Dr Elsie Inglis.* London, 1918.

Bell, Enid Moberly. *Storming the Citadel: The Rise of the Woman Doctor.* London, 1953.

Bennett, A. H. *English Medical Women: Glimpses of Their Work in Peace and War.* London, 1915.

Blake, Catriona. *The Charge of the Parasols: Women's Entry to the Medical Profession.* London, 1990.

Bland-Sutton, Sir John. *The Story of a Surgeon.* London, 1930.

Bourke, Joanna. *Dismembering the Male: Men's Bodies, Britain and the Great War.* London, 1996.

Brereton, Frederick Sadleir. *The Great War and the R.A.M.C.* London, 1919.

Brett, Maurice V., ed. *Journals and Letters of Reginald, Viscount Esher*, 4 vols. London, 1934–1938.

Brittain, Vera. *Testament of Youth*. London, 2014 [1933].

Brock, Claire. *British Women Surgeons and Their Patients, 1860–1918*. Cambridge, 2017.

Castle, Ian. *The First Blitz: Bombing London in the First World War*. Oxford, 2015.

———. *London, 1914–17: The Zeppelin Menace*. Oxford, 2008.

Cohen, Susan. *Medical Services in the First World War*. Oxford, 2014.

Crawford, Elizabeth. *Enterprising Women: The Garretts and Their Circle*. London, 2002.

———. *The Women's Suffrage Movement: A Reference Guide, 1866–1928*. London, 1999.

Davis, Kenneth S. *Invincible Summer: An Intimate Portrait of the Roosevelts, Based on the Recollections of Marion Dickerman*. New York, 1974.

Faderman, Lillian. *Surpassing the Love of Men: Romantic Friendship and Love Between Women from the Renaissance to the Present*. New York, 1981.

Fara, Patricia. *A Lab of One's Own: Science and Suffrage in the First World War*. Oxford, 2018.

Finzi, Kate John. *Eighteen Months in the War Zone: The Record of a Woman's Work on the Western Front*. London, 1916.

Furse, Dame Katharine. *Hearts and Pomegranates: The Story of Forty-Five Years, 1875–1920*. London, 1940.

Geddes, Jennian. *"Knowledge and Practice of Needlework a Great Asset": British Women in Surgery, 1873 to 1939*. London, 2011.

———. "Louisa Garrett Anderson (1873–1943), Surgeon and Suffragette." *Journal of Medical Biography* 16 (2008): 205–214.

———. "'Women as Army Surgeons': The Women's Hospital Corps, 1914–1919." MA thesis, London Metropolitan University, 2005.

Gilbert, Martin. *First World War*. London, 1994.

Glynn, Jennifer. *The Pioneering Garretts: Breaking the Barriers for Women*. London, 2008.

Graves, Robert. *Goodbye to All That*. London, 2000 [1929].

Hacker, Carlotta. *The Indomitable Lady Doctors*. Toronto, 1974.

Hale, Grace. "The Women's Hospital Corps." *League News* (magazine of St Bartholomew's Hospital) 4 (1917): 755–758.

Hallett, Christine E. *Containing Trauma: Nursing Work in the First World War*. Manchester, 2009.

———. "'Emotional Nursing': Involvement, Engagement and Detachment in the Writings of First World War Nurses and VADs." In Hallett and Alison S. Fell, eds., *First World War Nursing: New Perspectives*. New York, 2013, 87–102.

Hamer, Emily. *Britannia's Glory: A History of Twentieth Century Lesbians*. London, 1996.

————. "Keeping Their Fingers on the Pulse: Lesbian Doctors in Britain, 1890–1950." In Franz X. Eder, Lesley Hall, and Gert Hekma, eds., *Sexual Cultures in Europe: Themes in Sexuality*. Manchester, 1999, 139–158.

Harraden, Beatrice. "Women Doctors in the War." *Windsor Magazine* (1915): 179–193.

Harrison, Mark. *The Medical War*. Oxford, 2010.

Hart, Peter. *The Great War, 1914–1918*. London, 2014.

Haslam, Sara. "Reading, Trauma and Literary Caregiving, 1914–1918: Helen Mary Gaskell and the War Library." *Journal of Medical Humanities*, March 28, 2018.

Hastings, Max. *Catastrophe: Europe Goes to War 1914*. London, 2013.

Hoare, Philip. *Spike Island: The Memory of a Military Hospital*. London, 2002.

John, Angela V. *Elizabeth Robins: Staging a Life, 1862–1952*. London, 1995.

————. *Evelyn Sharp: Rebel Woman, 1869–1955*. Manchester, 2009.

————. *War, Journalism and the Shaping of the Twentieth Century: The Life and Times of Henry W. Nevinson*. London, 2006.

Koch, Theodore Wesley. *Books in Camp, Trench and Hospital*. London, 1917.

Leneman, Leah. *Elsie Inglis: Founder of Battlefront Hospitals Run Entirely by Women*. Edinburgh, 1998.

————. "Medical Women at War, 1914–1918." *Medical History* 38 (1994): 160–177.

MacDonagh, Michael. *In London During the Great War*. London, 1935.

MacLaren, Barbara. *Women of the War*. London, 1917.

MacPherson, W. G., ed. *History of the Great War Based on Official Documents: Medical Services*, 4 vols. London, 1921–1924.

Manton, Jo. *Elizabeth Garrett Anderson*. London, 1965.

Marwick, Arthur. *Women at War, 1914–1918*. London, 1977.

Mayhew, Emily. *Wounded: From Battlefield to Blighty, 1914–1918*. London, 2013.

Miles, Hallie. *Untold Tales of War-Time London*. London, 1930.

Mitchell, Ann M. *Medical Women and the Medical Services of the First World War*. Melbourne, 1978.

Mitchell, T. J., and G. M. Smith. *History of the Great War, Medical Services, Casualties and Medical Statistics of the Great War*. London, 1931.

Murray, Flora. *Women as Army Surgeons*. London, 1920.

Pankhurst, Christabel. *Unshackled: The Story of How We Won the Vote*. London, 1959.

Pankhurst, E. Sylvia. *The Home Front: A Mirror to Life in England During the First World War*. London, 1987 [1932].

Pankhurst, Emmeline. *My Own Story*. London, 1914.

Philo-Gill, Samantha. *The Women's Army Auxiliary Corps in France, 1917–1921: Women Urgently Wanted*. Barnsley, 2017.

Pratt, Edwin. *British Railways and the Great War*, 2 vols. London, 1921.

Raeburn, Antonia. *Militant Suffragettes*. London, 1973.

————. *The Suffragette View*. Newton Abbot, 1976.

Reznick, Jeffrey S. *Healing the Nation: Soldiers and the Culture of Caregiving in Britain During the Great War*. Manchester, 2004.

———. "Work-Therapy and the Disabled British Soldier in Great Britain in the First World War: The Case of Shepherd's Bush Military Hospital, London." In David A. Gerber, ed., *Disabled Veterans in History*. Ann Arbor, MI, 2000, 185–203.

Robins, Elizabeth. *Ancilla's Share: An Indictment of Sex Antagonism*. London, 1924.

Scotland, Thomas, and Steven Heys, eds. *War Surgery, 1914–18*. Solihull, 2012.

Scott, Jean. "Women and the GMC." *British Medical Journal* 289 (1984): 1764–1767.

Sheard, Heather. *A Heart Undivided: The Life of Dr Vera Scantlebury Brown*. Melbourne, 2016.

———. "'They Will Both Go to Heaven and Have Crowns and Golden Harps': Dr Vera Scantlebury Brown and Female Leadership in a First World War Military Hospital." In Fiona Davis, Nell Musgrove, and Judith Smart, eds., *Founders, Firsts and Feminists: Women Leaders in Twentieth Century Australia*. Melbourne, 2011, 90–104.

Sheard, Heather, and Ruth Lee. *Women to the Front: The Extraordinary Australian Women Doctors in the Great War*. Sydney, 2019.

Shipton, Elisabeth. *Female Tommies: The Frontline Women of the First World War*. Stroud, 2017.

Stephen, Guy. "Notes on the History of Boulogne as a Military Medical Base." *Royal United Services Institution Journal* 63, no. 454 (1919): 271–287, published online 2009.

Vivian, E. Charles. *With the Royal Army Medical Corps (R.A.M.C.) at the Front*. London, 1914.

White, Jerry. *Zeppelin Nights: London in the First World War*. London, 2015.

Notes

Sources cited only once are given here in full. Other sources are listed in full in the selected bibliography.

Abbreviations

BJN British Journal of Nursing
BMJ British Medical Journal
BRCS British Red Cross Society
EGA Elizabeth Garrett Anderson
FL Fales Library, New York
FM Flora Murray
IWM Imperial War Museum
LGA Louisa Garrett Anderson
LMA London Metropolitan Archives
LSMW London School of Medicine for Women
MH Mardie Hodgson
MWF Medical Women's Federation
ODNB Oxford Dictionary of National Biography
TNA The National Archives
WL Women's Library, London School of Economics

Chapter One: A Good Feeling

1. Details of the departure are from Murray 1920, 13–14. FM gives the date as Tuesday, September 14, but from LGA's letters to her mother and other accounts it is clear that it was Tuesday, September 15.

2. Adrian Gregory, "Railways Stations: Gateways and Termini," in Jay Winter and Jean-Louis Robert, *Capital Cities at War: Paris, London, Berlin, 1914–1919*, vol. 2 (Cambridge, 1997), 23–56.

3. Elsie Knocker quoted in Atkinson 2010, 4.

4. Pratt 1921, 1:197. The first batch of wounded arrived on August 30.

5. Alberti 1989, 38–39; Raeburn 1973, 256; David Mitchell, *Women on the Warpath: The Story of the Women of the First World War* (London, 1966), 34.

6. Jane Robinson, *Hearts and Minds: Suffragists, Suffragettes and How Women Won the Vote* (London, 2018), 245, citing Fawcett in *Common Cause*, August 7, 1914.

7. Atkinson 2010, 3; E. Sylvia Pankhurst 1987 [1932], 38.

8. "Women's Hospital Corps in Paris," *Magazine of the RFHLSMW* 9, no. 59 (November 1914): 139–140. This was probably written by LGA.

9. Family history of LGA is from Manton 1965, esp. 234–295; Geddes 2008; Anderson 1939. LGA was born on July 28, 1873.

10. Manton 1965, 276.

11. Details of LGA's childhood are from her letters to her parents, 1881 to 1887, Ipswich RO, HA436/1/3/2. The earliest letter is dated July 28, 1881, her eighth birthday.

12. Background on St Leonard's School from Julia M. Grant, Katharine H. McCutcheon, and Ethel F. Sanders, eds., *St. Leonard's School, 1877–1927* (Oxford, 1927). She was admitted on May 4, 1888, according to the school register.

13. LGA to her mother, March 7, 1891, Ipswich RO, HA436/1/3/2.

14. Biography of Elizabeth Garrett Anderson from Anderson 1939; Manton 1965; Crawford 2002; Glynn 2008. Background on women's entry into medicine from Blake 1990; Bell 1953.

15. Blake 1990, 42–43. Her name was added to the Medical Register on January 1, 1859. EGA met her later that year.

16. Sir William Jenner, cited in Bell 1953, 103.

17. Blake 1990, 66, 75.

18. Crawford 2002, 85. The bill was known as Gurney's Enabling Bill.

19. Scott 1984.

20. Geddes 2011. See also Mary Ann Elston, "'Run by Women (Mainly) for Women': Medical Women's Hospitals in Britain 1866–1948," in Anne Hardy and Lawrence Conrad, eds., *Women and Modern Medicine* (Amsterdam, 2001), 73–107.

21. Manton 1965, 296. Unless otherwise noted, underlining is in the original.

22. LGA worked at Plaistow Maternity Charity in 1898 and Camberwell Workhouse Infirmary in 1899–1900. She was appointed house surgeon at the Royal Free Hospital in 1901. *Magazine of the RFHLSMW*, 1898 to 1901.

23. Anderson 1939, 245. For more on Scharlieb and other women surgeons, see Brock 2017.

24. Letter from LGA to her mother, 1899–1901, Ipswich RO, HA436/1/3/6. The letter is undated.

25. LGA described her experiences in America in *Magazine of the RFHLSMW*, vol. 3 (January and May 1902): 887–900, 26–37.

26. Bell 1953, 145.

27. Annual reports of the New Hospital for Women, 1902–1907 and 1908–1913, LMA, H13/EGA/06/1-6. She was appointed surgical assistant in 1902, senior assistant to outpatients in 1903, surgeon to outpatients (assistant surgeon) from 1904. The hospital was renamed the Elizabeth Garrett Anderson Hospital in 1917. Facilities and patient statistics from Bennett 1915, 57–63.

28. Described by Elsie Inglis, who worked at the New Hospital in 1892, in Balfour 1918, 67.

29. LGA and Kate Platt, "Malignant Disease of the Uterus: A Digest of 265 Cases Treated in the New Hospital for Women," in *Journal of Obstetrics and Gynaecology of the British Empire* 14, no. 6 (December 1908): 381–392, cited in Brock 2017, 191.

30. Will of James Skelton Anderson, 1906, WL, 7EGA/12. Her father refers to having recently bought and furnished the house at 114a Harley Street. She also received an annuity of £800 per annum (worth about £88,000 today).

31. John M. T. Ford, "Medical Memorials: Florence Nightingale, OM (1820–1910)," *Journal of Medical Biography* 12, no. 2 (May 2004): 120; death certificate of Florence Nightingale, August 16, 1910.

32. Geddes makes this point well in Geddes 2005.

33. Atkinson 2018, 6. Further background on the women's suffrage movement is from Atkinson 2018 and Raeburn 1973, 1976.

34. Ada Flatman, quoted in Atkinson 2018, 117.

35. Crawford 1999, 13–14; Geddes 2005, 19.

36. LGA to Millicent Fawcett, June 22, 25, and 27, 1908, WL, microfilm M50/2/1/246-8. The originals are in the Papers of Millicent Garrett Fawcett at Manchester Archives and Local Studies.

37. Cheryl R. Jorgensen-Earp, ed., *Speeches and Trials of the Militant Suffragettes: The Women's Social and Political Union, 1903–1918* (Madison, NJ, 1999), 58–59.

38. Margaret Kineton Parkes, "The Tax Resistance Movement in Great Britain," c. 1910–1911, Records of the Women's Tax Resistance League, WL, 2WTR/4/9.

39. LGA to A. Gordon Pollock, November 14, 1910, LMA, H13/EGA/228/1-22. She had expected the deputation to take place the next day, but it was postponed until November 18.

40. Hertha Ayrton cited in Raeburn 1973, 170.

41. *Daily Telegraph*, March 6, 1912; *Morning Leader*, March 6, 1912. Millicent Fawcett's condemnation was in *The Times*, March 6, 1912.

42. LGA to EGA, eight letters from Holloway dated March 6 to 29, 1912, WL, 7LGA/1/2/1-8.

43. Winefred Rix quoted in Atkinson 2018, 307; Papers of Katie Gliddon, WL, 7KGG/1/1.

44. Alan Anderson to the Prison Commissioners, April 1, 1912, and notes from the Home Office, WL, 7LGA/1.

45. Crawford 1999, 13–14.

46. Background on Flora Murray's family is from *Burke's Landed Gentry Scotland* (2001): 620; "Sons of the South" (re: her brother), in *The Gallovidian Annual*, December 1921, 1–8; Jennian Geddes, "Murray, Flora (1869–1923), Physician and Suffragette," ODNB, https://doi.org/10.1093/ref:odnb/56304; *Scotsman*, March 14, 1888; will of John Murray, 1872, National Records of Scotland.

47. Murray, "Ethyl Chloride as an Anaesthetic for Infants," *Lancet* 166, no. 4291 (November 25, 1905): 1542–1543; *Times*, July 15, 1908.

48. LGA, *Medical Women's Federation Newsletter*, 1923, 42–43.

49. FM, "The Position of Women in Medicine and Surgery," *New Statesman*, November 1, 1913. According to one source, either FM or LGA was refused a staff appointment at a London hospital. *Morning Advertiser*, June 3, 1915, LMA, H24/SLW/Y6/1.

50. Crawford 1999, 432.

51. Diary of Gertrude Setchfield, WL, 7GLS; Christabel Pankhurst 1959, 251. The house was run with Catherine Pine in Pembridge Gardens.

52. Murray, "Torture in the Twentieth Century," WL, pamphlets 7EIJ/2.

53. Kitty Marion's memoir, WL, 7KMA; "on stretchers": Frances Bartlett, "My Suffrage Work," Museum of London, MS 57.113/5, 37–43. FM and LGA also jointly nursed Mary Richardson back to health after she was released on license from Holloway and before she went on to slash the Rokeby Venus in the National Gallery in 1914. Mary Richardson, *Laugh a Defiance* (London, 1953), 154.

54. *The Suffragette*, June 27, 1913, also published as a pamphlet, "'Cat & Mouse' Act," WL, pamphlets 7EIJ/2.

55. They included Mrs. Pankhurst in 1913, cited in Christabel Pankhurst 1959, 251, and Olive Wharry in 1914, cited in Crawford 1999, 707.

56. Raeburn 1976, 66–67; Dover: Emmeline Pankhurst 1914, 328.

57. Emmeline Pankhurst 1914, 240.

58. Kitty Marion's memoir, WL, 7KMA.

59. *Times*, April 2, 1914; Crawford 1999, 115–116.

60. Jennian Geddes, "Culpable Complicity: The Medical Profession and the Forcible Feeding of Suffragettes, 1909–1914," *Women's History Review* 17, no. 1 (February 2008): 79–94.

61. E. Sylvia Pankhurst 1987 [1932], 119; unpublished memoir of Sir Colin Skelton Anderson (private papers); Diary of Henry Nevinson, Oxford, Bodleian Library, MSS.Eng.misc.e.618/3, September 1, 1914; "tender and gentle": obituary in *The Workers' Dreadnought*, August 4, 1923, 5; Vera Scantlebury, "Women as Army Surgeons: A Record of Splendid Service," *The Woman's World* 1, no. 6 (1922): 11–12.

62. The Women's Hospital for Children, Harrow Road, Annual Reports 1913 and 1914, LMA, King Edward's Fund Collection, SC/PPS/093/080; Bennett 1915, 66–73; *The Hospital*, January 31, 1914, 481–482. The hospital was based in three adjoining cottages at 688 Harrow Road near Kensal Rise. *The Hospital* magazine was critical of the LSMW too. Brock 2017, 243.

63. Photograph, WL, 7LGA/6/13.

64. Land Registry, January 11, 1913; Electoral Register 1914. Murray kept up the lease on her apartment in Campden Hill Road, while Anderson retained her consulting rooms in Harley Street. LGA mentioned the Penn cottage to Evelyn Sharp c. 1910: LGA to Sharp, n.d. [c. 1910–1911), Oxford, Bodleian Library, MSS.Eng.lett.d.277.113/4. The couple had bought a smaller property, Stone Lodge, in Penn before jointly buying land to build their cottage, Paul End, in 1912.

65. Background on lesbian relationships from Hamer 1999, 1996; Faderman 1981. Hamer 1999 says Murray had her "first serious lesbian relationship" with Elsie Inglis, the Scottish surgeon, but gives no source for this, and there appears to be no evidence to back it up. Women doctors unmarried: Blake 1990, 160.

66. Isabel Hutton, *Memories of a Doctor in War and Peace* (London, 1960), 131–132.

67. Dedication in Murray 1920; LGA to Ivy Anderson, November 17, 1914, WL, 7LGA/2/1/22.

68. Diary of Evelyn Sharp, Oxford, Bodleian Library, MSS.Eng.misc.e.635, vol. 3, November 1, 1943; "great happiness": LGA to Sharp, n.d. [c. 1910–1911), Oxford, Bodleian Library, MSS.Eng.lett.d.277.113/4; "appealing, passionately loving letter": Nevinson diary, Oxford, Bodleian Library, MSS.Eng.misc.e.618/2, January 22, 1914.

Sharp also describes the Scottish trips in her memoir, *Unfinished Adventure: Selected Reminiscences from an Englishwoman's Life* (London, 1933), 123–125. Sharp and Nevinson were devoted to each other throughout their lives, though the relationship is thought to have been unconsummated until their marriage in 1933.

69. The lead-up to war is described in White 2015, 1–25.

70. Emmeline Pethick-Lawrence, *My Part in a Changing World* (London, 1938), 305.

71. Margot Lawrence, *Shadow of the Swords: A Biography of Elsie Inglis* (London, 1971), 97–98. There are various versions of this comment, but Lawrence's version was apparently confirmed by Inglis's niece.

72. Murray 1920, 5. Details of the unit's organization are from Murray 1920, 5–12; Hale 1917. FM describes the uniform on p. 10.

73. Gazdar, Judge, and Cuthbert are named in Murray 1920; details of their careers are from the LSMW student register in 1911 and the annual report of Harrow Road in 1913 at LMA. The nurses are named in *BJN*, September 19, 1914, 223, as Misses Wicks, Robellaz, Bryan, Cleavling, Brown, Pratt, Pearson, and Mrs. Lawrence.

74. Murray 1920, 10. A jacket belonging to Endell Street orderly Nina Last survives. WL, 7NLA.

75. LGA to EGA, n.d. [September 1914], WL, 7LGA/2/1.

76. Nevinson diary, Oxford, Bodleian Library, MSS.Eng.misc.e.618/2, September 15, 1914.

77. LGA to EGA, September 15, 1914, and September 16, 1914, WL, 7LGA/2/1; grocery boy: LGA to A. Gordon Pollock, chair of the managing committee of the New Hospital for Women, printed in *St Leonard's School Gazette*, March 1915.

78. Murray 1920, 4.

Chapter Two: A Sort of Holiday

1. The main sources for the WHC's work in Paris are Murray 1920; letters from Mardie Hodgson [MH] to her mother, Alice Maitland-Heriot [AM-H], from France, September 16, 1914, to January 9, 1915, courtesy of Andrew Wells; LGA letters from France to her family, WL, 7LGA/2/1/1-29; Hale 1917; Harraden 1915; contemporary news cuttings.

2. History of Claridge's is from Patrice de Moncan, *Les Belles Heures du Claridge* (Paris, 2000). There appears to be no connection with the London Claridge's Hotel, and it seems likely the French owners adopted the name simply as a symbol of luxury.

3. Hale 1917.

4. Biography of Mardie Hodgson: information from Andrew Wells (her grandson); family album; letters to her mother.

5. MH to AM-H, n.d. [September 16, 1914]. Misspellings and other errors from quoted letters and diaries have been retained throughout.

6. Murray 1920, 19. Beatrice Harraden said that FM kept a diary, although it has not survived. Harraden 1915.

7. LGA to EGA, September 17, 1914, WL, 7LGA/2/1/6.

8. MH to AM-H, September 17, 1914.

9. LGA to EGA, September 17, 1914, WL, 7LGA/2/1/6.

10. Captain Eugene Ginchereau, "The American Ambulance in Paris, 1914–1917," *Military Medicine* 180 (2015): 1201–1202. The term "ambulance" was used to mean the entire medical operation.

11. Murray 1920, 27.

12. Main sources on medical care are Harrison 2010; Scotland and Heys 2012; Cohen 2014; Mayhew 2013. Contemporary sources include Brereton 1919; Vivian 1914; MacPherson 1921–1924; H. S. Souttar, *A Surgeon in Belgium* (London, 1915).

13. Mitchell and Smith 1931, 8.

14. MacPherson 1921–1924, 2:195; anesthetized with chloroform: Brereton 1919, 99.

15. Vivian 1914, 138–139.

16. Brett 1934–1938, 3:189.

17. Ibid.

18. LGA to EGA, September 17, 1914, WL, 7LGA/2/1/6.

19. LGA to Ivy Anderson, September 17, 1914, WL, 7LGA/2/1/7.

20. Murray 1920, 27.

21. Their lack of experience is discussed in Geddes 2005. Brock 2017 points out that surgeons at the New Hospital for Women had experience performing abdominal surgery, including hysterectomies, through their gynecological and other work, and that FM and LGA held a weekly orthopedic clinic at the Children's Hospital. Brock 2017, 191. This was still little preparation for war surgery.

22. The medical problems are described in Mayhew 2013; Scotland and Heys 2012; Cohen 2014; Vivian 1914.

23. H. M. W. Gray, *The Early Treatment of War Wounds* (London, 1919), 1.

24. Bland-Sutton 1930, 87.

25. LGA to EGA, September 22, 1914, WL, 7LGA/2/1/8.

26. MH to AM-H, September 22, 1914.

27. The trip to Braisne: Murray 1920, 45–48; LGA to EGA, September 28, 1914, WL, 7LGA/2/1/10; LGA to AGA, September 27, 1914, WL, 7LGA/2/1/17; MH to AM-H, September 28 and 30, 1914.

28. "Women's Hospital Corps in Paris," *Magazine of the RFHLSMW* 9, no. 59 (November 1914): 139–140.

29. LGA to EGA, October 4, 1914, WL, 7LGA/2/1/12. The source of the ambulance or ambulances is confusing because LGA refers to Miss Ellis and her brother who brought the ambulance and lorry across; Hodgson describes a "well off" woman who bought them an ambulance in Paris, who could have been the same Miss Ellis. She was probably Christobel Ellis, an experienced motorist who offered her services to the French Red Cross in September 1914 and also worked for the British Red Cross in Paris. She went to Serbia at the end of 1914 and later became head of the motor branch of the WAAC. MacLaren 1917, 136. FM says two "Paris friends," Mlle. Block and Miss Grey, provided two ambulances. Hazel Cuthbert also refers to the corps having "two ambulances of its own." "Women Doctors and the War," *BMJ* 1, no 2825 (February 20, 1915): 354. It seems there were several ambulances being driven by various people at different times.

30. MH to AM-H, September 28 and 30, 1914, and undated note, "An expedition to Rheims."

31. LGA to EGA, September 22 and 27, 1914, WL, 7LGA/2/1/8 and 9.

32. MH to AM-H, September 22, 1914, and n.d. [c. September 1914].

33. LGA to EGA, n.d. [October 1914], WL, 7LGA/2/1/15.

34. Murray 1920, 38–39; "off his head": MH to AM-H, n.d. [c. September 1914].

35. Murray 1920, 41.

36. MH to AM-H, September 28 and 30, 1914.

37. MH to AM-H, n.d. [c. September 1914].

38. The writer Vera Brittain, who became a VAD in a British hospital in 1915, wrote that "the free-and-easy movements of girl war-workers had begun to modify convention." Brittain 2014 [1933], 154.

39. MH to AM-H, September 22, 1914; "bad jaw wounds": ibid., September 28 and 30, 1914.

40. MH to AM-H, September 22, 1914; "suffragetty": ibid., September 28 and 30, 1914; "jolly little party": ibid., n.d. [c. September 1914].

41. "Women's Hospital Corps in Paris," *Magazine of the RFHLSMW* 9, no. 59 (November 1914): 139–140. Blandy's career is discussed in Sarah Lefanu, "Majorie Blandy (1887–1937)," in Biddy Passmore, ed., *Breaking Bounds: Six Newnham Lives* (Cambridge, 2014), 53–65.

42. Diary of Gertrude Setchfield, September 26, 1914, Papers of Gertrude Lind Setchfield, WL, 7GLS. The meeting was held in London on September 24, 1914; NUWSS and Elsie Inglis: Balfour 1918, 147–151.

43. Murray 1920, 31; "chic": ibid., 11.

44. Murray 1920, 74.

45. Deaths: MH to AM-H, September 22, 1914; LGA to EGA, September 27, 1914, WL, 7LGA/2/1/9; "five men had died": MH to AM-H, September 28 and 30, 1914. The death rate at the American Hospital was recorded as 4.5 per 1,000 in its first year. Annual report for American Hospital 1915, Field Service, www.ourstory .info/library/2-ww1/AmHosp15/ahp1915.html.

46. Murray 1920, 41; MH to AM-H, October 24, 1914.

47. *St Andrew's Citizen*, September 26, 1914.

48. LGA to EGA, n.d. [October 1914], WL, 7LGA/2/1/15.

49. LGA to EGA, October 4, 1914, WL, 7LGA/2/1/12.

50. *Magazine of the RFHLSMW* 14 (July 1919): 115–116.

51. "Letter from the Doctors at the Front," Harrow Road children's hospital, annual report, 1914, LMA; Murray 1920, 74–75; "on the way to church": LGA to EGA, October 4, 1914, WL, 7LGA/2/1/12; "bathed in soft lights": LGA to A. Gordon Pollock, printed in *St Leonard's School Gazette*, March 1915; "poor little wifes sake": MH to AM-H, October 10, 1914.

52. "Letter from the Doctors at the Front."

53. LGA to EGA, September 27, 1914, WL, 7LGA/2/1/9; "full of horrors": LGA to EGA, September 22, 1914, WL, 7LGA/2/1/8; homey and cheerful: "Letter from the Doctors at the Front"; "comfort & friendly spirit": MH to AM-H, n.d. [c. October 1914].

54. LGA to EGA, September 22, 1914, WL, 7LGA/2/1/8; "years of unpopularity": LGA to EGA, September 27, 1914, WL, 7LGA/2/1/9; "a sort of holiday": LGA to AGA, September 27, 1914, WL, 7LGA/2/1/17.

55. Murray 1920, 39; "broken children": LGA to EGA, October 4, 1914, WL, 7LGA/2/1/12; "boys go back to school": Murray 1920, 40; LGA to A. Gordon Pollock, *St Leonard's School Gazette*, March 1915.

56. Murray 1920, 58–59.

57. British newspapers: *Daily Sketch*, October 17, 1914; untitled news cutting, n.d., photo album of Mardie Hodgson, courtesy of Andrew Wells; untitled news cutting, Millicent Fawcett's press cuttings album, WL, 7MGF/E/5; *Sheffield Weekly Telegraph*, February 6, 1915; *Globe*, October 23, 1914; *Daily Mail*, October 16, 1914; *BMJ* 2, no. 2809 (October 31, 1914): 767.

58. Bennett 1915, 118–122.

59. LGA to EGA, September 27, 1914, WL, 7LGA/2/1/9.

60. Murray 1920, 48–51; LGA to EGA, September 27, 1914, WL, 7LGA/2/1/9, and to AGA, September 27, 1914, WL, 7LGA/2/1/17; MH to AM-H, September 30, 1914; uniform: J. A. Spender, *Men and Things* (London, 1937), 39.

61. Brett 1934–1938, 3:190; "admirable hospitals": Lord Esher's War Journals, memo for Lord Kitchener, undated, Churchill Archive Centre, Cambridge.

62. Murray 1920, 52–53.

63. LGA to EGA, October 4, 1914, WL, 7LGA/2/1/12; "I wish the whole organisation": LGA to EGA, September 27, 1914, WL, 7LGA/2/1/9.

64. MH to AM-H, September 28 and 30, 1914.

65. Murray 1920, 34–36.

66. Ibid., 81–85.

67. LGA to EGA, October 11, 1914, WL, 7LGA/2/1/14; "getting very slack": MH to AM-H, October 24, 1914.

68. X-ray apparatus: untitled news cutting, n.d., photo album of Mardie Hodgson, courtesy of Andrew Wells; MH to AM-H, October 10, 1914.

Chapter Three: Sunshine and Sweetness

1. Details about the corps' work in Boulogne are mainly from Murray 1920; letters from Mardie Hodgson [MH] to her mother, Alice Maitland-Heriot [AM-H], from France, September 16, 1914, to January 9, 1915, courtesy of Andrew Wells; LGA letters from France to her family, WL, 7LGA/2/1/1-29; Hale 1917; Harraden 1915; and contemporary news cuttings. Background on Boulogne is from Finzi 1916; Stephen 1919; A. L. Walker [Adelaide Louisiana Walker], "Experiences at a Base Hospital in France, 1914–1915," from Scarletfinders, www.scarletfinders.co.uk/156 .html. FM said she and LGA arrived on November 1, but letters from LGA and MH make clear it was October 31.

2. Walker, "Experiences"; "city of hospitals": Finzi 1916, 47.

3. Background on the Flanders front in the autumn of 1914 is from Hastings 2013; MacPherson 1921–1924, vol. 2; Gilbert 1994. Some French, Belgian, and German wounded also arrived in Boulogne, although most French casualties were sent to Dunkirk.

4. Murray 1920, 86–87. This is also described by Finzi 1916; Walker, "Experiences."

5. Finzi 1916, 40.

6. Murray 1920, 90–91; "The Women's Hospital Corps," *The Ladies' Field*, February 13, 1915, 513. The Château Mauricien was originally built for Maurice Ulcoq, a banker and merchant born in Mauritius who had settled in London. I am indebted for information to Jérôme and Sandrine Lanoy, the current owners of the house, and to Jérôme's research, privately published as *Château Mauricien* (2016).

7. Finzi 1916, 21. No. 14 General Hospital was set up in the Hôtel Splendid and its casino, according to Stephen 1919, and No. 14 Stationary Hospital was located in a hotel on the seafront. FM refers to this as the Grand Hôtel. Murray 1920, 93. Both hotels were on the esplanade. Bathing huts: Stephen 1919; Baccarat Room: Arthur Stanley, MP, who chaired the British Red Cross Society's executive committee, quoted in "Red Cross Work in France," *The Times*, January 18, 1915.

8. Murray 1920, 91; "not ideal": LGA to AGA, October 30, 1914, WL, 7LGA /2/1/20; "sunshine and sweetness": Murray 1920, 91. The mayor was a local builder named Eugène Leroy.

9. Murray 1920, 91.

10. MH to AM-H, Saturday [October 31, 1914]; LGA to AGA, October 30, 1914, WL, 7LGA/2/1/20.

11. MH to AM-H, n.d. [early November 1914]; Thursday [November 7, 1914], Saturday [October 31, 1914].

12. The nurses are named in *Nursing Times*, January 4, 1915, as Breen, Clemow, Clevely [Cleavely], D'Arcy, Watkin, Platt, Stevens, Robertson, Collins, Comer, and Fowler. Fenn and Goodwin: Murray 1920, 94. Twenty Belgian refugees: LGA to AGA, n.d. [November 15, 1914], WL, 7LGA/2/1/21.

13. James Arthur Campbell to Keir Campbell, November 12, 1914, courtesy of Diarmid Campbell (Olga's nephew); background on Arthur Campbell is from Ian M. Campbell, *Some Notes on the Campbells of Inverawe* (1951), expanded by Diarmid Campbell with help from Niall Campbell (privately published 1988).

14. Murray 1920, 63–64; MH to AM-H, September 28 and 30, 1914, and November 15, 1914.

15. Murray 1920, 96–97. Another account of the meeting, apparently quoting from FM's lost diary, says it took place on "Monday," i.e., November 2, 1914. Harraden 1915.

16. MacPherson 1921–1924, vol. 2; Stephen 1919. Sloggett arrived on October 28, 1914 [Stephen 1919 says October 27] with his deputy, Burtchaell, and set up headquarters in the Hôtel Dervaux.

17. Harrison 2010, 37.

18. For more background on other women medical workers, see Leneman 1994 and 1998; Atkinson 2010.

19. LGA to AGA, November 15, 1914, WL, 7LGA/2/1/21.

20. Murray 1920, 96.

21. MH to AM-H, Thursday and Sunday [November 5 and 8, 1914].

22. MH to AM-H, Thursday and Sunday [November 5 and 8, 1914]. FM said the first patients arrived on November 6. As the trains generally arrived very late at night or early in the morning, it is possible the casualties were not admitted until the early hours of November 6. Murray 1920, 98.

23. Stephen 1919. A total 37,798 sick and wounded were carried by ambulance trains from the front to Boulogne and other base hospitals between October 15 and November 23, 1914, according to MacPherson 1921–1924, 2:331.

24. Lady Priscilla Norman, "Our Hospital in France," Private Papers of Sir Henry and Lady Norman, IWM, 01/15/1. The Normans opened their British Hospital, as it was known, in the former Hotel Bellevue, overlooking the Wimereux River, on November 12, 1914. It had eighty staff members, including four surgeons, and a fleet of seven ambulances. The hospital requisitioned bathing huts for its stores and had a "very nice mortuary" in the garage.

25. LGA to AGA, November 15, 1914, WL, 7LGA/2/1/21.

26. LGA to AGA, October 30, 1914, WL, 7LGA/2/1/20.

27. LGA to Ivy Anderson, November 17, 1914, WL, 7LGA/2/1/22.

28. Postcard, MH to AM-H, n.d. [probably November 11, 1914]. It is likely the hotel "guest" pictured was the original owner, Maurice Ulcoq. Private information, Jérôme Lanoy.

29. Hale 1917.

30. Finzi 1916, 30; "trench-haunted look": ibid., 50.

31. Stephen 1919.

32. Harrison 2010, 24; Stephen 1919. The ambulance trains were adapted from French rolling stock. The first purpose-built ambulance trains did not arrive in France until April 1915.

33. Stephen 1919.

34. LGA to AGA, November 15, 1914, WL, 7LGA/2/1/21.

35. LGA to Ivy Anderson, November 17, 1914, WL, 7LGA/2/1/22.

36. *The Vote*, February 12, 1915.

37. Murray 1920, 98–99.

38. LGA to Ivy Anderson, November 17, 1914, WL, 7LGA/2/1/22.

39. "The Women's Hospital Corps," *The Ladies' Field*, February 13, 1915, 513.

40. LGA to AGA, December 12, 1914, WL, 7LGA/2/1/25, and January 17, 1915, WL, 7LGA/2/1/28.

41. MH to AM-H, December 6, 1914.

42. Murray 1920, 100.

43. Ibid., 99.

44. LGA to AGA, c. November 28, 1914, WL, 7LGA/2/1/23, enclosing letter from Jack Canham, n.d., Manchester.

45. Patients: Corporal David Watt, *Todmorden and District News*, November 20, 1914; Lance Corporal Frank Reynolds, *Banbury Advertiser*, December 31, 1914, also *Sunday Post*, December 20, 1914.

46. Murray 1920, 100. FM refers to "a suffragette friend" who met the policeman, but the story that it was LGA was handed down within the family. Personal communication, Jennian Geddes. The cartoon was published in *Punch* on August 4, 1915.

47. LGA to AGA, January 17, 1915, WL, 7LGA/2/1/28, enclosing letter from Mrs. E. Toms to LGA, n.d.

48. Sir Henry Norman, "A Voluntary Hospital," Private Papers of Sir Henry and Lady Norman, IWM, 01/15/1.

49. This was Elizabeth Exell, a nursing sister who trained at Bath Royal United Hospital and joined the corps on September 20, 1914. 1914 Star Medal Roll, WO329/2504. Her brother Edward was killed in action at St Yves. "The Exell War Heroes," Thornbury Roots, www.thornburyroots.co.uk/families/exell-war-heroes.

50. Wilder Penfield, "Sir Gordon Morgan Holmes (1876–1965)," rev. ODNB, online ed., May 2006, https://doi.org/10.1093/ref:odnb/33954. The hospital is now called the National Hospital for Neurology and Neurosurgery.

51. LGA to AGA, c. November 28, 1914, WL, 7LGA/2/1/23.

52. Ibid.

53. Olga Campbell to Keir Campbell, November 27, 1914, private collection.

54. Nevinson diary, Oxford, Bodleian Library, MSS.Eng.misc.e.618/3, October 23, 1914; Walking to Wimereux: ibid., November 27, 1914; "Get things out": ibid., December 8, 1914. Background on Nevinson is from John 2006.

55. Evelyn Sharp, *Unfinished Adventure* (London, 1933), 160; John 2009, 82.

56. LGA to AGA, c. November 28, 1914, WL, 7LGA/2/1/23; Lord Esher to LGA, January 14, 1915, enclosed with letter, LGA to AGA, January 17, 1915, WL, 7LGA/2/1/28.

57. LGA to Ivy Anderson, December 16, 1914, WL, 7LGA/2/1/26.

58. Sir Frederick Treves, "Red Cross Work in the North of France," in Joint War Committee Summaries of Work, summary of work for week ending December 14, 1914, appendix 1, London Joint War Committee of the British Red Cross Society and the Order of St John of Jerusalem in England, 1914.

59. MH to AM-H, November 21, 1914 [Paris].

60. MH to AM-H, December 6, 1914 [Paris]; Murray 1920, 102.

61. MH to AM-H, n.d. [c. December 2, 1914 [Paris].

62. MH to AM-H, November 21, 1914.

63. MH to AM-H, November 28, 1914.

64. Ancestry.com, various pages.

65. MH to AM-H, December 2, 1914.

66. MH to AM-H, n.d. [early December 1914].

67. MH to AM-H, November 21, 1914.

68. MH to AM-H, November 28, 1914.

69. MH to AM-H, December 6, 1914.

70. MH to Sir William Maitland-Heriot [her stepfather], November 24, 1914.

71. FM to AM-H, December 9, 1914; LGA to AM-H, November 23, 1914, in letters of Mardie Hodgson.

72. LGA to Ivy Anderson, November 17, 1914, WL, 7LGA/2/1/22.

73. LGA to Ivy Anderson, n.d., [c. December 1914], WL, 7LGA/2/1/29.

74. LGA to Ivy Anderson, December 16, 1914, WL, 7LGA/2/1/26.

75. LGA to AGA, December 12, 1914, WL, 7LGA/2/1/25.

76. LGA to Ivy Anderson, December 16, 1914, WL, 7LGA/2/1/26; "The Women's Hospital Corps," *The Ladies' Field*, February 13, 1915, 513.

77. MH to AM-H, n.d. [c. December 19, 1914].

78. LGA to AGA, December 12, 1914, WL, 7LGA/2/1/25; "go right on": LGA to Ivy Anderson, December 16, 1914, WL, 7LGA/2/1/26.

79. FM to AM-H, December 9, 1914, in letters of Mardie Hodgson.

80. Murray 1920, 103–108; Harraden 1915. Harraden says the Christmas detail is taken from Murray's (lost) journal.

81. Nevinson diary, Oxford, Bodleian Library, MSS.Eng.misc.e.618/3, January 3, 1915.

82. Murray 1920, 110–111.

83. MH to AM-H, n.d. "Friday" [December 1, 1915]; "great success": MH to AM-H, January 9, 1915; "closed Claridge": LGA to AGA, January 17, 1915, WL, 7LGA/2/1/28. FM says Claridge's closed on January 18, 1915, but it is clear from Hodgson's letters that it was January 8. Murray 1920, 111.

84. A few of these medals survive, including one awarded to nurse Evelyn Clemow, now at RCN archives, Edinburgh, and another to Olga Campbell, in family ownership.

Chapter Four: Good God! Women!

1. Murray 1920, 114. History of the War Office from *The Old War Office Building: A History* (London, 2001). Background on London in early 1915 from MacDonagh 1935; MacLaren 1917. Main sources for the early days of Endell Street are Murray 1920; the Endell Street Scrapbook, WL, 7LGA/3 (Scrapbook hereafter).

2. Mark Harrison, "Keogh, Sir Alfred (1857–1936)," ODNB, https://doi.org /10.1093/ref:odnb/34296. Keogh had replaced Sloggett as director general of army medical services, and Sloggett had become head of medical services in France.

3. "Women's Work in the War (I)," *The Times History of the War* 4 (July 1915): 251.

4. LGA to A. Gordon Pollock, printed in *St Leonard's School Gazette*, March 1915.

5. Murray 1920, 116–117.

6. *Times*, February 19, 1915.

7. Keogh to unknown correspondent, March 2, 1915, Edith Barling album, University of Birmingham special collections, EB/37. The letter is addressed to "My dear Master" and was previously cataloged as being to "Marsh(?)." It was probably to Frederick Howard Marsh, professor of surgery at Cambridge University and master of Downing College, who had written a supportive article in the *Cambridge Review* published on February 24, 1915. "Scorn and ridicule": Keogh letter reproduced in Murray 1920, 166–167.

8. *BMJ* 1, no. 2980 (February 9, 1918): 179. The figure included doctors both in the RAMC and in general combat. Background on the medical workforce in 1915 is from Cohen 2014, 11; Mitchell 1978, 2; MacPherson 1921–1924, 1:145–146.

9. Vivian 1914, 172.

10. *Lancet* 185, no. 4774 (February 27, 1915): 451.

11. Letter, "Women Doctors and the War," *Times*, December 8, 1914.

12. *Times*, December 5, 1914.

13. Letter, Asquith, July 15, 1915, *Daily Telegraph*, reprinted in *Magazine of the RFHLSMW* 10, no. 62 (November 1915).

14. Murray 1920, 119.

15. Ibid., 123–126.

16. Ibid., 124. This assertion is repeated by various staff members at different times, although it is probably apocryphal. My thanks for advice to Ruth Richardson and Peter Higginbotham.

17. MacLaren 1917, 1–4.

18. Flora Murray, "A Woman's Hospital in War," *The Common Cause*, January 23, 1920.

19. Murray 1920, 129.

20. Hale 1917.

21. Murray 1920, 128.

22. Their names are given in ibid., 227. They are described by Louisa's nephew Colin Anderson as a Black Aberdeen and a White West Highland. Note by Colin Anderson regarding embroidered shoebag, WL, 7LGA/2/3. Garrett was the black dog.

23. Interview with Marion Dickerman, Marion Dickerman Papers, National Park Service, Hyde Park, New York.

24. Murray 1920, 137–138.

25. Hale 1917. The doctors, nurses, and some of the other staff members are variously named in Murray 1920, 134–136; Murray, "A Woman's Hospital in War," *The Common Cause*, January 23, 1920; "Recent Appointments," *Magazine of the RFHLSMW* 10, no. 61 (July 1915): 99; *BJN*, June 12, 1915; Buckley, Wellcome Library, SA/MWF/C168. Amy Sheppard: obituary, *British Journal of Ophthalmology* 20, no. 11 (November 10, 1936). Helen Chambers: Peter D. Mohr, "Chambers, Helen (1879–1935)," ODNB, https://doi.org/10.1093/ref:odnb/60892. The names (and

total number) of the first doctors vary in different accounts. They certainly included Murray, Anderson, Louisa Woodcock (physician), Amy Sheppard (ophthalmologist), Eva White (radiographer), Helen Chambers (pathologist), and Eva Handley-Read (dental surgeon) and assistant surgeons Gertrude Gazdar, Rosalie Jobson, Morna Rawlins, Gertrude Dearnley, Winifred Buckley, and Margaret Fraser. The accounts by FM and Buckley were written later so may be less accurate. Much original research on the careers of the Endell Street doctors was carried out by Jennian Geddes. The first twenty-nine nursing sisters are named in the *BJN*, June 12, 1915.

26. Buckley obituary, *Journal of the MWF* (Medical Women's Federation) 42, no. 3 (July 1959): 170–171. The egg drink is mentioned in an interview with Dr. Elizabeth Hamilton-Browne, September 27, 1978, University of Sydney, university archives, A14.

27. The vital work nurses performed in the First World War is described in Hallett 2009.

28. Reference for Clemow by LGA, January 27, 1915, Papers of Evelyn Clemow, RCN archives, C716. Family information from her great-nephew Christopher Haviland.

29. *BJN*, November 1926; letter, R. Cox-Davies to Miss Sidney Browne, February 1, 1915, TNA, WO/399/11745.

30. Abel-Smith 1960, 82–99; Hallett 2013.

31. *BJN*, June 12, 1915.

32. Letter in *Sydney Daily Telegraph*, November 19, 1915, Scrapbook, WL, 7LGA/3, and other newspaper reports. Churchill did not have a direct niece of a suitable age at the time so she may have been a distant relative, if true. Barbara Last, however, referred to a fellow orderly named Churchill.

33. Murray 1920, 198–199.

34. Interview with Marion Dickerman, Marion Dickerman Papers, National Park Service, Hyde Park, New York; memoir of John Wells (Hodgson's son), private communication, Andrew Wells.

35. *New Zealand Herald*, November 3, 1916.

36. *Illustrated London News*, March 21, 1915.

37. Background on Elizabeth Robins from John 1995.

38. Diary of Elizabeth Robins, FL, May 10, 1915.

39. Elizabeth Robins, "Dr. Flora Murray: Reminiscences of Her War Work," *Observer*, August 5, 1923.

40. Haslam 2018. Reading as therapy is also discussed in Reznick 2004, 68.

41. Koch 1917; library background from Murray 1920, 193–197; "finest" library: cutting, n.d. [end of 1916], Scrapbook, WL, 7LGA/3.

42. Robins, "Dr. Flora Murray: Reminiscences."

43. Murray 1920, 143.

44. Ibid.

45. Robins diary, FL, May 14, 1915; "made hay of our library": May 15, 1915.

46. Military operations in 1915: Hew Strachan, *The Illustrated History of the First World War*; Hart 2014.

47. Hallett 2009, 59.

48. Cynthia Asquith, quoted in White 2015, 121. Wounded in restaurants: Ethel M. Bilbrough, *My War Diary, 1914–1918* (London, 2014), 159. The entry was May 1915.

49. MacPherson 1921–1924, 1:372.

50. White 2015, 122, 301n.

51. Based on figures from *List of the Various Hospitals Treating Military Cases in the United Kingdom* (London, 1917), with thanks to Charlie Forman and Pete Starling for advice.

52. Nurse Claire Tisdall with the London Ambulance Column, quoted in Mayhew 2013, 198–208.

53. Nina Last, War Memories, Papers of Nina Courage (née Last), WL, 7NLA/1/1b and 2b (Nina Last, 7NLA/1/1b and 2b, hereafter); Murray 1920, 145. Other details of the convoys come from "'Manned' Exclusively by Women," *New Zealand Press*, January 3, 1918, Papers Past.

54. Vera Scantlebury, Letter Diaries, May 4, 1917, VSB Papers. FM describes the method for handling the stretchers in her evidence to the committee for the organization of women's service at Board of Education, Whitehall, December 8, 1916, IWM Women's Work Collection MUN 18.6.

55. Harraden, *Where Your Treasure Is* (London, 1918), 157–159. Harraden is said to have based one of the novel's nurses on Evelyn Clemow, to whom she gave a signed copy of her book inscribed with, "In memory of The Military Hospital, Endell St": Papers of Evelyn Clemow, RCN archives, C716.

56. Pratt 1921, 1:211.

57. Buckley, Wellcome Library, SA/MWF/C168.

58. Murray 1920, 146–147.

59. LGA and Helen Chambers, "Treatment of Septic Wounds, with Special Reference to the Use of Salicylic Acid," *Lancet* 187, no. 4840 (June 3, 1916).

60. Murray 1920, 168–169.

61. "Soldiers as Patients," *Daily Telegraph*, May 18, 1915.

62. Newspaper reports: *Daily Chronicle*, April 25, 1916; *Daily Sketch*, July 12, 1916 [both Scrapbook, WL, 7LGA/3]; *Pall Mall Gazette*, June 30, 1915; *The Suffragette*, April 16, 1915, 13; *BJN*, June 12, 1915, 501–502.

63. Quoted in Harraden 1915, 179–193.

64. *The Times History of the War* 4 (July 1915): 250–256.

65. *Girl's Own Paper*, March 1915 [Scrapbook, WL, 7LGA/3].

66. *Manchester Courier*, July 1, 1915 [Scrapbook, WL, 7LGA/3]; *The Hospital*, May 29, 1915.

67. "Women and War," *Lancet* 186, no. 4794 (July 17, 1915): 134–136.

68. Murray 1920, 143–144; "little as possible": ibid., 127; "sink or swim": ibid., 156; "failure and disaster": ibid., 217; Buckley: Wellcome Library, SA/MWF/C168.

69. Keogh to LGA, January 19, 1918, reprinted in Murray 1920, 166–167.

70. Robins diary, May 17, 1915, FL; hopeless cases: Robins, "Dr. Flora Murray: Reminiscences," and Robins, "Soldiers Two," *Reveille*, February 1919, 378–382.

71. Harraden, preface to Murray 1920, viii.

72. Leneman 1994.

73. Robins diary, May 10, 1915, FL. Robins said LGA made this comment at their first meeting at Endell Street on May 10.

Chapter Five: The Laughing Cure Theory

1. The main sources for details about the library and Robins's time at Endell Street are her diary and letters from Beatrice Harraden to Elizabeth Robins, both at the Fales Library (FL), and Koch 1917. Koch's book devotes a chapter to Endell Street.

I'm indebted to Sara Haslam for her advice on First World War hospital libraries. For further information, see Haslam 2018.

2. *Bristol Times*, January 5, 1916. Harraden gave a talk on running the library to the National Home Reading Union on January 4, 1916, which was widely reported in the national and regional press.

3. *Manchester Guardian*, January 5, 1916; "pigeon's blood ruby": Harraden to Robins, August 22, 1915, FL.

4. Harraden quoted in "Hospital Libraries," *Yorkshire Post*, November 30, 1923.

5. Robins diary, May 26 and June 24, 1915, FL.

6. Fred Hunter, "Harraden, Beatrice (1864–1936)," ODNB, https://doi.org /10.1093/ref:odnb/33720; Crawford 1999, 276–277.

7. Eleanor Bourne, "Twenty Eight Years Ago," Bourne Papers, State Library of Queensland.

8. Ethel Hill in *The Vote*, November 11, 1909, cited in Lis Whitelaw, *The Life and Rebellious Times of Cicely Hamilton* (London, 1990), 82.

9. Wilberforce to Robins, April 19, 1916, FL.

10. Harraden's anxieties: Robins diary, June 21 and 25, July 1 and 8, 1915, FL.

11. Robins diary, July 22, 1915, FL.

12. Harraden to Robins, August 30, 1915, FL.

13. Robins 1924, 254.

14. Interview with Marion Dickerman, Marion Dickerman Papers, National Park Service, Hyde Park, New York.

15. Vera Scantlebury, April 18, 1918, Letter Diaries, vol. A10, VSB Papers.

16. Bourne, "Twenty Eight Years Ago."

17. Nina Last, WL, 7NLA/1/1b and 2b.

18. Brock 2017, 186.

19. H. G. Wells, *Mr. Britling Sees It Through* (Oxford, 2016 [1916]), 377–380. My thanks to Sara Haslam for directing me to Wells's book.

20. Murray 1920, 160–163.

21. Ibid., 148. My thanks to Mick Crumplin for advice.

22. One Canadian officer reported that a butler came around before dinner to take orders, and alcohol was available upon request. Reznick 2004, 55.

23. *Newcastle Journal*, July 13, 1915 (also reported in other newspapers, including the *New Zealand Herald*, August 28, 1915).

24. Robins diary, June 2, 1915, FL.

25. William Glen: *Scotsman*, June 16, 1915; John Noel Pinnington: *Scotsman*, July 19, 1915 and armed forces service records, TNA; Thomas Miller: *Newcastle Daily Journal*, June 9, 1915.

26. Harraden to Robins, August 14 and 22, 1915, FL.

27. Murray 1920, 150–153; dawn: FM, "A Woman's Hospital in War," *The Common Cause*, January 23, 1920. Background on Gallipoli: Hart 2014, 167–186; Mitchell and Smith 1931, 198–207.

28. Max Arthur, *Forgotten Voices of the Great War* (London, 2003), 118–119.

29. John 2006, 150.

30. Ian M. Campbell, *Some Notes on the Campbells of Inverawe (1951), Expanded by Diarmid Campbell with Help from Niall Campbell* (privately published, 1988); Diarmid Campbell, *Keir Arthur Campbell DSO FRGS (1892–1955) Sometime at Rhu in Caol Slate & His Family, Some Biographical Notes* (privately published, 2009).

31. Murray 1920, 150–152. Medical assessments of British Army recruits in the First World War revealed a scale of malnutrition and poor health that shocked public authorities. More than 40 percent of the recruits in 1917–1918 were five foot five or shorter and there were clear class differences in height and weight. J. M. Winter, "Military Fitness and Civilian Health in Britain During the First World War," *Journal of Contemporary History* 15, no. 2 (1980): 211–244.

32. Robins diary, September 6, 7, and 8, 1915, FL. Bushranger stories: *Manchester Guardian*, January 5, 1916.

33. Harraden to Robins, n.d. [postmarked December 17, 1915], FL.

34. Murray 1920, 157.

35. *Tatler*, July 1916, 96; "no vexatious rules": *New Zealand Star*, April 14, 1916, accessed via Papers Past, National Library of New Zealand.

36. Robins diary, September 27 and 28, 1915, FL. She talked to the *Scotsman* later, on October 8, 1915.

37. Miles 1930, 71. She was describing her husband, Eustace, watching the airship. "Electric blue cigar": Kitty Marion's memoir, WL, 7KMA; "great rushing sound": Robins diary, September 8, 1915, FL. Background on the Zeppelin raids is from Castle 2008.

38. *Sun*, September 9, 1915, via Papers Past. The Endell Street entertainment program is described in Murray 1920, 159, 188–192. For entertainment and nurturing approaches in other war hospitals, see Reznick 2004.

39. Untitled newspaper cuttings, January 1916, Scrapbook, WL, 7LGA/3.

40. *Daily Graphic*, January 5, 1916, Scrapbook, WL, 7LGA/3.

41. *New Zealand Star*, October 14, 1915, Papers Past.

42. *Times*, n.d. [February 1916], Scrapbook, WL, 7LGA/3; Murray 1920, 179.

43. Robins diary, November 19, 1915, FL.

44. Murray 1920, 192–193. Embroidered shoebag: WL, 7LGA/2/3; Elmy: war service records, Ancestry.com. Elmy was wounded on April 14, 1917, and created the picture in June. The picture is in the possession of Jennian Geddes. On the reverse a note states: "This piece of work was done by Gunner W. T. Elmy, with one arm." Murray quote and "soldier needle-workers": *Mataura Ensign* (New Zealand), January 23, 1918, Papers Past.

45. Christmas decorations and activities in Murray 1920, 189–190; Harraden to Robins, various letters, December 1915, FL; Robins diary, December 1915–January 1916, FL.

46. The pantomime script was written by Alix Augusta Grein, described by Murray as Mrs. J. T. Grein, although she usually went by the penname Michael Orme. Both the Greins were keen suffragists.

47. Murray and Harraden arguments in Harraden to Robins, December 14, 16, 29, and 30, 1915, FL.

48. Pageant: *The Times*, December 29, 1915; *The Queen*, January 8, 1916; *The Lady*, January 8, 1916; *Lady's Pictorial*, January 8, 1916, all Scrapbook, WL, 7LGA/3.

49. *The Times*, January 1, 1916.

50. Harraden to Robins, December 29, 1915, FL.

51. Robins' resignation: Robins diary, January 25 and 26, 1916, FL; Harraden to Robins, January 24 and 29, 1916, FL.

52. Elizabeth Robins, ed., *Theatre and Friendship: Some Henry James Letters with a Commentary by Elizabeth Robins* (London, 1932), 301–311. The *New York Times* article, published March 11, 1916, appears as an appendix. Robins had lunch with

her friend Sir Edward Grey, the foreign secretary, a few days before she left for America. Grey had met House several times during his British visit to discuss American policy, so it is tempting to speculate that Grey may have primed Robins to use her persuasive talents on House during their voyage. Robins refers to sailing on the SS *New Amsterdam*, but biographies of House make clear it was the SS *Rotterdam*, which sailed on February 24, 1916. Background on House: Charles E. Neu, *Colonel House: A Biography of Woodrow Wilson's Silent Partner* (New York, 2015); Godfrey Hodgson, *Woodrow Wilson's Right Hand: The Life of Colonel Edward M. House* (New Haven, CT, 2006).

Chapter Six: Almost Manless

1. Nina Last's experiences are from Nina Last, "War Memories," two auto-biographical accounts, and a biography by her granddaughter Annie Fox, all in Papers of Nina Last, WL, 7NLA/1/1b and 2b (Nina Last, WL, 7NLA/1/1b and 2b, hereafter); and personal information from Annie Fox. Nina was born September 1, 1895. Her accounts were written c. 1950 and her uniform is preserved at the WL. Barbara Last: personal information from her daughter Nancy Prentis. Barbara was born March 21, 1897, and baptized Mary Barbara Last. It is not clear exactly when Nina began working at Endell Street, but since she spent a year at Ashridge House following Christmas 1914, February 1916 seems the likeliest date.

2. MacDonagh 1935, 93.

3. Background on the VAD scheme is from Abel-Smith 1960, 81–99; Reports by Joint War Committee and the Joint War Finance Committee of the British Red Cross Society and the Order of St John of Jerusalem in England on Voluntary Aid rendered to the Sick and Wounded at Home and Abroad, 1921.

4. Furse 1940, 292.

5. Ibid., 300; rest station at Boulogne: ibid., 310–319.

6. Ibid., 332. Prominent VADs included Venetia Stanley, confidante of Prime Minister Herbert Asquith, and Lady Cynthia Asquith, his daughter-in-law.

7. Abel-Smith 1960, 86–87.

8. Yvonne McEwen, *"It's a Long Way to Tipperary": British and Irish Nurses in the Great War* (Dunfermline, 2006), 116.

9. Furse 1940, 355.

10. Hallett 2013, 87–102.

11. Brittain 2014 [1933], 186–187. Her fiancé, Roland Leighton, was killed in action in December 1915. Brittain became a pacifist after the war.

12. Background on Frances Lyndall Schreiner is from "War Work, 1914–1918," album at Newnham College Cambridge, compiled by Edith Margaret Sharpley and transcribed by Laura Archer-Hind, 1922, 10; Newnham College Register, 1907, 202. She worked at Endell Street in 1918 and 1919. Her book of short stories, *Hospital Sketches*, was published in 1918. In 1923 she became the first woman to be called to the bar in South Africa.

13. Nina Last's typical day is from WL, 7NLA/1/1b and 2b.

14. Brittain 2014 [1933], 187 and 341.

15. MacDonagh 1935, 118–120.

16. Nina Last, WL, 7NLA/1/1b and 2b. His name was Wallie St. John-Mildmay, only son of the Reverend Arundell St. John-Mildmay and his wife, Alys. Wallie was

killed in action on April 16, 1918. Du Ruvigny's Roll of Honour, 1914–1924, via Ancestry.com, www.ancestry.co.uk/search/collections/ukderuvhonourroll.

17. Annual report of New Hospital for Women, 1917, LMA, H13/EGA/08/4. A temporary assistant surgeon was appointed in her stead in 1916, but in January 1917 she became a member of the consulting staff. Harrow Road: mentioned by Vera Scantlebury, September 18, 1918, Letter Diaries, vol. A13, VSB Papers.

18. Wilberforce to Robins, March 8, 1916, FL. Wilberforce described LGA as having "red hair, red nose."

19. Vera Scantlebury, "Women as Army Surgeons, a Record of Splendid Service," *The Woman's World* 1, no. 6 (May 1922): 11–12. Visited once a week: *Manchester Guardian*, February 12, 1917, Scrapbook, WL, 7LGA/3.

20. Murray 1920, 227–229. Murray devotes more words to the couple's dogs than to the professional nurses.

21. Unpublished memoir of Sir Colin Skelton Anderson (private papers).

22. Murray 1920, 204–206.

23. Furse 1940, 320.

24. Murray 1920, 181–182.

25. Rosalie Slaughter Morton, *A Woman Surgeon: The Life and Work of Rosalie Slaughter Morton* (London, 1937), esp. 200–201. Her work is also described in Shipton 2017, 103–104.

26. Murray 1920, 217–220.

27. *The Play Pictorial*, April 1916, 65. He was Benjamin William Findon, the magazine's editor.

28. Details of the auxiliary hospitals are from Murray 1920, 176–177; County of London Branch Reports, 1914–1919 and 1920, BRCS; *BJN*, March 11, 1916; *Tatler*, September 12, 1917; Byculla and Crosfield VAD Hospital: Lost Hospitals of London, https://ezitis.myzen.co.uk/byculla.html; Holly Park: Lost Hospitals of London, https://ezitis.myzen.co.uk/hollypark.html.

29. News cutting, unknown newspaper, July 24, 1916, Scrapbook, WL, 7LGA/3; Dollis Hill House Trust, www.dollishillhouse.org.uk/history.htm; *Sunday Pictorial*, June 24, 1917.

30. Buckley, Wellcome Library, SA/MWF/C168.

31. Murray 1920, 230–231; *Daily News and Leader*, July 24, 2016; *Manchester Guardian*, November 8, 2016, both Scrapbook, WL, 7LGA/3.

32. Letitia Fairfield, "Medical Women in the Forces," *Journal of the MWF* (Medical Women's Federation) 49, no. 2 (1967): 99–107, Wellcome Library, SA/MWF/C168.

33. Untitled news cutting, November 8, 1916, Scrapbook, WL, 7LGA/3. The cutting refers to 1,100 women. Woman beat man to post: *Northern Daily Telegraph*, June 17, 1916, LMA, South London Hospital news cuttings, H24/SLW/Y6/1.

34. Cutting, no title, n.d. [c. July 1916], Scrapbook, WL, 7LGA/3; *Official Journal of the British Red Cross Society*, January 1916.

35. Fawcett to Asquith, May 4, 1916, and his reply, May 6, 1916, reprinted in Millicent Fawcett, *What I Remember* (London, 1924), 232–233.

36. *Daily News and Leader*, July 24, 1916, Scrapbook, WL, 7LGA/3; "never be closed": *Daily Telegraph*, January 1, 1916, cited in Brock 2017, 256.

37. Photographs, January 1916, Scrapbook, WL, 7LGA/3.

38. *Daily Chronicle*, April 25, 1916, Scrapbook, WL, 7LGA/3.

39. Letter to editor and reply, May 25, 1916, Scrapbook, WL, 7LGA/3.

40. *Daily Telegraph*, August 12, 1916, Scrapbook, WL, 7LGA/3; 400–800 patients per month: Murray 1920, 175.

41. Harry Barter: *Daily Mail*, February 11, 1916, Scrapbook, WL, 7LGA/3; armed forces service records, TNA; Tony Rea, *South Devon in the Great War* (Barnsley, 2016), 38; Bostock: "Edwin Francis Bostock (1878–1961)," Red Herrings and White Lies, www.redherringsandwhitelies.co.uk/edwin_f_bostock.html; armed forces service records, TNA.

42. Murray 1920, 144–145, 221–223.

43. *Daily Telegraph*, June 7, 1916, Scrapbook, WL, 7LGA/3.

44. News cutting, untitled, n.d. (c. June 1916), Scrapbook, WL, 7LGA/3. River trips: *Morning Post*, June 6, 1916, Scrapbook, WL, 7LGA/3.

45. The staff changes are described by Buckley, Wellcome Library, SA/MWF/C168. Magill was born May 1, 1881, and graduated from LSMW in 1906.

46. The first woman to qualify as a doctor in Australia earned her license in 1891. Newspaper notice: Sheard and Lee 2019, 1–2; Jacqueline Bell, "Bourne, Eleanor Elizabeth (1878–1957)," *Australian Dictionary of Biography* 7 (1979), http://adb .anu.edu.au/biography/bourne-eleanor-elizabeth-5305; Eleanor Bourne, "Reminiscence, 1916–1918," Eleanor Elizabeth Bourne Papers, OM81-130/1, State Library of Queensland; letter from George Bourne to Eleanor Bourne, October 30, 1915, George Herbert Bourne Papers, State Library of Queensland, OM68-25. On Rachel Champion Shaw, see Dick Shaw, *Which Way Is Home*, privately published [c. 2005]; Mary P. Shaw, *The Shaws of Tullyvallin* (privately published, 1976).

47. On Elizabeth Hamilton-Browne, see John Atherton Young, Ann Jervie Sefton, and Nina Webb, eds., *Centenary Book of the University of Sydney Faculty of Medicine* (Sidney, 1984), 235–236; letter from EHB to Sir Thomas Street, February 21, 1916, University of Sydney archives. My thanks to Heather Sheard for helping to pinpoint her arrival.

48. Staff photograph, August 1916, WL, 7NLA/2/0. Nina has been identified on the top row, sixth from the left, by her granddaughter Annie Fox, while Barbara sits in the third row, second from left. Eleanor Bourne has been identified in the second row, tenth from the right, by the Geoffrey Kaye Museum, Melbourne, Australia, and Elizabeth Hamilton-Browne has been identified as thirteenth from the left in the second row by Heather Sheard.

49. Brittain 2014 [1933], 246.

Chapter Seven: Pioneers, O Pioneers!

1. Background on the Somme battle is from Hart 2014, 209–241; Martin Middlebrook, *The First Day of the Somme* (London, 2003 [1971]); Leo van Bergen, *Before My Helpless Sight: Suffering, Dying and Military Medicine on the Western Front, 1914–1918* (London, 2009), 77–81; MacPherson 1921–1924, 3:11–51. Information on the Lincolnshire regiment is from Major General C. R. Simpson, ed., *The History of the Lincolnshire Regiment, 1914–1918* (London, 1931), 159–176; Unit war diary, 1st battalion, Lincolnshire Regt, TNA WO 95/2154/1, July 1–3, 1916. The regiment became the Royal Lincolnshires after the Second World War. William Bilton: *Daily Sketch*, July 6, 1916, Scrapbook, WL, 7LGA/3; war service records via Ancestry.com. The *Sketch* refers to "W. Bilton." Records have survived for two soldiers named William Bilton in the Lincolnshire Regiment, but one is described as 4'11½" tall on enlistment while the other, more likely, candidate was 5'7".

2. MacPherson 1921–1924, 3:41. The figure is based on a sample between July 26 and August 11, 1916.

3. White 2015, 166–168.

4. MacPherson 1921–1924, 2:375.

5. Brittain 2014 [1933], 247–258.

6. Mayhew 2013, 66.

7. MacPherson 1921–1924, 3:50.

8. *Daily Mail*, August 22, 1916, Scrapbook, WL, 7LGA/3.

9. Barbara Last to her mother, September 24, 1916, WL, 7NLA/1/5.

10. Harraden to Robins, August 14, 1916, FL.

11. Various news cuttings, July 31 and August 26 and 27, 1916, Scrapbook, WL, 7LGA/3.

12. Background on John Joseph O'Donoghue is from Lives of the First World War, https://livesofthefirstworldwar.org/lifestory/3304497. My thanks to his granddaughter Kate Kendall for sharing his story.

13. *Fife Free Press*, October 14, 1916.

14. Mayhew 2013, 8.

15. Murray 1920, 173–174.

16. Ana Carden-Coyne, "Gendering the Politics of War Wounds Since 1914," in Carden-Coyne, ed., *Gender and Conflict Since 1914: Historical and Interdisciplinary Perspectives* (Basingstoke, 2012), 83–97; Louise Bell, "Physical Disability and the First World War," talk at TNA, December 14, 2016, and blog post, "Diamond Cutting for Disabled Servicemen," TNA, November 22, 2017, https://blog.nationalarchives .gov.uk/blog/diamond-cutting-disabled-servicemen.

17. Bell, "Diamond Cutting"; Bourke 1996, 33, 37; Mitchell and Smith 1931, 320. Scotland says that by 1930 more than 1.6 million people were receiving pensions or other gratuities as a result of war injuries or sickness. Thomas R. Scotland, "Developments in Orthopaedic Surgery," in Scotland and Heys 2012, 149–177.

18. Bourke 1996, 75.

19. A full table is given in Bourke 1996, 66.

20. Reznick 2000. His work is also described in Reznick 2004.

21. Graves 2000 [1929], 188. Others spoke of wanting to forget: Bourke 1996, 22.

22. *Daily Mail*, August 22, 1916.

23. *Mitchell's Newspaper Press Directory*, 1916, with thanks to the British Library Newsroom. The *Sketch* later merged with the *Daily Mail*.

24. Press coverage: *Tatler*, July 19, 1916; *Daily Star*, July 22, 1916; *Daily Mail*, August 22, 1916; *Daily Telegraph*, August 12, 1916, all in Scrapbook, WL, 7LGA/3.

25. Advances in medicine: Harrison 2010; Mayhew 2013; Scotland and Heys 2012.

26. MacPherson 1921–1924, 1:115–116.

27. Murray 1920, 162–164.

28. Nina Last, WL, 7NLA/1/1b and 2b. Bland-Sutton worked as a military surgeon at the 3rd London General Hospital, Wandsworth, for two years at the start of the war before asking to be relieved. He was also a supporter of the Harrow Road Hospital for Children. Background on head surgery from David Currie, "Wounds of the Skull and Brain," in Scotland and Heys 2012, 234–236.

29. Brock 2017, 66.

30. *Common Cause*, June 30, 1916, 151. She had a school in Gloucester Place, London, and wrote a textbook on electricity as medical therapy: Magill, *Notes on*

Galvanism and Faradism, 2nd ed. (London, 1919). Electrotherapy was little used before 1915. On the growth of physical therapy during the First World War, see Jean Barclay, *In Good Hands: The History of the Chartered Society of Physiotherapy, 1894–1994* (Oxford, 1994).

31. Wound management: Robin Reid, "Pathology," in Scotland and Heys 2012, 116–133; "The Treatment of Septic Wounds: Carrel's Sterilisation Method," *Lancet* 188, no. 4862 (November 4, 1916); Jaclyn Gaydos, "History of Wound Care: A Solution to Sepsis: The Carrel-Dakin Method," *Today's Wound Clinic* 11, no. 2, (February 2017), www.todayswoundclinic.com/articles/history-wound-care-solution -sepsis-carrel-dakin-method. Scotland points out that while Dakin's solution may have reduced mortality, it was no substitute for effective surgery to remove all the dead tissue. Thomas R. Scotland, "Developments in Orthopaedic Surgery," in Scotland and Heys 2012, 149–177.

32. Background on the BIPP trial from LGA, "The Treatment of Infected Suppurating War Wounds," *Lancet* 188, no. 4853 (September 2, 1916): 447; LGA and Helen Chambers, "The Treatment of Septic Wounds with Bismuth-Iodoform-Paraffin Paste," *Lancet* 189, no. 4879 (March 3, 1917): 331–334; Murray 1920, 164–166; James Rutherford Morison, *BIPP Treatment of War Wounds* (London, 1918).

33. LGA, "Bismuth and Iodoform Paste in Gunshot Wounds," *Lancet* 189, no. 4879 (March 3, 1917): 331. She was speaking to the Association of Registered Medical Women.

34. Murray 1920, 165–166. A photograph of the visit is included in Mardie Hodgson's album.

35. James Rutherford Morison, "Remarks on the Treatment of Infected, Especially, War Wounds," *Journal of the Royal Army Medical Corps* 30, no. 3 (March 1918): 306–319. I am indebted to Mick Crumplin for directing me to this paper and for his advice generally on BIPP.

36. BIPP use elsewhere: various articles in *BMJ* and other journals, including C. Gordon Watson, "Treatment of Wounds with Bipp," *BMJ* 1, no. 4179 (February 8, 1941): 211; J. A. Gunn, "Lessons from War Surgery," *Canadian Medical Association Journal* 10, no. 4 (April 10, 1920): 354–361; editorial, "Listerism and War Wounds," *BMJ* 2, no. 3339 (December 27, 1924): 1205; Col. A. G. Butler, *The Official History of the Australian Army Medical Services in the War of 1914–1918,* vol. 2, *The Western Front* (Melbourne, 1940), 323–324. BIPP today: G. J. Crosland and A. P. Bath, "Bismuth Iodoform Paraffin Paste: A Review," *Journal of Laryngology & Otology* 125 (2011): 891–895. My thanks to Mick Crumplin and Pete Starling for advice.

37. Barbara Last to her mother, September 3, 1916, and Nina Last to her mother, n.d. [September 1916], WL, 7NLA/1/5; Eleanor Bourne, "Twenty Eight Years Ago," Bourne Papers, State Library of Queensland. Background on Zeppelin raids: Castle 2008; White 2015, 169–172.

38. Barbara Last to her father, October 15, 1916, WL, 7NLA/1/5.

39. Ibid.

40. Harraden to Robins, November 1 [1916] and December 6, 1916, FL.

41. Harraden to Robins, December 16, 1916, FL.

42. Background on Frances Evelyn Windsor from Hacker 1974, 184–191; obituary in *Canadian Medical Association Journal* 95 (November 26, 1966): 1164; personal information from her grandson Michael Fellows and other family members. An alternative story suggests she joined the CMAC as a doctor because recruiting officers had assumed from her name that she was male, but when she arrived on ship and the

mistake was discovered, she was switched to the RAMC. Her service record, however, makes plain she enlisted as a nurse.

43. Ross Davies, *Three Brilliant Careers: Nell Malone, Miles Franklin, Kath Ussher* (Queensland, 2015); transcript of interview with Kath Ussher, Liddle Collection, Leeds University, Liddle/WW1/W0125. The interview, by Peter Liddle, was conducted in 1975. My thanks to Ross Davies.

44. Kath Ussher, *The Cities of Australia* (London, 1928), 101, 19.

45. Flora Murray, evidence to committee for the organization of women's service at Board of Education, Whitehall, December 8, 1916, IWM Women's Work Collection MUN 18.6. The number of remaining men was variously given by FM as six and eight. The larger figure probably included the special constable and the RAMC detachment CO.

46. "Women Doctors," *Daily Telegraph*, October 3, 1916, Scrapbook, WL, 7LGA/3.

47. "50 Women Doctors Wanted for Army," untitled news cutting, November 8, 1916, Scrapbook, WL, 7LGA/3.

48. *Daily Chronicle*, November 24, 1916, Scrapbook, WL, 7LGA/3.

49. *Common Cause*, December 8, 1916, Scrapbook, WL, 7LGA/3; Scott 1984.

50. Jubilee of New Hospital for Women: *Daily News*, December 13, 1916; *Daily Telegraph*, December 16, 1916; "Women in Medicine, 1866–1916," *The Hospital*, December 23, 1916.

51. "Women Doctors," *Daily Telegraph*, October 3, 1916, Scrapbook, WL, 7LGA/3.

52. *Manchester Guardian*, November 8, 1916, Scrapbook, WL, 7LGA/3.

53. Elizabeth Robins letter, *Daily Chronicle*, October 6, 1916, Scrapbook, WL, 7LGA/3.

54. *The Hospital*, December 23, 1916.

55. FM, evidence to committee for the organization of women's service at Board of Education, Whitehall, December 8, 1916, IWM Women's Work Collection MUN 18.6.

56. Fara 2018, 195–213; Dame Helen Gwynne-Vaughan, *Service with the Army* (London, 1941); Murray 1920, 232–233.

57. Christmas 1916: news cuttings and photographs, December 1916, Scrapbook, WL, 7LGA/3; Bourne, "Twenty Eight Years Ago."

58. *Manchester Guardian*, February 12, 1917, Scrapbook, WL, 7LGA/3.

Chapter Eight: The March of the Women

1. Biographical details of Vera Scantlebury are from Sheard 2016, 2011. I am indebted to Heather Sheard for help and advice. Scantlebury describes her time at Endell Street in the nineteen volumes of her Letter Diaries to her family as well as in letters to her friend Dorothy Stevenson and to her fiancé, Dr. Frank Kingsley Norris. Vera Scantlebury Brown Papers, University of Melbourne Archives, Melbourne (VSB Papers hereafter). Scantlebury wrote her Letter Diaries on carbon-copy pads so she could send the top sheet to her family and keep the bottom sheet as her diary. Her brother was baptized George Clifford Scantlebury but was known as Cliff.

2. VS Letter Diaries, vol. A2, April-May 1917; letter to Dorothy Stevenson, April 1917, VSB Papers.

3. Murray 1920, 207; obituary, *Lancet* 189, no. 4880 (March 10, 1917): 390–391.

4. Western front in 1917: Hart 2014, 326–351; MacPherson 1921–1924, 3:54–200. The first Russian Revolution took place in February according to Russian calendars but March by the Gregorian calendar.

5. Scantlebury's typical day: Sheard 2016, 59.

6. Scantlebury's doubts: Sheard 2011; Sheard 2016, 37–38; VS Letter Diaries, vol. A2, May 10, 1917; VS to Frank Norris, May 5, 1917, VSB Papers.

7. Descriptions of Murray, Anderson, and other Endell Street doctors: VS Letter Diaries, vol. A2, May 2 and 10, 1917, VSB Papers.

8. Sheard 2011.

9. On suffragettes: Sheard 2016, 40–41; VS Letter Diaries, May 13 and 18, 1917, vol. A2; May 19, 22 and 28, 1917, vol. A3, VSB Papers.

10. VS Letter Diaries, May 15, 1917, vol. A2, VSB Papers.

11. VS Letter Diaries, July 7, 1917, vol. A3, VSB Papers.

12. Trip to Penn: VS Letter Diaries, May 18, 1917, vol. A2, VSB Papers.

13. Return visits to Penn: VS Letter Diaries, June 9 and 21, 1917, vol. A3, VSB Papers.

14. VS Letter Diaries, May 11, 1917, vol. A2, VSB Papers.

15. Empire Day and Whit Monday: VS Letter Diaries, May 24, 1917, vol. A2, and May 28, 1917, vol. A3, VSB Papers.

16. Sheard 2016, 62, and VS Letter Diaries, November 29, 1917, vol. A7, VSB Papers.

17. VS Letter Diaries, June 20, 1917, vol. A3, VSB Papers.

18. Military surgery: VS Letter Diaries, June 21 and 25, 1917, vol. A3, VSB Papers.

19. VS Letter Diaries, June 4, 1917, vol. A3, VSB Papers.

20. VS Letter Diaries, June 13, 1917, vol. A3, VSB Papers.

21. VS to Frank Norris, June 29, 1917, VSB Papers, via Adam Matthew database, Gender: Identity and Social Change, www.amdigital.co.uk/primary-sources/gender-identity-and-social-change.

22. VS Letter Diaries, May 24, 1917, vol. A2, and August 15, 1917, vol. A4, VSB Papers. Men "progressing quite well": VS Letter Diaries, June 6, 1917, vol. A3, VSB Papers.

23. VS Letter Diaries, January 14, 1918, vol. A8, VSB Papers.

24. VS Letter Diaries, June 12, 1917, vol. A3, VSB Papers.

25. VS Letter Diaries, June 26, 1917, vol. A3, VSB Papers.

26. VS Letter Diaries, July 26, 1917, vol. A4, VSB Papers.

27. Evelyn Windsor wedding: VS Letter Diaries, June 30, 1917, vol. A3, VSB Papers; Hacker 1974, 185; information from her family via her grandson Michael Fellows.

28. MacPherson 1921–1924, 1:372. The total wounded shipped from France to the United Kingdom in 1917 was 700,562, even higher than for 1916 at 523,153. In August a total of 88,798 arrived.

29. Pratt 1921, 1:211.

30. White 2015, 203–206; MacDonagh 1935, 244.

31. VS Letter Diaries, August 2, 1917, vol. A4, VSB Papers.

32. White 2015, 212–215; Castle 2015, 119–133.

33. VS Letter Diaries, June 13 and July 7, 1917, vol. A3, VSB Papers.

34. Eleanor Bourne, "Twenty Eight Years Ago," Bourne Papers, State Library of Queensland.

35. VS Letter Diaries, September 27, 1917, vol. A6, VSB Papers.

36. VS Letter Diaries, August 15, 1917, vol. A4, VSB Papers.

37. VS Letter Diaries, August 27, 1917, vol. A5, VSB Papers.

38. VS Letter Diaries, July 12, 1917, vol. A5, VSB Papers.

39. Donald Creighton, *Harold Adams Innis: Portrait of a Scholar* (Toronto, 1957); William J. Buxton, Michael R. Cheney, and Paul Heyer, eds., *Harold Innis Reflects: Memoir and WWI Writings/Correspondence* (Lanham, MD, 2016).

40. "The Great War, 1914–1919," Kent Fallen website, n.d., www.kentfallen.com /PDF%20REPORTS/HYTHE%20UNITED%20REFORM.pdf; war service records, TNA.

41. The Wartime Memories Project, https://wartimememoriesproject.com/great war/view.php?uid=222979.

42. Searching Ancestry.com reveals twelve men who died at Endell Street in 1917. Their details are recorded under "UK, Army Registers of Soldiers' Effects, 1901– 1929," www.ancestry.co.uk/search/collections/ukarmyregisterseffects.

43. Murray 1920, 233–235. The hospital provided beds for members of the WAAC—renamed the Queen Mary's Army Auxiliary Corps in April 1918—until the QMAAC Hospital opened at Isleworth in early 1919. Background on military women from Shipton 2017, 198–214.

44. LGA to Ethel May, May 14, 1917, and LGA to Dr. May, September 24, 1917, Papers of Ethel May, Royal London Hospital Archives and Museum, RLHPP/MAY/3 and 4. She was awarded a Royal Red Cross in the honors' list in August 1917.

45. Barbara Last to her mother, October 24, 1917, WL, 7NLA/1/5.

46. VS Letter Diaries, September 10, 1917, vol. A5, VSB Papers.

47. Various news cuttings, including *The Times*, September 28; *Sphere*, October 6; *Nursing Mirror*; October 6; photographs in the *Sketch*, October 3, 1917, and VS Letter Diaries, September 27, 1917, vol. A6, VSB Papers; Bourne, "Twenty Eight Years Ago."

48. VS Letter Diaries, October 3, 1917, vol. A6, VSB Papers; Dick Shaw, *Which Way Is Home*, privately published [c. 2005]. Dick was the five-year-old boy, Champion's second son.

49. Barbara Last to her mother, July 18 and October 24, 1917, WL, 7NLA/1/5.

50. VS Letter Diaries, October 16, 1917, vol. A6, VSB Papers. The "October" Russian Revolution began on November 7, 1917, according to the Gregorian calendar.

51. VS Letter Diaries, November 7 and 13, 1917, vol. A7, VSB Papers.

52. VS Letter Diaries, November 15, 1917, vol. A7, VSB Papers.

53. VS Letter Diaries, December 6, 1917, vol. A8, VSB Papers.

54. VS Letter Diaries, January 24, 1918, vol. A8, VSB Papers.

55. *The Times*, December 18, 1917; *Pall Mall Gazette*, December 22, 1917; VS Letter Diaries, December 22, 1917, vol. A8, VSB Papers.

56. LGA to A. Gordon Pollock, January 22, 1918, LMA, H13/EGA/228/4. Alan had been knighted in the August 1917 honors' list at the same time that Anderson was awarded the CBE; he had become controller of the admiralty.

57. LGA address to LSMW, October 1, 1917, *Magazine of the RFHLSMW* 12, no. 68 (November 1917). LGA advised the War Office to hand over management of the Bombay hospital entirely to women, but although it was staffed by women doctors, it was managed by men. Murray 1920, 236–237.

58. LGA address to LSMW, October 1, 1917, *Magazine of the RFHLSMW* 12, no. 68 (November 1917).

59. Typescript of note by Agnes Conway, December 7, 1917, IWM, BRCS 24.1/1. Background on Conway from Fara 2018, 147–149.

60. Murray 1920, 239–249.

61. VS Letter Diaries, December 22 and 29, 1917, vol. A8, VSB Papers; Murray, "A Woman's Hospital in War," *The Common Cause*, January 23, 1920.

62. VS Letter Diaries, January 1, 1918, vol. A8, VSB Papers.

63. Murray 1920, 206–207; VS Letter Diaries, January 11 and 20, 1918, vol. A8, VSB Papers.

Chapter Nine: Darkest Before Dawn

1. Background on the Odhams bomb: Castle 2015, 169–173; W. J. B. Odhams, *The Story of the Bomb, Dropped on the Premises of Messrs Odhams, Jan 29 1918* (London, 1919); MacDonagh 1935, 251–258; Frank Morison, *War on Great Cities* (London, 1937), 158–161. VS estimated that two hundred people were sheltering, but the Odhams booklet says it was about six hundred, a figure repeated elsewhere. Both VS and Hallie Miles said some people drowned. Miles 1930, 145. I am grateful to Ian Castle for advice.

2. VS Letter Diaries, January 29, 1918, vol. A8, VSB Papers.

3. Hart 2014, 410–440.

4. Miles 1930, 147.

5. White 2015, 255.

6. White 2015, 258; Judith R. Walkowitz, *Nights Out: Life in Cosmopolitan London* (New Haven, CT, 2012), 64–91.

7. Nina Last, WL, 7NLA/1/1b and 2b.

8. Keir Campbell to Olga Campbell, February 5, 1918, transcribed in Diarmid Campbell, *Keir Arthur Campbell DSO FRGS (1892–1955) Sometime at Rhu in Caol Slate & His Family, Some Biographical Notes* (privately published, 2009), 140–141.

9. Margaret Elizabeth Murray (known as Elizabeth) to her mother, March 17, 1918, private family papers, Murraythwaite. The event must have been the Pankhursts' appearance on March 16, 1918. FM had three nieces, her brother William's daughters Elizabeth, Vivian, and Eleanor.

10. VS Letter Diaries, February 11, 1918, vol. A9, VSB Papers.

11. VS Letter Diaries, February 26 and March 6, 1918, vol. A9, and March 21, 1918, vol. 10, VSB Papers. Scantlebury's relationship with Norris had cooled by May 1918 and ended soon thereafter. Sheard 2016.

12. Elizabeth Murray to her mother, June 19, 1918, private family papers, Murraythwaite.

13. Shipton 2017, 207–209; Philo-Gill 2017; Papers of Helen Gwynne-Vaughan, National Army Museum, 9401-253-17 and 20. The number of pregnancies was found to be twenty-one, a ratio of less than 3:1000, and two of these women were married; there were also twelve cases of venereal disease noted. Marwick 1977, 128. The WAAC was renamed Queen Mary's Army Auxiliary Corps (QMAAC) in April 1918, but I've kept the title WAAC to avoid confusion.

14. MacDonagh 1935, 186.

15. "Wounded W.A.A.C.'S," *The Times*, June 10, 1918; "Wounded WAACS," *Sunday Pictorial*, June 9, 1918; "First Women 'Casualties' from France," cutting, journal unknown, IWM, Endell Street Scrapbook, LBY 89/1782. *The Times* refers to "about a dozen" WAACs; Philo-Gill says it was eleven. Philo-Gill 2017, 114.

16. Information from Ancestry.com. She was born in Termon, County Donegal, and died on July 19, 1918. Her name is recorded in *Ireland's Memorial Records, 1914–1918*, vol. 2 (Dublin, 1923), 4.

17. VS Letter Diaries, March 30, 1918, vol. A10, VSB Papers.

18. VS Letter Diaries, April 18, 1918, vol. A10, VSB Papers.

19. VS Letter Diaries, May 19, 1918, vol. A11, VSB Papers.

20. VS Letter Diaries, May 6, 1918, vol. A10, VSB Papers.

21. VS, Case Notes, May 1, 1918, VSB Papers, via Adam Matthew database, Gender: Identity and Social Change, www.amdigital.co.uk/primary-sources/gender-identity-and-social-change.

22. VS Letter Diaries, May 11, 1918, vol. A11, VSB Papers.

23. Interview with Dr. Elizabeth Hamilton-Browne, September 27, 1978, University of Sydney, university archives.

24. VS Letter Diaries, May 5, 1918, vol. A10, VSB Papers.

25. Personal information from her grandson Michael Fellows and other family members. According to VS, Windsor left on April 27. Her son, Peter Windsor Leacock, was born on June 17, 1918. Family members remember Windsor saying that Queen Mary visited the operating theater, but it was most likely Queen Alexandra, who visited twice in the early months of 1918. Queen Mary did not visit until June.

26. Nina Last, WL, 7NLA/1/1b and 2b.

27. Murray 1920, 208; *BJN*, January 12, 1918, 22. She died on January 5, 1918.

28. First signs of Spanish flu: VS Letter Diaries, June 25 and 28 and July 4 and 15, 1918, vol. A11, VSB Papers; Murray 1920, 208–209.

29. Murray 1920, 250–251.

30. Letter from Dr. Dulcie Staveley, August 7, 1987, reproduced in *The Invisible Light, Journal of the Radiology History and Heritage Charitable Trust* 13 (May 2000): 8–9; Christopher M. Staveley, "The Staveley Family," unpublished account, 1999. My thanks to Kate Staveley Down, great-niece of Dulcie Staveley, for personal information.

31. VS Letter Diaries, July 30, 1918, vol. A12, VSB Papers. Scantlebury did not name the orderly. Queen Alexandra's visit was August 1, 1918.

32. American orderlies: Murray 1920, 249–250; *Syracuse Herald*, April 26, May 26, July 1, August 25, September 5, September 15, and October 18, 1918, and March 9, 1919.

33. Brittain 2014 [1933], 384.

34. Davis 1974; interview with Marion Dickerman, Marion Dickerman Papers, National Park Service, Hyde Park, New York.

35. Nina Last, WL, 7NLA/1/1b and 2b.

36. VS Letter Diaries, August 8 and 13, 1918, vol. A12, VSB Papers.

37. VS Letter Diaries, August 19, 1918, vol. A12, VSB Papers.

38. VS Letter Diaries, August 26, 1918, vol. A12, VSB Papers.

39. VS Letter Diaries, September 2, 1918, vol. A13, VSB Papers.

40. *Syracuse Herald*, September 15, 1918.

41. Nina Last to her mother, September 8, 1918, WL, 7NLA/1/5.

42. Private information from Barb Angus, whose son is Larry's grandson, and service records.

43. VS Letter Diaries, September 3, 1918, vol. A13, VSB Papers.

44. Nina Last to her mother, October 13, 1918, WL, 7NLA/1/5.

45. VS Letter Diaries, October 27, 1918, vol. A14, VSB Papers.

46. VS Letter Diaries, October 17, 1918, vol. A13, VSB Papers.

47. VS Letter Diaries, October 24, 1918, vol. A14, VSB Papers.

48. VS Letter Diaries, September 2, 1918, vol. A13, VSB Papers.

49. VS Letter Diaries, October 25, 1918, vol. A14, VSB Papers.

50. Leneman 1994.

51. "Medical Women and Income Tax," LGA to the editor of *The Times*, October 12, 1918; and W. Leonard Thackrah, *The Times*, October 15, 1918.

52. VS Letter Diaries, October 24, 1918, vol. A14, VSB Papers.

53. Robin Reid, "Pathology," in Scotland and Heys 2012, 116–133.

54. *Scotsman*, October 5, 1918.

55. London on Armistice Day: White 2015, 267–269; MacDonagh 1935, 327–331; VS Letter Diaries, November 11, 1918, vol. A14, VSB Papers; interview with Marion Dickerman, Marion Dickerman Papers, National Park Service, Hyde Park, New York.

56. White 2015, 271; Hart 2014, 468.

57. Cited in Brock 2017, 186.

58. VS Letter Diaries, November 12, 1918, vol. A14, VSB Papers.

59. Nina Last to her father, November 16, 1918, WL, 7NLA/1/5.

60. VS Letter Diaries, November 30, 1918, vol. A14, VSB Papers; Murray 1920, 226–227.

Chapter Ten: Full of Ghosts

1. Graves 2000 [1929], 234–235. Graves fell ill during the third wave of the pandemic in February 1919.

2. Background on Spanish flu from Laura Spinney, *Pale Rider: The Spanish Flu of 1918 and How It Changed the World* (London, 2018); John M. Barry, *The Great Influenza: The Story of the Deadliest Pandemic in History* (New York, 2005); Mark Honigsbaum, *Living with Enza: The Forgotten Story of Britain and the Great Flu Pandemic of 1918* (London, 2009).

3. Deaths in Britain and London: "Influenza Death Rate in England and Wales, 1918–1919," Registrar General 1920, table reproduced in Steve Duffy, "Spanish Flu Pandemic 1918—Could It Happen Again?," BBC News, October 15, 2018, www.bbc.co.uk/news/uk-wales-45798623; Honigsbaum, *Living with Enza*, 128; White 2015, 265.

4. Background on flu impact in London: White 2015, 264–266; Honigsbaum, *Living with Enza*, passim.

5. VS Letter Diaries, October 19, 1918, vol. A13, and October 29, 1918, vol. 14, VSB Papers.

6. Flu patients at Endell Street: Murray 1920, 172–173; VS Letter Diaries, November 18, 1918, vol. 14, VSB Papers.

7. Murray 1920, 172.

8. Nina Last, WL, 7NLA/1/1b and 2b.

9. Interview with Marion Dickerman, Marion Dickerman Papers, National Park Service, Hyde Park, New York.

10. Nina Last, WL, 7NLA/1/1b and 2b; *The Times*, February 22, 1919. According to *The Times*, Endell Street was one of a small number of British military hospitals to pioneer the segregation of patients and wearing masks.

11. Notice in *Annandale Observer*, n.d. [December 1918], with thanks to Alison Ramsay and the Devil's Porridge Museum, Dumfries and Galloway.

12. Anderson, Murray, Grace Hale, and Winifred Buckley were all listed on the electoral register as living at Endell Street in 1919.

13. *Hartlepool Northern Daily Mail*, April 17, 1919. Pankhurst had been narrowly beaten in the 1918 General Election and announced she was standing again for the next.

14. VS Letter Diaries, December 24, 1918, vol. 15, VSB Papers.

15. Christmas 1918: Murray 1920, 252–253; VS Letter Diaries, December 24 and 26, 1918, vol. 15, VSB Papers; *Globe*, December 18, 1918; *Daily Mirror*, December 27, 1918; *The Times*, December 27, 1918.

16. VS Letter Diaries, December 30, 1918, vol. 15, VSB Papers.

17. Cited in Honigsbaum, *Living with Enza*, 126.

18. Nina Last, WL, 7NLA/1/1b and 2b.

19. Staff who died in 1919: Murray 1920, 208–210; Nina Last to her mother, January 10 and March 2, 1919, WL, 7NLA/1/5; Nina Last, 7NLA/1/1b and 2b. There are no details of Mary Graham's background.

20. Murray 1920, 209. Helen was a pupil at the progressive Bedales School from 1912 to 1914. Her death is commemorated in the Bedales School Memorial Library. My thanks to staff at Bedales.

21. Murray 1920, 209; Nina Last to her mother, March 2, 1919, WL, 7NLA/1/5; .P. Campion, *The Honourable Women of the Great War and the Women's (War) Who's Who* (Bournemouth, 1919); *Yorkshire Post*, July 30, 1936.

22. Nina Last to her mother, March 2, 1919, WL, 7NLA/1/5.

23. Australian Red Cross Society, Wounded and Missing Enquiry Bureau files, 1914–1918 War, 1DRL/0428.

24. Excerpts from Vic Jones's diary for 1919, courtesy of his family, with thanks to Mrs. Reece King (née Jones), his daughter, and Miles King, his grandson.

25. Murray 1920, 171. She trained at the LSMW and qualified in 1909.

26. Murray 1920, 211 and 252–256.

27. Nina Last, WL, 7NLA/1/1b and 2b.

28. "Demobilisation in Britain, 1918–20," TNA, www.nationalarchives.gov.uk /pathways/firstworldwar/spotlights/demobilisation.htm.

29. Murray 1920, 155.

30. Interview with Marion Dickerman, Marion Dickerman Papers, National Park Service, Hyde Park, New York.

31. Murray 1920, 154–155.

32. Ibid., 203–204. She was Joyce Ward, who stayed until November 1919.

33. Ibid., 211–212.

34. *Syracuse Herald*, March 9, 1919.

35. Grace Hale, *British Journal of Nursing*, May 24, 1919, 355–357.

36. *Daily Telegraph*, May 25, 1919.

37. Annual Report of the Medical Officer of Health, Fulham, 1919, 45.

38. Murray 1920, 242–245; Winston Churchill to Jane Walker, president of MWF, MWF archives, Wellcome Library, SA/MWF/C/253.

39. *The Times*, March 19, 1919; *Feilding Star* (New Zealand), May 29, 1919, Papers Past.

40. *The Times*, November 1, 1919.

41. *Manchester Guardian*, January 4, 1919.

42. *Standard and St James's Gazette*, July 18, 1919, Scrapbook, WL, 7LGA/3.

43. FM says the order to close came in October, but LGA refers to this on September 17, 1919. Murray 1920, 256–257 and 261–263; LGA to Winifred Buckley, September 17, 1919, cited in Buckley, Wellcome Library, SA/MWF/C168. Nina said Endell Street was the last wartime hospital in London. Nina Last, WL, 7NLA/1/1b and 2b.

44. Nina Last to her mother, October 19, 1919, WL, 7NLA/1/5.

45. Nina Last to her mother, October 26, 1919, WL, 7NLA/1/5.

46. BH to ER, September 26 and October 1 and 7, 1919, Elizabeth Robins Collection 1897–1938, box 1.9, Harry Ransom Center, University of Texas.

47. Grace Hale demobilization papers and letters, WO/399/3437.

48. Murray 1920, 146; Buckley, Wellcome Library, SA/MWF/C168. Buckley refers to thirty-two thousand patients who "passed through the hospital," presumably both inpatients and outpatients.

49. *Daily Sketch*, July 6, 1916, Scrapbook, WL, 7LGA/3; *The Times*, July 30, 1923.

50. Murray 1920, 166–167.

Chapter Eleven: The Soft Long Sleep

1. Jennian Geddes, "Artistic Integrity and Feminist Spin: A Spat at the Endell Street Military Hospital," *Burlington Magazine* 147 (2005): 617–618; Geddes 2005; IWM archives.

2. The sketch is in the IWM, Art.IWM ART 2767; the photograph on which it is based is in the WL. The other portraits show two Endell Street orderlies (Art.IWM ART 2853 and 2854) and the hospital dispenser (Art.IWM ART 2765).

3. The picture is described in a list of IWM pictures as "The Operating Theatre, Endell St Hospital—Dr Garrett-Anderson [*sic*] operating": IWM EN1/3/COR/007.

4. FM to Col. Brereton, February 22, 1920; FM to Lady Norman, March 3, 1920, Papers of the IWM women's work subcommittee, EN1/3/HOSP/005; minutes of the subcommittee, April 1919 to July 1920, IWM EN1/3/GEN/011.

5. Lady Norman to FM, May 22, 1920, IWM EN1/3/HOSP/005; Norman to Francis Dodd, May 28, 1920, and other correspondence with Dodd, IWM ART/WA1/107.

6. Claire Buck, *Conceiving Strangeness in British First World War Writing* (2015), 189, quoting Agnes Conway; details of exhibits from *Guide to IWM and Great Victory Exhibition* (1920), IWM archives, EN1/1/MUS/041/4. Background on the origins of the IWM and its women's work section are from Buck and Gaynor Kavanagh, *Museums of the First World War: A Social History* (London, 1994).

7. The oil painting is in storage at the IWM: Art.IWM ART 4084; a preliminary chalk drawing for the picture, showing seven women, is in the Wellcome Library (Wellcome Library no. 45014i); a charcoal sketch of LGA operating exists in the archives of the Elizabeth Garrett Anderson Hospital, University College London Hospitals National Health Service Foundation Trust.

8. LGA to Lady Norman, January 25, 1921, IWM EN1/3/HOSP/005. Spare's picture went to an outer London military hospital but was missing by 1969. Geddes, "Artistic Integrity and Feminist Spin."

9. Leonore Davidoff and Belinda Westover, *Our Work, Our Lives, Our Words: Women's History and Women's Work* (Basingstoke, 1986); Arthur Marwick, *Women at War, 1914–1918* (London, 1977).

10. Millicent Fawcett, *The Women's Victory—and After: Personal Reminiscences, 1911–1918* (London, 1920), 106.

11. Philip Gibbs, cited in Susan Kingsley Kent, *Making Peace: The Reconstruction of Gender in Interwar Britain* (Princeton, NJ, 1993), 100.

12. Alberti 1989, 148–149. The figure was 56 percent.

13. Kate Adie, *Corsets to Camouflage: Women and War* (London, 2003), 135.

14. Letter to *The Times*, cited in Robins 1924, 233–234.

15. Kent, *Making Peace*, esp. chap. 5.

16. Alberti 1989, 99; report of speech by Ray Strachey in *Magazine of the RFHLSMW* 14, no. 74 (July 1919): 100–102. The total rose from 4.5 million before the war to an estimated 6 million after.

17. David Reynolds, *The Long Shadow: The Great War and the Twentieth Century* (London, 2013), 209.

18. Geddes 2005; Bell 1953, 168–189; Leneman 1994; Lesley A. Hall, "A Century of Struggle: Women Advancing in the Medical Profession," paper presented at the Medical Women's Federation centenary conference, May 12, 2017.

19. MacAlister: Scott 1984; VD hospital: *Time and Tide*, May 28, 1920.

20. Women doctors offered posts: They were Gladys Wauchope and Ida Mann, cited in Carol Dyhouse, "Driving Ambitions: Women in Pursuit of a Medical Education, 1890–1939," *Women's History Review* 7, no. 3 (1998): 321–341.

21. She was Isabel Hutton, cited in Hall, "A Century of Struggle."

22. "Women Medics and the First World War," St George's Library Blog, November 24, 2014, https://stglibrary.wordpress.com/2014/11/24/women-medics-and -the-first-world-war.

23. Letter to *The Times*, March 10, 1922.

24. Elsie M. Lang, *British Women in the Twentieth Century* (London, 1929), 71–73; Women doctors' marriage rate: Louisa Martindale, *The Woman Doctor and Her Future* (London, 1922), 129.

25. *Magazine of RFHLSMW* 14, no. 74 (July 1919): 126–133.

26. Much original research on the women's careers after the war was done by Jennian Geddes. My thanks to her for sharing these details. Other information has been gleaned from medical directories and other sources.

27. Peter D. Mohr, "Chambers, Helen (1879–1935)," ODNB, https://doi.org /10.1093/ref:odnb/60892; obituary *The Times*, July 21, 1935.

28. "Hazel Haward Chodak-Gregory," Royal College of Physicians, Lives of the Fellows, "Munk's Roll," vol. 5, http://munksroll.rcplondon.ac.uk/Biography/Details /842. She had married a fellow doctor, Alexis Chodak-Gregory, in 1917.

29. Sarah Lefanu, "Majorie Blandy (1887–1937)," in Biddy Passmore, ed., *Breaking Bounds: Six Newnham Lives* (Cambridge, 2014), 53–65. She died of breast cancer in 1937, aged fifty.

30. Information from Royal College of Obstetrics and Gynaecology. My thanks to Suzy Boyd and Carly Randall. Dearnley also became the first female consultant at Queen Charlotte's Hospital, London.

31. Obituary, *The Times*, December 29, 1955.

32. Winifred Buckley, response to questionnaire, Newnham College archives.

33. Sheard 2016.

34. John Atherton Young, Ann Jervie Sefton, and Nina Webb, eds., *Centenary Book of the University of Sydney Faculty of Medicine* (Sydney, 1984), 235–236; interview with Dr. Elizabeth Hamilton-Browne, September 27, 1978, University of Sydney, university archives.

35. Hacker 1974, 192–197; obituary in *Canadian Medical Association Journal* 95 (November 26, 1966): 1164; personal information from her grandson Michael Fellows and other family members.

36. Mary Byatt, "Olga Byatt," in Susan Bennett, Mary Byatt, Jenny Main, Anne Oliver, and Janet Trythall, *Women of Moray* (Edinburgh, 2012), 169–176; letters from Olga Campell to Marion Dickerman, September 15, 1919, March 16, 1920, December 24, 1920, and March 6, 1921, Marion Dickerman Papers, National Park Service, Hyde Park, New York; information from family members Robin and Jilly Byatt, Fiona Byatt, and Lucy Byatt.

37. Information from Andrew Wells (her grandson).

38. Davis 1974; obituary for Marion Dickerman, *New York Times*, May 18, 1983.

39. Nina Last, WL, 7NLA/1/1b and 2b; information from Nina's granddaughter Annie Fox. The daughters were Margaret, known as Peggy, and Barbara.

40. Information from Barbara's daughter Nancy Prentis. Barbara died in 1952.

41. *Yorkshire Post*, September 17, 1920.

42. Murray 1920, 259–261; FM, "A Woman's Hospital in Peace," in *Common Cause*, January 30, 1920; annual report of The Women's Hospital for Children, 1920, LMA.

43. Interview with Dr. Elizabeth Hamilton-Browne, September 27, 1978, University of Sydney, university archives.

44. Harraden to Robins, August 4 [1920], Elizabeth Robins Collection 1897–1938, box 1.9, Harry Ransom Center, University of Texas; preface, Murray 1920, iix–x. She wrote to Robins the same day she wrote the preface. Despite her carping, two months earlier Harraden had been treated by FM, who visited her "every day for nearly a month." Harraden to Robins, May 6, 1920, Elizabeth Robins Collection 1897–1938, box 1.9, Harry Ransom Center, University of Texas.

45. Murray 1920, v, 212; the lines are from "In Memory of Barry Cornwall."

46. *Lancet* 197, no. 5079 (January 1, 1921); *Scotsman*, November 27, 1920.

47. Alberti 1989, passim.

48. Crawford 1999, 432, 513.

49. Letter to the editor, signed Flora Murray, *The Times*, June 30, 1921; lunch event, *The Times*, December 16, 1921. The Six Point Group was founded by Margaret Mackworth, Viscountess Rhondda. It initially demanded specific changes, such as equal pay for teachers, but later this widened into more general aims.

50. FM to William Murray, September 19 and 30, 1922, private papers of Murray family. In the second letter she mentions visiting Paris by airplane.

51. Funeral expenses of William Murray, private papers of Murray family.

52. Flora Murray, death certificate, July 30, 1923; will, dated December 6, 1921, executed August 30, 1923; funeral details in *Lancet* 202, no. 5215 (August 11, 1923); *Woman's Leader*, August 10, 1923.

53. Nina Last, WL, 7NLA/1/1b and 2b.

54. Murray obituaries: *The Vote*, August 10, 1923; *Observer*, August 5, 1923; LGA, in *Newsletter of the Medical Women's Federation*, 1923; *Northern Advocate* (New Zealand), October 6, 1923. Adelaide Anderson (Louisa's cousin) read news of Murray's death in Australia. A memorial was erected in Dalton parish church near Murray's home in Dumfriesshire.

55. Geddes 2008.

56. *The Vote*, March 6, 1925.

57. Anderson 1939. Colin Anderson referred to LGA burning her parents' letters afterward. Unpublished memoir of Sir Colin Skelton Anderson (private papers).

58. LGA tribute to Millicent Fawcett, *Woman's Leader*, November 15, 1929; David Rubinstein, *A Different World for Women: The Life of Millicent Garrett Fawcett* (New York, 1991), 263.

59. VS Letter Diaries, n.d. [November 1928], vol. B3, VSB Papers.

60. *Sydney Morning Herald*, November 30, 1928, accessed via Trove.

61. Rubinstein, *A Different World*, 282.

62. Annual reports of the Elizabeth Garrett Anderson Hospital, 1939 and 1943, LMA, H13/EGA/12/1 and 5.

63. LGA to Kenneth Anderson, January 7, 1940, Ipswich RO, HA436/5/2/2.

64. Unpublished memoir of Sir Colin Skelton Anderson (private papers).

65. She was diagnosed with retroperitoneal sarcoma, according to the death certificate.

66. LGA to Evelyn Sharp, October 30, 1943, MS.Eng.lett.d.279.56/57, Oxford, Bodleian Library.

67. *The Times*, November 24, 1943; Evelyn Sharp diary, November 23, 1943, MS.Eng.lett.d.279.56/57, Oxford, Bodleian Library; obituaries: *New York Times*, November 17, 1943; LGA's will, signed October 4, 1943, WL, 7lga/5/1.

68. Hall, "A Century of Struggle"; UK figures from General Medical Council, 2017; British Medical Association, *Equality and Diversity in UK Medical Schools*, October 2009, posted on National Health Service History website, www.nhshistory .net/bmastudentreport2009.pdf; British Medical Association, Equality Lens, updated December 6, 2018, www.bma.org.uk/about-us/equality-diversity-and-inclusion/equality -lens/trend-1. Global figures from *OECD Health Statistics*, 2016.

Index

Index

compound fractures, 47, 130, 185, 186

disabilities from, 179, 181, 265,

gangrene, 43, 51, 52, 74–75, 112, 115, 185, 255

head injuries, 43, 130, 185, 186

septic, 43, 47, 75, 115, 133, 153, 187, 188–189, 218, 219, 235, 236

Wright, Charles, 288

Wright, Sir Almroth, 188

Wright method, 188

X-ray department, 15, 28, 99, 162–163, 169, 187, 237–238

X-ray equipment, 28, 41–43, 61, 130–131, 167, 185, 190

Yorkshire Post, 168

Ypres, Belgium, 267

First Battle (1914), 64, 72, 79–80, 84, 90–91, 105

Second Battle (1915), 110, 120, 132–133, 168

Third Battle (1917), 213–217, 229, 267

Zeppelins, 137–138, 191–192, 194, 295

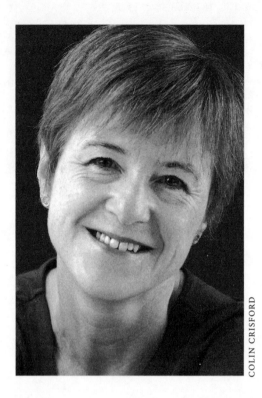

COLIN CRISFORD

WENDY MOORE is a journalist and author of several previous books, including *How to Create the Perfect Wife* and *Wedlock*, a *Sunday Times* best seller. Her writing has appeared in *The Times*, *The Guardian*, *The Observer*, and the *Sunday Telegraph*. She lives in London.